Placental Pathology

ATLAS OF NONTUMOR PATHOLOGY

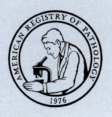
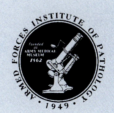

ATLAS OF NONTUMOR PATHOLOGY

First Series
Fascicle 3

Placental Pathology

Frederick T. Kraus, MD

Raymond W. Redline, MD

Deborah J. Gersell, MD

D. Michael Nelson, MD, PhD

Jeffrey M. Dicke, MD

Published by the
American Registry of Pathology
Washington, DC
in collaboration with the
Armed Forces Institute of Pathology
Washington, DC

2004

ATLAS OF NONTUMOR PATHOLOGY

EDITOR
Donald West King, MD

ASSOCIATE EDITORS
Leslie H. Sobin, MD
J. Thomas Stocker, MD
Bernard Wagner, MD

EDITORIAL ADVISORY BOARD
Ivan Damjanov, MD
Cecilia M. Fenoglio-Preiser, MD
Fred Gorstein, MD
Daniel Knowles, MD
Virginia A. LiVolsi, MD
Florabel G. Mullick, MD
Juan Rosai, MD
Fred Silva, MD
Steven G. Silverberg, MD

Manuscript Reviewed by:
Rebecca N. Baergen, MD
David R. Genest, MD

Available from the American Registry of Pathology
Armed Forces Institute of Pathology
Washington, DC 20306-6000
www.afip.org
ISBN: 1-881041-89-1

Copyright © 2004 The American Registry of Pathology

All rights reserved. No part of this publication may be reproduced or transmitted in any form or by any means: electronic, mechanical, photocopy, recording, or any other information storage and retrieval system without the written permission of the publisher.

INTRODUCTION TO SERIES

This is the third Fascicle of the Atlas of Nontumor Pathology, a complementary series to the Armed Forces Institute of Pathology (AFIP) Atlas of Tumor Pathology, first published in 1949.

For several years, various individuals in the pathology community have suggested the formation of a new series of monographs concentrating on this particular area. In 1998, an Editorial Board was appointed and outstanding authors chosen shortly thereafter.

The purpose of the atlas is to provide surgical pathologists with ready expert reference material most helpful in their daily practice. The lesions described relate principally to medical non-neoplastic conditions. Many of these lesions represent complex entities and, when appropriate, we have included contributions from internists, radiologists, and surgeons. This has led to some increase in the size of the monographs but the emphasis remains on diagnosis by the surgical pathologist.

Previously, the Fascicles have been available on CD-ROM format as well as in print. In order to provide the widest possible advantages of both modalities, we have formatted the print Fascicle on the World Wide Web. Use of the Internet allows cross-indexing within the Fascicles as well as linkage to PubMed.

Our goal is to continue to provide expert information at the lowest possible cost. Therefore, marked reductions in pricing are available to residents and fellows as well as to pathology faculty and other staff members purchasing the Fascicles on a subscription basis.

We believe that the Atlas of Nontumor Pathology will serve as an outstanding reference for surgical pathologists as well as an important contribution to the literature of other medical specialties.

Donald West King, MD
Leslie H. Sobin, MD
J. Thomas Stocker, MD
Bernard Wagner, MD

PROLOGUE

This atlas of placental pathology is organized into chapters that in general follow the standard categories of disease in any organ, such as inflammation or vascular-coagulation problems. It is intended to be concise enough to serve as a practical guide at the bench for pathology residents, and for diagnostic surgical pathologists whose contact with placentas is relatively infrequent. Some novel aspects of placental pathology require emphasis.

The placenta is a unique multifunctional organ and therefore unlike any other pathologic specimen.

The placenta is intimately connected to two different people. Problems that affect the placenta may affect each person in very different ways. Furthermore, when problems occur, mother and child will likely come under the care of two very different physician-specialists, each of whom is interested in the implications of placental pathology for a specific—and different—individual. A truly responsive report can become a significant challenge for the pathologist.

Another important distinction between a placenta and other organs is the kind of clinical data available to the pathologist at the time the placenta is examined. Important information about the mother is usually known and can be provided with the placenta, but some of the most significant events affecting an injured newborn have yet to occur at the time of delivery. Although data about the intrapartum fetal heart rate often accompany the placenta to the laboratory, the chances that such an abnormality will actually lead to significant injury is about 1 in 100. However, significant data about the neonate, such as prolonged respiratory difficulty or seizures that occur between 6 and 12 hours postdelivery, although known to the baby's physician, rarely get communicated to the pathologist in time to influence the preparation of the pathology report.

Even in recent years the pathology report for a placenta, a *fetal* organ, most commonly is placed with the *mother's* hospital record. As the mother usually leaves the hospital after about 2 days, the pathology report is often inserted into the record after she is discharged. The obstetrician who sees the report soon after delivery may not share it with the pediatrician.

An optimal analysis of an abnormal placenta requires collaboration between pathologist, obstetrician, and pediatrician.

Without adequate clinical information even an experienced pathologist may underestimate subtle changes that might require a more extensive examination. If mother or baby are sick, both the obstetrician and the pediatrician need to examine the pathology report of the placenta to confirm that the problems of their patient have been adequately addressed. If a more complete examination is required, they must convey this to the pathologist for immediate attention. Unless the pathologist is informed in a timely manner, the fixed placental tissue will be discarded, and the opportunity to convert histologic hints into solid conclusions by more extended study will be lost. This is a common state of affairs, noticed acutely if a lawsuit is filed. The apparent lack of an explanation, or a serious search for an explanation, when the newborn is injured or stillborn can be a factor in the decision to file a lawsuit in the first place.

Adequate regular communication between obstetricians, pediatricians, and pathologists will be necessary to achieve optimal understanding of perinatal injury and thereby improve approaches to treatment. The challenge will be met best by those who recognize the unique difficulties posed by analyzing and reporting the results of placental pathologic examinations.

The organization of this text is intended to facilitate a pathologist's understanding of the different concerns of obstetricians and pediatricians.

While all physicians interested in perinatal injury have similar goals and overlap in approach to problems, there are differences in emphasis by different specialists that may be confusing. In recognition of this, two different approaches to understanding how placental pathology may be viewed are presented. Overlap between these approaches is intentional.

A more fundamental approach is set forth in chapter 2, Basic Pathways of Prenatal and Perinatal Injury: A Pathogenic Approach to Placental Interpretation. Most of current placental research is focused on the different pathways that lead to injury, such as genetic mutations or abnormal immune responses. The pediatrician is especially concerned with these *mechanisms* of injury, and with *adverse outcomes*, for example, premature delivery and hypoxic-ischemic injury.

Chapter 3, Clinical Syndromes and Their Pathologic Correlates in the Placenta, presents the problem of conducting a placental examination in the context most familiar to a pathologist. The clinical settings of the pregnancy, labor, and delivery are of paramount importance to the understanding of the obstetrician, who in current practice is the individual who decides that the placenta should undergo pathologic study. Such information as maternal diabetes mellitus, preeclampsia, or potential infection represent the data available to the obstetrician. These important data are generally supplied to the pathologist with the form that requests pathologic examination of the placenta. This chapter presents a guide for the pathologist less frequently involved with placental pathology in the use of this type of clinical information to conduct an informed search for the more likely or more significant lesions.

Chapter 14, Diagnostic Ultrasound in Obstetrics, presents a brief review of placental and fetal ultrasound imaging. Prenatal ultrasound studies are employed increasingly to evaluate fetal growth and development, and also represent something of a preview of both fetal and placental morphology. A pathologist engaged in evaluating a placenta should be aware of the information already known about the placenta well before it is delivered. Grossly evident structures such as clots may be documented, and Doppler imaging may direct interest in histologic explanations for fetal vascular pathology within the placenta of a growth-restricted newborn.

An informative placental examination in the context of maternal illness or neonatal morbidity must be a cooperative venture. Insights into clinical problems (seizures, pulmonary hypertension, renal failure) that become evident hours or days after delivery will not occur unless the problems are addressed by a pathologist who is aware that they have occurred. The placental pathology report is often a work in progress that may not be "final" until many days after delivery.

Frederick T. Kraus, MD
Department of Obstetrics and Gynecology
Washington University School of Medicine

Raymond W. Redline, MD
Department of Pathology and Reproductive Biology
University Hospitals of Cleveland and Case School of Medicine

Deborah J. Gersell, MD
Department of Pathology
St. John's Mercy Medical Center

D. Michael Nelson, MD, PhD
Department of Obstetrics and Gynecology
Washington University School of Medicine

Jeffrey M. Dicke, MD
Department of Obstetrics and Gynecology
Washington University School of Medicine

ACKNOWLEDGMENTS

I would like to thank Dr. Thomas Applewhite for supplying the ultrasound and radiographic images for figures 5-1C and D, 6-45, 6-47, 6-52, and 9-11; Dr. Kurt Benirschke for reviewing chapter 6; and Drs. Baergen and Genest for reading the entire manuscript. I would also like to express my sincere appreciation to The Sisters of Mercy at St. John's Mercy Medical Center, St. Louis, Missouri, for their longstanding support of pathology research as well as this atlas.

Frederick T. Kraus, MD

We would like to recognize Jennifer Ackerman Arndt and Dianne Welter, who took many of the gross photographs, especially for chapters 6, 7, 8, 9, and 12. We are also very grateful for Marie Wolinski's assistance with typing and administrative tasks.

Deborah J. Gersell, MD and Frederick T. Kraus, MD

I would like to thank Kurt Benirschke, Carlos Abramowsky, Beverly Dahms, and especially Shirley Driscoll for guidance and encouragement over the years.

Raymond W. Redline, MD

Diagrams 2-1, 2-2, 4-1, 6-1–6-5, 7-1, 8-1, 13-1–13-3, 12-1, 12-13, 12-50, and 12-51 were prepared by Vicki Friedman, Director, Department of Medical Photography, Illustration, and Computer Graphics at the Washington University School of Medicine, St. Louis, Missouri.

Permission to use copyrighted illustrations has been granted by:

BMJ Publishing Group
    British Medical Journal 1999;319:1054-9. For table 3-1.

College of American Pathologists
    Archives of Pathology and Laboratory Medicine 2002;126:157-64. For figures 6-61A and 6-61B.

Elsevier
    European Journal of Obstetrics & Gynecology and Reproductive Biology 1999;83:131-5. For appendix 10.

    Human Pathology 1987;18:387-91. For appendix 6.

    Placenta 1983;4:423-6. For appendix 9.

Lippincott Williams & Wilkins
    Obstetrics and Gynecology 1992;80:575-84. For appendix 8A.

    Obstetrics and Gynecology 1992;80:585-92. For appendix 8B.

    International Journal of Gynecological Pathology 2001;20:284-8. For figure 11-1.

    International Journal of Gynecological Pathology 1998;17:241-4. For figure 11-3.

Springer-Verlag
    Pathology of the Human Embryo and Previable Fetus: An Atlas, 1990. For appendices 1A and 1B.

    Pediatric and Developmental Pathology 2000;3:462-71. For appendix 11.

    Pediatric and Developmental Pathology 1998;1:538-42. For figure 11-6.

Taylor & Francis
    Pediatric Pathology & Laboratory Medicine 1996;16:901-7. For appendices 3A, 3B, 4, and 5.

    Pediatric Pathology & Laboratory Medicine 1995;15:51-6. For figure 11-5.

PLACENTAL PATHOLOGY

1. Anatomy, Structure, and Function ... 1
   - Introduction ... 1
   - Gross and Microscopic Anatomy ... 1
     - Amnion and Membranous Chorion ... 1
     - Umbilical Cord ... 3
     - Chorionic Plate and Stem Villi ... 4
     - Terminal Villous Unit and Interhemal Membrane ... 5
     - Basal Plate and Anchoring Villi ... 6
     - Placental Margin and Membranes ... 8
   - Developmental Anatomy ... 9
     - Blastocyst Trophectoderm (Days 18 to 20 of Menstrual Cycle) ... 10
     - Nidation and Maternal Capillary Circulation (Days 20 to 28 of Menstrual Cycle) ... 10
     - Chorionic Plate and Body Stalk (4 to 5 Weeks from Last Menstrual Period [LMP]) ... 10
     - Villous Stromal Vasculogenesis (5 to 6 Weeks from LMP) ... 10
     - Elaboration of Mesenchymal Villi (6 to 8.5 Weeks from LMP) ... 11
     - Development of Stem Villi (8.5 to 11.5 Weeks from LMP) ... 12
     - Early Implantation and Arterial Plugs (6 to 12 Weeks from LMP) ... 12
     - Late Implantation and Arterial Remodeling (12 to 20 Weeks from LMP) ... 14
     - Membrane Formation and Peripheral Expansion (9 to 18 Weeks from LMP) ... 15
     - Trophoblast Proliferative Units and Placental Growth (13 to 40 Weeks from LMP) ... 16
     - Terminal Villogenesis (22 to 30 Weeks from LMP) ... 16
   - Functional Anatomy ... 17
     - Fetoplacental Arterial Perfusion ... 17
     - Fetoplacental Venous Return ... 17
     - Maternal Arterial Perfusion/Placental Lobule ... 17
     - Maternal Venous Drainage/Marginal Sinus ... 18
     - Umbilical Cord Dynamics ... 18
     - Membranes and Labor ... 18
     - Syncytiotrophoblast and Maternal Physiology ... 19
2. Basic Pathways of Prenatal and Peripartum Injury: A Pathogenic Approach to Placental Interpretation ... 23
   - Introduction ... 23
   - Primary Adverse Outcomes of Prenatal and Peripartum Injury ... 23
     - Preterm Delivery ... 24
     - Fetal Growth Restriction ... 25

	Hypoxic-Ischemic Injury	26
	Placental Lesions	27
	Subcategorization	28
	Physiologic Consequences	29
	Pathways of Injury	29
3.	Clinical Syndromes and Their Pathologic Correlates in the Placenta	33
	Clinical Diagnoses Based Primarily on Maternal History or Maternal Examination	33
	Pregnancy-Induced Hypertension, Preeclampsia, and Eclampsia	33
	Acute Fatty Liver of Pregnancy	34
	Essential Hypertension	34
	Maternal Thrombophilia (Including Maternal Deep Vein Thromboses, Pulmonary Infarcts, Cerebral Vascular Accidents)	34
	Diabetes Mellitus	35
	Maternal Anemias	35
	Recurrent Spontaneous Abortion (Recurrent Pregnancy Loss, Habitual Abortion)	36
	Primarily Fetal Conditions	36
	Clinical Chorioamnionitis (Versus Histologic Chorioamnionitis)	36
	Preterm Birth, Preterm Labor, Premature Rupture of Membranes	37
	Post-term Pregnancy	37
	Intrapartum Electronic Fetal Monitoring: Nonreassuring Fetal Heart Rate, Bradycardia, Decelerations	37
	Fetal Growth Restriction, Intrauterine Growth Restriction, and the Small for Gestational Age Newborn	38
	Erythroblastosis: Nucleated Red Blood Cells in the Fetal Circulation of the Placenta	41
	Fetal or Neonatal Thrombocytopenias	41
	Meconium-Stained Amniotic Fluid and the Meconium Aspiration Syndrome	42
	Abnormal Amniotic Fluid Volume	42
4.	Disorders of Placental Development	47
	Introduction	47
	Disorders of Membrane Development	47
	Placental Membranacea	47
	Circumvallation/Circummargination	47
	Disorders of Uterine Implantation	49
	Placenta Previa	49
	Placenta Accreta, Increta, Percreta	51
	Superficial Implantation	53
	Disorders of Placental Migration	54
	Shape Abnormalities	54

	Peripheral Cord Insertion	57
	Disorders of Villous Development	59
	Distal Villous Hypoplasia with Placental Undergrowth (Peripheral Villous Hypoplasia, "Terminal Villous Deficiency")	59
	Distal Villous Immaturity with Placental Overgrowth ("Delayed Villous Maturation")	60
	Disorders of Fetal Vascular Development	61
	Chorangioma and Localized Chorangiomatosis	61
	Villous Chorangiosis (Hypercapillarization)	62
	Diffuse Multifocal Chorangiomatosis	64
	Genetic and Chromosomal Disorders	65
	Metabolic Storage Diseases	65
	Mesenchymal Dysplasia	66
	Chromosomal Abnormalities	68
5.	Inflammation and Infection	75
	Introduction	75
	Infections	75
	Acute Chorioamnionitis (Histologic)	75
	Subacute Chorioamnionitis	84
	Acute Chorioamnionitis with Peripheral Funisitis	86
	Acute Intervillositis with Intervillous Abscesses	87
	Acute Villitis	90
	Active Chronic Villitis and Intervillositis with Villous Necrosis	90
	Chronic Placentitis, TORCH Type	92
	Chronic Intervillositis with Malarial Pigment	96
	Perinatal Infections with Minimal or No Placental Inflammation	99
	Idiopathic Inflammatory Lesions	101
	Chronic Villitis (Villitis of Unknown Etiology)	101
	Chronic (Histiocytic) Intervillositis (Massive Chronic Intervillositis)	107
	Chronic Chorioamnionitis	107
	Chronic Deciduitis	108
	Eosinophilic/T-Cell Vasculitis	109
	Chronic Decidual Periarteritis	110
6.	Circulatory Problems: Thrombi and Other Vascular Lesions	117
	Introduction	117
	Circulatory Relationships in the Placenta and the Varied Effects of Intraplacental Clotting	117
	Maternal Circulation: Thrombi, Hematomas, and Decidual Vascular Lesions	118
	Decidual Vasculopathy: Acute Atherosis and Spiral Artery Thrombi	118

	Infarcts	123
	Intraplacental Hematomas (Intervillous Thrombi) and Massive Subchorial Hematomas	127
	Retroplacental Hematomas, Marginal Hematomas, and Placental Abruption	128
	Maternal Circulation: Nonvascular Lesions	135
	Massive Perivillous Fibrin Deposition (Gitterinfarcts) and Maternal Floor Infarct	135
	Fetal Circulation: Thrombi and Hematomas	141
	Fetal Stem Vessel (Large Vessel) Thrombi and Fetal Thrombotic Vasculopathy	141
	Fetal Vascular Narrowing and Increased Umbilical Vascular Resistance	151
	Hemorrhagic Endovasculitis	151
	Endothelial Cushions of Fibrinous Vasculosis	156
	Fetal Circulation: Other Lesions	157
	Subamnionic Hematoma	157
	Stasis Problems	157
7.	Normal Structure and Pathology of the Membranes	163
	Anatomy and Physiology	163
	Meconium Staining	164
	Inflammation	168
	Squamous Metaplasia	168
	Amnion Nodosum	169
	Amnionic Bands	171
	Extramembranous Pregnancy	172
	Gastroschisis	175
	Cysts (Subamnionic Fibrin Cysts)	175
8.	Embryonic Development and Pathology of the Umbilical Cord	179
	Embryonic Development	179
	Normal Umbilical Cord	179
	Vestigal Remnants	180
	Allantoic Remnants	180
	Omphalomesenteric Remnants	180
	Insertion Anomalies	182
	Velamentous Insertion and Membranous Vessels	182
	Marginal Insertion	185
	Furcate Insertion	186
	Tethered Insertion ("Amnionic Webs")	187
	Cord Length	187
	Short Cord	187
	Long Cord	188

	Cord Diameter	189
	Numerical Variation in Umbilical Vessels	189
	Single Umbilical Artery	189
	Supernumerary Vessels	192
	Focal Lesions	192
	Knots	192
	Abnormal Torsion	193
	Stricture	196
	Hematoma	196
	Hemangioma	197
	Abnormalities in Umbilical Cord Vessels	197
	Aneurysms	197
	Segmental Thinning	197
	Meconium-Induced Necrosis	198
	Ulceration	198
	Thrombosis	198
	Rupture	199
9.	Abortion, Stillbirth, and Intrauterine Fetal Death	207
	Introduction	207
	Early Spontaneous Abortion, Products of Conception, and Embryonic Death	207
	Late Spontaneous Abortion (Miscarriage, Stillbirth, and Intrauterine Fetal Death)	222
10.	Fetal and Placental Hydrops	229
	Introduction	229
	Immune Hydrops (Erythroblastosis Fetalis, Hemolytic Disease of the Newborn)	229
	Nonimmune Hydrops	232
	Cardiovascular	232
	Fetal Anemias	232
	Fetal Infections	235
	Pulmonary Lesions and Other Intrathoracic Causes	236
	Major Chromosomal Disorders	236
	Other Congenital Anomalies and Genetic Metabolic Diseases	236
	Fetal Tumors	236
11.	Tumor-Like Lesions and Metastatic Neoplasms	239
	Putative Primary Placental Neoplasms	239
	Hemangioma (Chorangioma)	239
	Intraplacental Leiomyoma	239
	Teratomas (or Acardiac Twins?)	240
	Adenoma (Choristoma?)	241
	Hepatocellular Adenoma (Heterotopic Liver)	241

	Heterotopic Adrenal Cortex	241
	Metastatic Neoplasms	241
	Fetal Primary Tumors Involving the Placenta	242
	Maternal Primary Tumors Involving the Placenta	243
12.	Multiple Pregnancy	249
	Twin Gestation	249
	Zygosity	249
	Frequency and Etiology	249
	Placentation	249
	Umbilical Cord, Chorionic Vascularity, and Placental Mass	258
	Monoamnionic Monochorionic Placentas	259
	Complications of Multiple Pregnancy	261
	Twin-Twin Transfusion Syndrome	261
	Asymmetric Growth	268
	Intragestational Fetal Loss	269
	Duplication Abnormalities	272
	Higher Multiple Births	276
13.	Examination Technique	283
	Pathologist-Clinician Relationship	283
	Approach to the Specific Clinical Scenario	283
	Stepwise Handling of the Specimen	285
	Gross Description	286
	Technique and Rationale for Tissue Sampling	286
	Multiple Pregnancy	287
	Alternative Approaches to Placental Examination	289
	Special Studies	290
14.	Diagnostic Ultrasound in Obstetrics	295
	Introduction	295
	Ultrasound Imaging of the Placenta and Umbilical Cord	295
	Ultrasound Imaging of the Fetus	300
	First Trimester Ultrasound Examination	300
	Second and Third Trimester Ultrasound Examination	300
	Doppler Ultrasound in Assessment of the Growth-Restricted Fetus	304
A.	Appendix: Placental Weights and Measures	311
	The Value of Placental Measurements	311
	Index	323

1
ANATOMY, STRUCTURE, DEVELOPMENT, AND FUNCTION

INTRODUCTION

In order to evaluate placentas for clinically significant abnormalities, pathologists need to have a thorough understanding of the basic anatomy, how it changes during development, and how it translates into organ function. Many of the concepts of structure-function and development in the placenta have undergone dramatic change over the past several years because of advances in developmental biology and antenatal monitoring. This chapter presents the basic gross and microscopic anatomy of the placenta, highlighting artifacts and normal variants that may be confused with pathologic lesions. Briefly discussed are the overlapping development sequences that act in concert to assemble a normal term placenta, placing them in temporal context and emphasizing their clinical relevance. Finally, the basic structure-function relationships that govern the maternal and fetal circulations, the onset and timing of labor, and the maternal physiologic accommodation to pregnancy are considered.

GROSS AND MICROSCOPIC ANATOMY

Amnion and Membranous Chorion

The amnion is a simple squamous epithelium with an underlying basement membrane and an associated band of loose connective tissue approximately 5 to 10 cells in thickness (fig. 1-1). It forms the inner lining of the amnionic cavity, covering the chorionic plate and its extension in the fetal membranes, the chorion laevae. An attenuated layer of amnionic epithelial cells also surrounds the umbilical cord. Amnion represents the extraembryonic extension of fetal skin, with which it shares a number of characteristics including pemphigoid antigens and cytokeratins (69). At areas of repetitive stress, such as at the umbilical cord insertion, amnion may undergo metaplasia to form plaques of keratinizing, stratified squamous epithelium, 0.5 to 2.0 cm in diameter, which may be seen by gross examination (see chapter 7, Squamous Metaplasia).

Amnion is easily separated from the underlying chorion in both membranes and chorionic

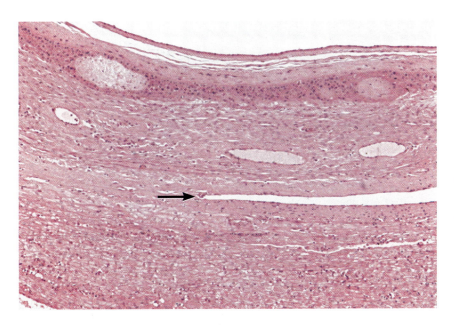

Figure 1-1

PLACENTAL MEMBRANES

The amnion (top) consists of simple cuboidal epithelium with a thin layer of underlying fibroblasts; it is separated from the underlying chorion by a narrow space. The chorion is composed of connective tissue with a subjacent band of eosinophilic, mononuclear trophoblast which contains a few hyalinized villi. Underlying the chorion is the maternal decidua, consisting of decidua capsularis and decidua vera from the opposite side of the uterus. A cleft-like space marks the point of fusion (arrow).

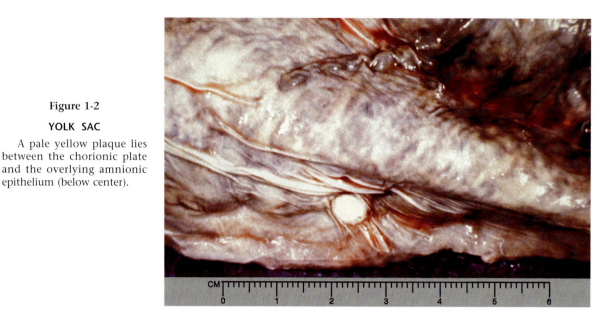

Figure 1-2

YOLK SAC

A pale yellow plaque lies between the chorionic plate and the overlying amnionic epithelium (below center).

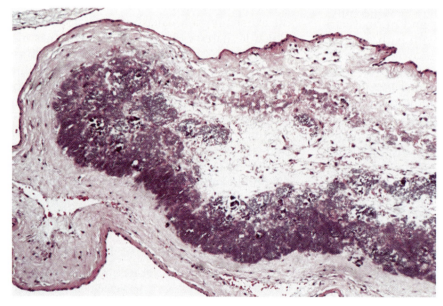

Figure 1-3

YOLK SAC

The yolk sac degenerates in late pregnancy to form a calcific plaque below the amnion.

plate, and once separated, is easily torn. Isolated tears in the amnion frequently occur during labor and delivery or at the time of placental examination, but infrequently prior to labor. It is important not to misinterpret shreds of torn amnion hanging off the umbilical cord as pathologic amnionic bands (see chapter 7, Amnionic Bands). The yolk sac, a vestigial organ in human pregnancies, may be seen immediately beneath the amnion as either a yellow plaque at the time of gross examination (fig. 1-2) or a calcified nodule at microscopic examination (fig. 1-3).

The membranous chorion (chorion laevae) is formed by the collapse of the placental intervillous space during membrane development (see below). It is composed of a heterogenous mixture of mononuclear trophoblastic cells, with either vacuolated or eosinophilic cytoplasm, plus a few widely scattered atrophic chorionic villi. Below the chorion laevae trophoblast is decidualized maternal endometrium; above is a layer of avascular connective tissue. The connective tissue of the chorion and amnion is distinct and held together by thin fibrils of collagen. Recent

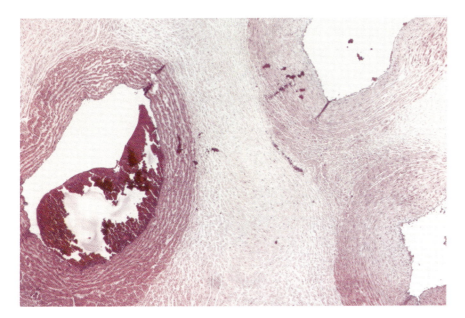

Figure 1-4

UMBILICAL CORD

The thin-walled vein is seen on the left and the two thick-walled arteries on the right. The vessels are surrounded by a hypocellular matrix known as Wharton's jelly. The inner circular layer of smooth muscle, which contracts to obstruct arterial flow at parturition, is best seen in the artery on the lower right.

data suggest that a fetal genetic polymorphism may lead to overexpression of a membrane collagenase in some patients with premature membrane rupture (29).

Umbilical Cord

The umbilical cord is the cable linking the fetus to the placenta (fig. 1-4). Within the cable are two muscularized arteries and a single, large, thin-walled vein embedded in a hydrated extracellular matrix gel known as Wharton's jelly. The cable is usually twisted to some degree, generally to the left (i.e., the diagonal twists run from upper left to lower right), with an average of 2.1 twists per 10 cm at term (76). On cut section, the paired arteries are distinguished from the vein by thicker walls and a smaller lumen. The thicker wall of the artery is composed of a tightly bundled outer circular layer of smooth muscle and an inner spiral longitudinal layer, which contracts to occlude the placental circulation at the time of delivery (folds of Hoboken) (71). An anastomosis between the two arteries (Hyrtyl's anastomosis) near their decussation at the chorionic plate acts to balance the two circulations and obviates any adverse consequences following involution or failure to develop of one of the two arteries (see chapter 8, Single Umbilical Artery) (64). The umbilical vein may be focally ectatic, forming varicosities that have been termed false knots. These varicosities are of no clinical significance.

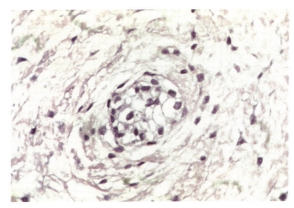

Figure 1-5

ALLANTOIC DUCT REMNANT

The allantoic duct lies between the two umbilical arteries which follow its course from the fetus to the chorionic plate. It arises from the roof of the bladder and is lined by transitional epithelium. In some species the allantoic sac plays an important role in fetal nutrition, but it is vestigial in man.

Two additional structures in the early umbilical cord, which may persist into the second and third trimesters, are the transitional epithelial-lined allantoic duct (fig. 1-5), lying directly between the two arteries, and the intestinal epithelial-lined vitelline duct (fig. 1-6), with or without its accompanying omphalomesenteric arteries (see chapter 8, Vestigial Remnants). The vitelline duct and its vessels communicate with the yolk sac in early pregnancy. The umbilical

Figure 1-6
VITELLINE DUCT REMNANT

The vitelline duct arises from the midileum (Meckel's diverticulum) and is sometimes flanked by vessels which connect the placental yolk sac to the primitive vitelline circulation of the embryo early in pregnancy. It is lined by intestinal-type epithelium with goblet cells. Occasionally, vitelline vessels give rise to umbilical hemangiomas. In some species (but not in man) the yolk sac plays an important role in fetal nutrition.

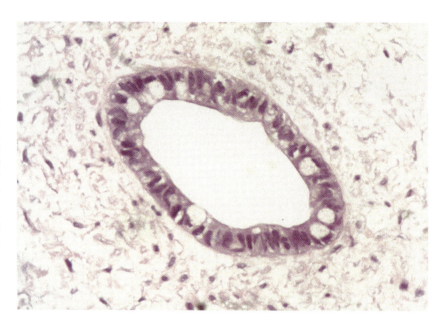

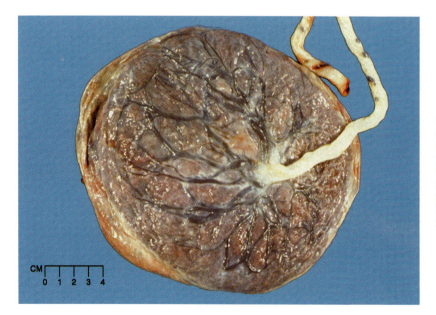

Figure 1-7
CHORIONIC PLATE (FETAL SURFACE)

The surface is covered by glistening, transparent amnion. Chorionic arteries and veins branch from the umbilical cord insertion. Arteries pass over veins. Plaques of yellow-white subchorionic fibrin bulge slightly upward. The normal color ranges from gray-blue to red. Membranes normally arise from the margin of the round-oval disc.

cord insertion is generally near the center of the placental disc (fig. 1-7), but may be displaced to any location on the chorionic plate or in the membranes because of asymmetry in the process of membrane formation (described below). The vessels within the umbilical cord that insert in the membranes may become occluded by torsion during gestation or torn at the time of membrane rupture, leading to fetal hemorrhage (see chapter 8, Insertion Anomalies).

Chorionic Plate and Stem Villi

The chorionic plate (fetal surface of the placenta) is normally covered by a layer of glistening amnion and undergirded by variable amounts of white-tan subchorionic fibrin (fig. 1-7). Viewed from above, it is generally reddish blue, with the plaques of subchorionic fibrin bulging slightly upward. The amount of subchorionic fibrin is of no clinical significance. Arteries and veins, approximately 8 to 10 each, branch from the umbilical vessels and extend in every direction, stopping at the peripheral margin of the placental disc; arteries travel over veins. Approximately 40 major primary stem villi, each measuring 0.5 to 1.5 mm in diameter, protrude perpendicularly downward from the chorionic plate (10). These in turn each separate into 4 to 8 secondary stem villi, which travel parallel to the chorionic plate.

Microscopically, the chorionic plate and stem villi, both primary and secondary, are composed of dense collagenized connective tissue surrounding thick-walled arteries and veins (fig. 1-8). It is difficult to distinguish whether any given vessel is an artery or vein, but veins generally have thinner walls than arteries. The trophoblast that originally surrounds stem villi is largely replaced by fibrin, which deposits as a consequence of vascular stasis. Since this fibrin is surrounding non-gas exchanging structures it has no clinical significance.

The more distal extensions of major stem villi include immature intermediate (anchoring) villi, which implant in the basal plate (see below), and mature intermediate (tertiary stem) villi, which develop early in the third trimester (16). Mature intermediate villi give rise to terminal villous units (discussed below). At the end of this process, each primary stem villus in the mature placenta has given rise to approximately 10 to 15 total branching generations of smaller villi (45). A more rigorous discussion of the process of villous morphogenesis, with illustrations, can be found elsewhere (4). At term, major stem villi may show remnants of a peripheral paravascular capillary net, more typical of earlier stem villi (fig. 1-9). This subtrophoblastic capillary net can proliferate to form chorangiomas or diffuse chorangiomatosis (see chapter 4) (61).

Terminal Villous Unit and Interhemal Membrane

The terminal villous unit consists of the most distal portion of the mature intermediate stem villus that contains a muscularized arteriole plus the terminal villi arising from it (fig. 1-10) (81). At this point, flow into gas exchanging villi is regulated by placental arteriolar tone. The terminal villi are composed of capillaries, fetal macrophages (Hofbauer cells), and a few perivascular fibroblasts without associated col-

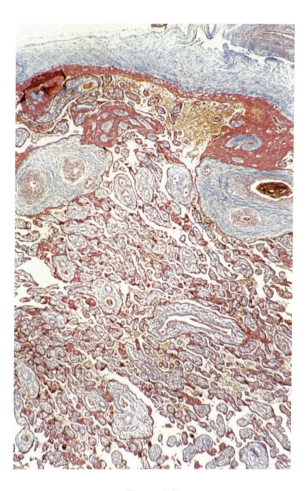

Figure 1-8

CHORIONIC PLATE AND STEM VILLI

The chorionic plate consists of blue-stained, heavily collagenized connective tissue containing thick-walled fetal vessels. The undersurface of the plate is lined by bright red-staining fibrin. Primary stem villi project vertically downward and have a similar appearance to the chorionic plate, while secondary stem villi are less densely collagenized and run horizontal to the chorionic plate (trichrome stain).

lagen. The surrounding trophoblast bilayer is stretched thin, so that only the outer syncytiotrophoblast layer is seen in most villi. Normal terminal villi contain one or more attenuated regions where capillaries are intimately applied to the trophoblast basement membrane. These regions, known as vasculosyncytial membranes, constitute the interhemal membrane, where the majority of gas exchange occurs (42). Focal aggregates of degenerating syncytiotrophoblast nuclei (syncytial knots), especially prominent in placentas with evidence

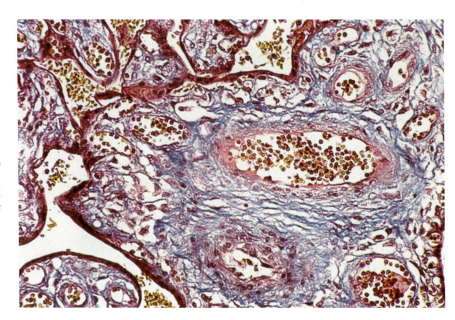

Figure 1-9

PARAVASCULAR CAPILLARY NET OF STEM VILLI

Stem villi may show a subtrophoblastic layer of capillaries surrounded by a prominent reticular network of fibrils. This capillary net can give rise to chorangiomas and chorangiomatosis (trichrome stain).

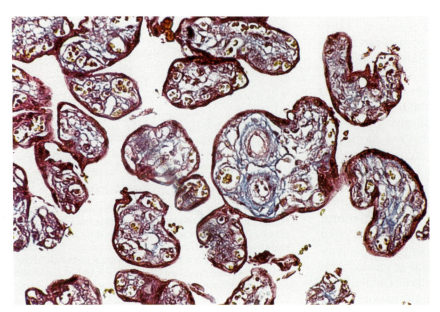

Figure 1-10

TERMINAL VILLOUS UNIT

A single tertiary stem villus, defined by its central arteriole and surrounding perivascular collagen, is surrounded by terminal villi. These mature terminal villi contain very little collagen and are composed of 4 to 6 capillaries closely applied to a thin syncytial layer of trophoblast that separates the fetal and maternal circulations (trichrome stain).

of maternal underperfusion, are seen in most term placentas. They may have adaptive significance by attenuating the cytoplasm of adjacent trophoblast, decreasing the thickness of the interhemal membrane, and maximizing gas exchange (80). The growth of terminal villi is driven by capillary proliferation (angiogenesis) (43). Imbalances between capillary and adjacent stromal growth can lead to hypercapillarization (see chapter 4, Villous Chorangiosis), another placental adaptation that may enhance gas exchange.

Basal Plate and Anchoring Villi

The basal plate (maternal surface) is dark red, with a smooth to pebbled texture attributable to sheets of extracellular matrix material corresponding to the so-called stria of Rohr and Nitabuch seen on microscopic examination (fig. 1-11). The surface of the basal plate and the immediately adjacent intervillous space often undergo variable amounts of calcification, which has no clinical significance. The contour of the basal plate is coarsely folded, forming clefts

Anatomy, Structure, Development, and Function

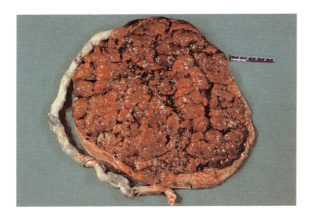

Figure 1-11

BASAL PLATE (MATERNAL SURFACE)

The maternal surface is opaque and coarsely folded into irregular lobulations. It is dark red, with a smooth to coarsely pebbled texture. Fine, speckled yellow calcifications are seen in the center of many of the lobules (trichrome stain).

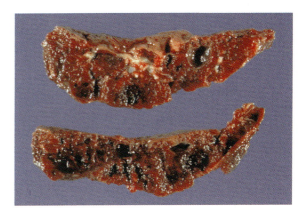

Figure 1-12

PLACENTAL SEPTAL CYST

The cyst is seen on the right side of the upper cross section of placenta. It is lined by a smooth wall and contains clear fluid.

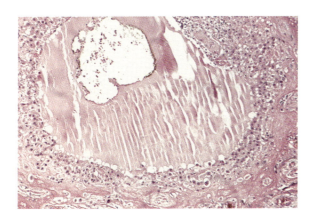

Figure 1-13

PLACENTAL SEPTAL CYST

Septal cysts are really pseudocysts formed by infoldings of the basal plate with intermediate trophoblast. The discohesive trophoblast secretes an eosinophilic fluid that is rich in major basic protein.

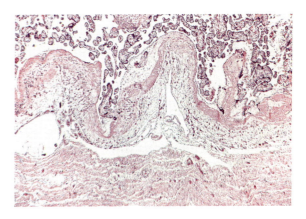

Figure 1-14

BASAL PORTION OF THE PLACENTA AND UNDERLYING UTERUS

The basal plate is the serpiginous horizontal layer across the mid-portion of the slide. It is composed of trophoblast with surrounding matrix-type fibrinoid (Nitabuch's layer) and underlying decidualized endometrium. The natural cleavage plane between placenta and the underlying uterus is just below the basal plate. Gas-exchanging terminal villi occupy the top of the figure.

known as placental septa that protrude into the parenchyma and can extend as far as the fetal surface. Septa form as a consequence of continuing radial placental growth after fixation of the membrane margin (sealing of the closure ring) and have no functional significance. Entrapped nests of basal plate trophoblast in the septa can secrete clear fluid to form septal cysts, which are of no clinical significance (figs. 1-12, 1-13).

Microscopically, the basal plate contains a variety of elements (fig. 1-14). Anchoring villi, the most distal extensions of the primary stem villi, insert in and are often surrounded by maternal endometrium. The trophoblast cells lining the endometrial aspect of the anchoring villi differentiate to form invasive intermediate trophoblast (fig. 1-15) (7,24). This intermediate trophoblast synthesizes copious amounts

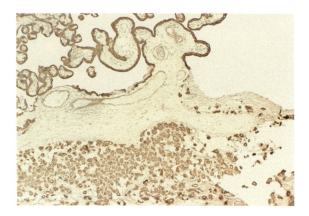

Figure 1-15
ANCHORING VILLUS WITH SUBJACENT INTERMEDIATE TROPHOBLAST

The villous trophoblast on the underside of the anchoring villus (in contact with endometrium) undergoes an epithelial-mesenchymal transformation to form an invasive intermediate trophoblast, which invades the uterus (bottom of slide). Free-floating terminal villi are seen at the top of the slide (cytokeratin immunostain).

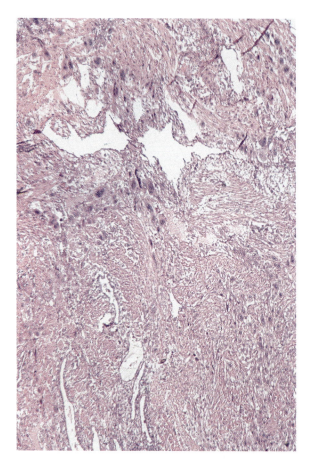

Figure 1-16
PLACENTAL SITE (TROPHOBLAST) GIANT CELLS

Intermediate trophoblast cells at the point of maximal invasion fuse to form multinucleate giant cells. The majority of these giant cells are normally found in the inner third of the myometrium. Exceptions are preeclamptic placentas with characteristic superficial implantation in which abundant giant cells may be found in the basal plate.

of extracellular matrix material, particularly enriched in a specific molecule known as oncofetal fibronectin, which accumulates between the trophoblast and the underlying endometrium (stria of Nitabuch) (27). Trophoblastic giant cells (placental site giant cells) form when the intermediate trophoblast achieves its maximum extent of invasion (fig. 1-16). Since this usually occurs within the myometrium, the finding of excessive giant cells in the basal plate may be an indication of abnormally superficial implantation. Occasionally, dilated maternal arteries lined by fibrinoid matrix and scattered endovascular trophoblast may be seen (see below). Maternal veins generally run parallel to the basal plate and are less conspicuous. These veins may also contain variable amounts of trophoblast and fibrinoid, particularly on the side facing the placenta (6,20).

A background population of mononuclear cells in the attached decidualized endometrium is common. Plasma cells are not normal in this location. Fragmentation of the maternal surface of the placenta (basal plate) may be associated with retained placenta and should be communicated to the clinician. The absence of an endometrial layer between the trophoblast and smooth muscle in the basal plate is indicative of placenta accreta (see chapter 4), while the presence of a few smooth muscle fibers within decidualized endometrium is not.

Placental Margin and Membranes

The placental margin is normally characterized by a sharply demarcated transition between the placental disc and the attached membranes. In some cases this transition zone may be less abrupt, or even markedly irregular, and the placenta may assume various nondiscoid shapes (see chapter 4, Disorders of Placental Migration). The transition zone is characterized histologically by the collapse of the intervillous space, leaving only a few atrophic villi and a band of trophoblast sandwiched between the fetal surface (fibrous chorion and amnion) and the maternal surface (decidualized endometrium with maternal blood vessels).

Formation of the placental margin is somewhat more complicated than simple atrophy. Since the gestational sac forms on one side of the uterus and eventually fuses with the opposite wall, it is clear that the margin must actually represent a fold, composed of the endometrium covering the implanting gestational sac and that of the opposite uterine wall. This fold creates a potential space where blood can accumulate, leading to the circumvallate placenta (see chapter 4). It has become apparent that the placenta grows laterally during early gestation by a process of villous attachment to and extension into large lateral uterine veins (discussed in more detail below) (22,59). This leads to the formation of a dilated marginal venous sinus which drains a substantial amount of the blood in the intervillous space (fig. 1-17). Transient increases in maternal venous pressure may lead to rupture of these engorged marginal veins (fig. 1-18) (33,67).

DEVELOPMENTAL ANATOMY

The purpose of this section is to simplify the complex subject of placental development by separating it into compartments, and considering processes and events in terms of when they occur relative to the last menstrual period (10,25,

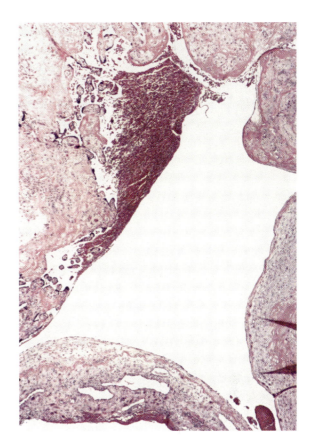

Figure 1-17

DILATED MARGINAL VEIN (MARGINAL SINUS)

A dilated, blood-filled marginal space is bounded by villi on the left, chorion and amnion on the top, and decidualized endometrium on the bottom.

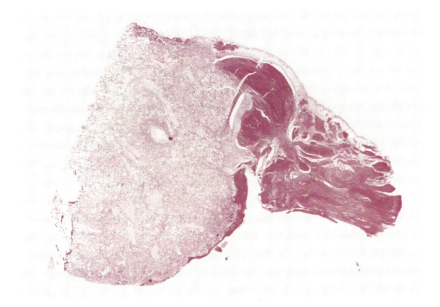

Figure 1-18

DISTENDED MARGINAL SINUS VEIN WITH EARLY MARGINAL ABRUPTION

The dilated marginal vein in the mid-portion of this whole mount histologic section is flanked on the right by fresh hemorrhage underlying the membranes.

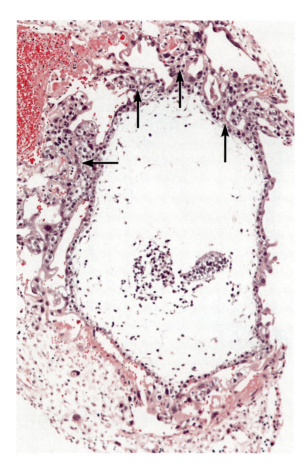

Figure 1-19

EARLY LACUNAR TROPHOBLAST PLAQUE WITH A FEW PRIMARY VILLI

The slide shows a proliferating primitive syncytial trophoblast surrounding the extraembryonic coelom with a thin layer of interposed extraembryonic mesoderm. The primitive trophoblastic syncytium has begun to organize into columns with cores of central mononuclear cytotrophoblast (arrows). Embryonic tissue is seen at the center and the plaque is surrounded by secretory endometrium.

36,62,65). Further details regarding the developmental biology of human and rodent placental development can be found in recent reviews (23,35).

Blastocyst Trophectoderm (Days 18 to 20 of Menstrual Cycle)

A morphologically evident trophoblast first becomes distinct from the embryonic inner cell mass at the 16-cell stage of development, prior to implantation. Experimental work in animals implicates a specific array of growth factors secreted by the embryonic inner cell mass that maintain the pluripotency of these trophoblast stem cells prior to contact with the maternal endometrium (77).

Nidation and Maternal Capillary Circulation (Days 20 to 28 of Menstrual Cycle)

Nidation, or apposition, refers to the binding of the blastocyst trophectoderm to the endometrial epithelium, a process that involves a number of growth factors, adhesion molecules, and cytokines (14). Within days of nidation, the blastocyst translocates across the epithelium to lodge in the endometrial stroma directly adjacent to one of the approximately 4,000 spiral arteries in the uterus. The placenta at this stage is referred to as a primitive trophoblast plaque. The trophoblast proliferates and differentiates to form a primitive syncytium, which erodes adjacent capillaries and venules to form intracellular lacunae (fig. 1-19). These lacunae eventually enlarge and become remodeled to form the definitive intervillous space. Columns of primitive syncytium, lying between the enlarging lacunar spaces, are invaded by cords of cytotrophoblastic cells which grow down from the primitive chorion to form "primary villi." It seems likely that the remnants of the primitive syncytium disappear or are overgrown by the mature syncytiotrophoblast, which forms by fusion and terminal differentiation of the invading cytotrophoblast (see below).

Chorionic Plate and Body Stalk (4 to 5 Weeks from Last Menstrual Period [LMP])

Mesoderm derived from the inner cell mass grows out from the allantois through the body stalk to form a sheet covering the primitive chorion. In rodents, fusion with the chorion depends on specific molecular interactions between the allantoic mesoderm and the trophoblast (31).

Villous Stromal Vasculogenesis (5 to 6 Weeks from LMP)

Vasculogenic villous stroma develops from extraembryonic mesoderm derived from the degenerating hypoblast of the primitive yolk sac (5). Downgrowth of this stroma into the recently formed primary villi forms "secondary villi" (fig. 1-20). Capillaries develop in situ from this extraembryonic mesoderm following induction by the adjacent trophoblast (fig. 1-21).

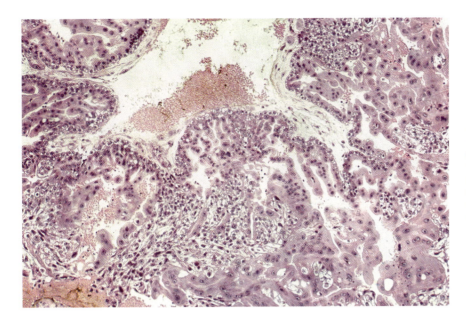

Figure 1-20

SECONDARY VILLUS FORMATION

Secondary villi form as extraembryonic mesoderm grows down the center of the primary villi. Connective tissue is separated from eosinophilic syncytial trophoblast by mononuclear cytotrophoblast with clear cytoplasm (center right).

Figure 1-21

VILLOUS CAPILLARY FORMATION

Villous stromal connective tissue adjacent to trophoblast is induced by vascular endothelial growth factors to form capillaries with nucleated red blood cells.

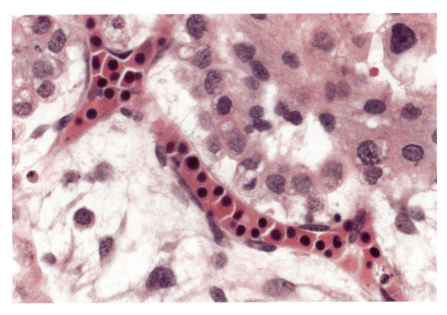

The formation of villous capillaries transforms secondary villi into primitive "tertiary villi" (fig. 1-22). The villous capillary network forms in parallel with, and independent of, the paired umbilical arteries that emanate from the iliac arteries along the allantois and the formation of a beating heart in the embryo. Anastomosis of capillaries with larger vessels in the placenta at about 6 weeks is contemporaneous with the same process in the central nervous system. Development of other organ vascular beds follows shortly thereafter. A practical implication of parallel development of capillaries and larger vessels is that capillaries may be seen within villi and below the chorion in gestations without a viable fetus, such as hydatidiform moles or other anembryonic pregnancies (44).

Elaboration of Mesenchymal Villi (6 to 8.5 Weeks from LMP)

The transition from unbranched, primitive tertiary villi to the finger-like mesenchymal villi seen most commonly in early elective terminations occurs through iterative cycles of

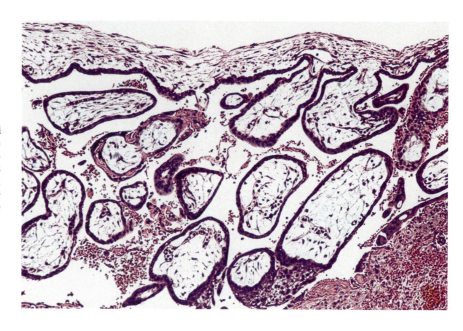

Figure 1-22

TERTIARY VILLUS FORMATION

Simple unbranched villi with subtrophoblastic capillaries mark the third stage of villous development. At this stage, the primitive syncytium has disappeared and the definitive intervillous space has formed.

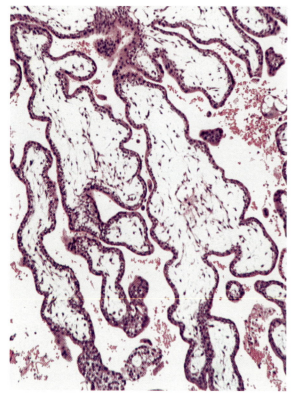

Figure 1-23

BRANCHING MESENCHYMAL VILLI

Prior to 10 weeks' gestation, chorionic villi branch as finger-like mesenchymal villi with abundant loose connective tissue stroma. From their origin in the chorionic plate to their terminal branches, the villi are uniform in appearance.

branching morphogenesis (fig. 1-23). Early mesenchymal villi are characterized by scant connective tissue and an absence of thick-walled fetal vessels. These features help the pathologist separate early to mid-first trimester placentas from later stages.

Development of Stem Villi
(8.5 to 11.5 Weeks from LMP)

Immature intermediate villi, characterized by more densely collagenized connective tissue stroma and thicker-walled fetal vessels, are formed in the late first trimester. They provide the enlarging placenta with greater structural support for the higher pressure circulation required to perfuse the enlarging villous tree (fig. 1-24).

Early Implantation and Arterial Plugs
(6 to 12 Weeks from LMP)

Early implantation is mediated by trophoblast derived from that portion of the anchoring villus in direct contact with maternal endometrium at the floor of the intervillous space. This trophoblast first proliferates to form a confluent sheet known as the cytotrophoblast shell at the floor of the placenta. Some trophoblast in the shell then undergoes an epithelial-mesenchymal transformation to form invasive intermediate trophoblast, which permeates the endometrium in the vicinity of the placenta (implantation site) (fig. 1-25).

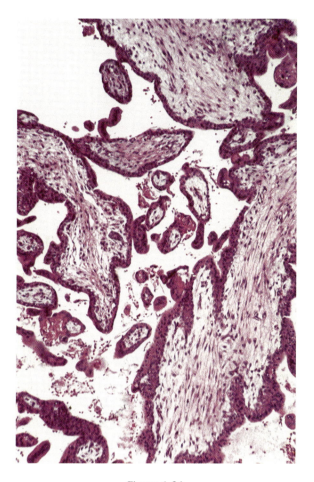

Figure 1-24

IMMATURE INTERMEDIATE STEM VILLI

After 10 weeks, as the placenta enlarges, villi near the chorionic plate acquire thick-walled vessels and a sheath of more cellular fibroblastic connective tissue.

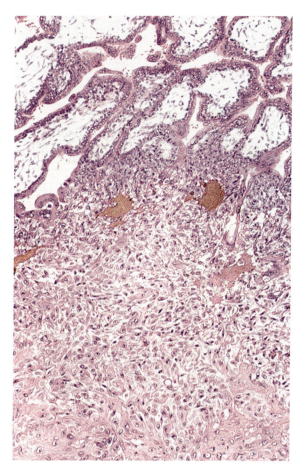

Figure 1-25

EARLY PRIMARY IMPLANTATION

Cellular trophoblast cells with clear cytoplasm form the cytotrophoblast shell immediately below the villi. As the trophoblast cells invade toward deeper levels, they first become larger and more discohesive (immature intermediate trophoblast), and later acquire eosinophilic cytoplasm (mature intermediate trophoblast).

A fascinating and still somewhat controversial aspect of placental development is that despite early invasion of the uterine arteries, arterial circulation to the intervillous space is not fully established until 10 to 12 weeks of gestation (15,39). Prior to this time, endovascular trophoblast derived from the cytotrophoblast shell adopts a pseudovasculogenic phenotype and grows down into the arterial lumens, forming loose cellular plugs which act as sieves to restrict arterial flow to the intervillous space (fig. 1-26) (86). Some believe that most of the circulation to the intervillous space at this stage is indirect, depending on anastomoses connecting capillaries and veins with arteries distant from the implanting placenta. Two hypotheses have been advanced for this peculiar developmental sequence: first, that the poorly supported, early intervillous space might be obliterated by the pressure associated with a direct maternal arterial circulation and second, that oxygen-free radicals generated at the oxygen tension of arterial blood are toxic to the developing trophoblast (40). The functional consequence of indirect perfusion is that many developmental sequences in the early placenta take place in an anaerobic environment. Some early abortions associated with marked intervillous hemorrhage may be the result of premature arterial perfusion of the intervillous space.

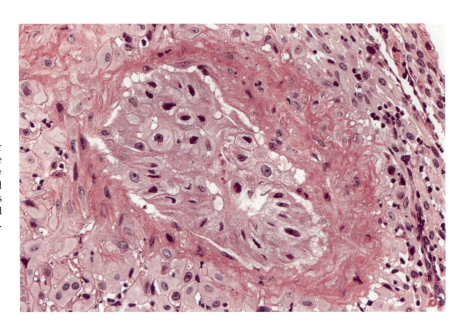

Figure 1-26

CYTOTROPHOBLAST PLUG IN SPIRAL ARTERY

Mononuclear endovascular trophoblast cells from the cytotrophoblast shell grow down the lumena of spiral arteries to form loose plugs which retard arterial blood flow to the intervillous space.

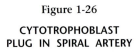

Figure 1-27

SECONDARY IMPLANTATION

Invasive intermediate trophoblast permeates the myometrium. Trophoblast cells at this location are spindle shaped with hyperchromatic nuclei.

Late Implantation and Arterial Remodeling (12 to 20 Weeks from LMP)

Implantation by the intermediate trophoblast has traditionally been separated into two distinct phases: primary, which is confined to the endometrium as described above and secondary, which involves extension of the trophoblast into the inner third of the myometrium (fig. 1-27) (63). Concurrent with secondary implantation, the endovascular trophoblast filling the lumens of uterine arteries invades the muscular wall, leading to dissolution of the muscular media and fixed vascular dilatation. This process creates a low pressure arterial circulation protected from vasospastic influences (figs. 1-28, 1-29). This trophoblast-dependent remodeling is supplemented by trophoblast-independent vascular remodeling, which has been shown in rodents to depend on cytokines secreted by uterine natural killer cells (2,21). Recent publications have deemphasized the separation of primary and secondary phases of implantation and consider the entire process of implantation as a continuum carefully regulated by factors such as ambient oxygen tension, growth factors, and cytokines (12,13,70,73). Deficient implantation and inadequate arterial remodeling predispose to the clinical disorder known as preeclampsia (see chapter 4, Distal Villous Hypoplasia with Placental Undergrowth and chapter 6, Decidual Vasculopathy).

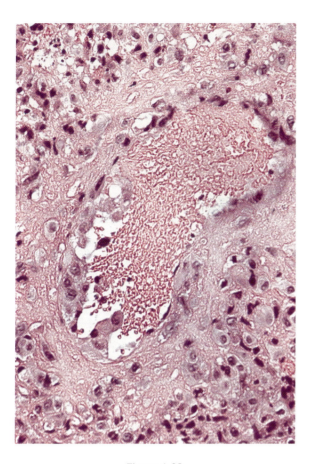

Figure 1-28

VASCULAR REMODELING IN THE DECIDUA

Endovascular trophoblast invades the vascular wall, replacing the smooth muscle with fibrinoid matrix material.

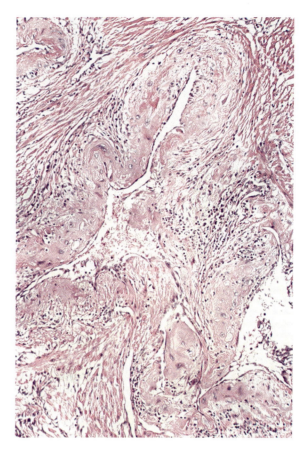

Figure 1-29

LARGE MYOMETRIAL ARTERY WITH TROPHOBLAST REMODELING

During secondary implantation, trophoblastic remodeling of spiral arterioles extends into large arteries in the myometrium. Failure of this deep remodeling is typical of preeclamptic gestations.

Membrane Formation and Peripheral Expansion (9 to 18 Weeks from LMP)

The formation of the placental membranes converts the placenta from a sphere protruding from one uterine wall to a disc surrounded by a thin sac that fills the uterine cavity. This process occurs in several stages. First, at about 9 to 11 weeks, the previously free amnionic sac fuses with the chorionic connective tissue, coincident with atrophy of the intervillous space at the periphery of the placenta. As the placenta grows and the sac enlarges, the remnants of intervillous trophoblast condense to form the chorion laevae, a layer that provides structural integrity for the adjacent and poorly supported fetal amnion and maternal decidua.

Recent data have shown that in addition to interstitial growth by elaboration of villous trees, the placenta also grows laterally by forming new anchoring villi in the open uterine veins that drain the intervillous space (21). Through serial rounds of attachment and new villous growth, the lateral placental veins enlarge, forming a marginal sinus surrounded by an investing layer of vascular smooth muscle (fig. 1-30) (59).

Between 17 and 20 weeks, the enlarging placenta/membrane sac comes in contact with and fuses with the endometrium of the opposite side of the uterus. Fusion provides the membranes with a maternal vascular supply that later assumes importance in the regulation of labor (see

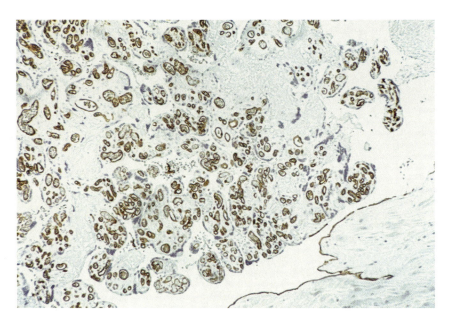

Figure 1-30

MARGINAL PLACENTA

CD34 stain highlights the vascular endothelial lining of the marginal intervillous space (lower right), which forms as a consequence of lateral placental growth into dilated uterine veins during early to mid-gestation.

below). One adverse consequence of filling the entire uterine cavity is exposure of the gestational sac to pathogenic microorganisms residing anywhere in the endometrium (chronic endometritis), lower uterine segment, or endocervix (see chapter 5, Chronic Deciduitis). The timing of endometrial fusion could explain the dramatically increasing incidence of preterm labor after 20 weeks' gestation (30).

Trophoblast Proliferative Units and Placental Growth (13 to 40 Weeks from LMP)

The trophoblastic epithelium of the terminal villi mediates the critical functions of gas exchange, substrate transport, waste elimination, and protection of the fetal vasculature. Growth of the villous trophoblast occurs at a constant rate throughout gestation by the process of hyperplasia without hypertrophy (75). The growth rate of the villous trophoblast lags behind that of the villous stroma, resulting in a dramatic thinning of the trophoblast layer by the third trimester. Recent work suggests that the villous trophoblast, like other epithelia, proliferates, differentiates, and undergoes renewal via a tightly regulated sequence (53). After 4 to 6 divisions, postmitotic villous cytotrophoblast cells fuse at a more or less constant nuclear ratio of 1 to 9 throughout gestation to form a multinucleate syncytiotrophoblast. Aberrations in the process of cytotrophoblast-syncytiotrophoblast fusion could potentially affect the function of trophoblast epithelium in terms of anticoagulant properties, integrity of the maternal-fetal vascular barrier, substrate transport, or hormone synthesis (72).

Aging syncytiotrophoblast nuclei undergo apoptosis to form syncytial knots and bridges, which are eventually extruded into the maternal circulation and cleared in the pulmonary circulation (see chapter 6, Decidual Vasculopathy) (53). Hypoxia and other stressors can accelerate the turnover of villous trophoblast by ischemic necrosis, leading to accelerated formation of syncytial knots and an increase in precursor cytotrophoblast (28,38,51). An excessive degree of syncytial knot extrusion can lead to exposure of villous connective tissue and the deposition of large amounts of intervillous fibrin-type fibrinoid (54,60).

Terminal Villogenesis (22 to 30 Weeks from LMP)

Terminal villogenesis, the final stage of placental morphogenesis, accommodates the dramatic increase in demand as the fetus enlarges from approximately 300 g at 20 weeks to over 3,000 g at term. Immature intermediate stem villi are replaced by mature intermediate stem villi, which give rise to terminal villi by a process of active longitudinal capillary growth and coiling (branching angiogenesis). Terminal villi, as described above, are specialized structures that bring fetal capillaries in close proximity to the oxygenated maternal blood in the intervillous space. Premature truncation of distal villous development (mature intermediate and terminal villous), with severe maternal underperfusion, can aggravate fetal hypoxia by decreasing the effective surface for fetal gas exchange. Overdevelopment of distal villi (continuous growth without maturation), as in fetoplacental growth disorders such as diabetes, can add mass at the expense of efficiency of placental function (see chapter 4).

FUNCTIONAL ANATOMY

Fetoplacental Arterial Perfusion

The distribution of fetal cardiac output to the various organ systems is regulated by the autonomic nervous system in response to the level of oxygen delivery from the placenta. Hypoxia leads to a redistribution of blood flow away from peripheral organs and toward the most critical organs, the heart and brain (34). Decreased flow in the middle cerebral artery and evidence of myocardial injury (increased fetal cardiac troponin levels) are late events in the hypoxic fetus and are harbingers of impending fetal death (52, 74). Prolonged hypoxia leads to decreased perfusion of the kidneys and oligohydramnios (83). Transient, often trivial, episodes of hypoxia in term and especially post-term fetuses can lead to shunting of blood away from the fetal gastrointestinal tract resulting in meconium release (41).

Unlike other fetal vascular beds, the placental arterial circulation lacks autonomic innervation and hence responds only to local signals such as pressure and flow (57). It is a low resistance circuit, normally receiving approximately 55 percent of the fetal cardiac output. The redistribution of blood flow that occurs with hypoxia has no immediate effect on placental vascular tone (37). However, severe longstanding hypoxia associated with a global decrease in cardiac output eventually leads to decreased placental perfusion, hypoplasia of distal placental villi, and a decrease in the overall placental vascular bed (79). This increases placental vascular resistance, decreases umbilical arterial blood flow, and results in abnormal umbilical pulsed-flow Doppler studies. Morphologic correlates of increased placental resistance and decreased umbilical artery flow are discussed in chapter 6. The consequences of segmental occlusion of fetal placental arteries are discussed in chapter 8.

Fetoplacental Venous Return

Oxygenated blood from the terminal villi is collected in stem villous veins and ultimately returned to the fetus via the umbilical vein. Compression or torsion of the umbilical cord or increased fetal central venous pressure can lead to transient or prolonged reductions in umbilical venous blood flow. Severely decreased venous return to the fetus can lead to hypoxia, redistribution of blood flow, and, ultimately, fetal cardiac failure and hydrops (see chapter 10). Obstruction to umbilical venous blood flow also causes stasis in the placental circulation, which can lead to thrombosis, premature involution of fetal stem vessels, and degeneration of the stroma and capillaries of the terminal villi (see chapter 8). Elevated venous pressure may contribute to fetal vascular thrombosis, umbilical or chorionic vessel rupture, or fetomaternal hemorrhage. The effects of increased pressure may be aggravated by other factors such as endothelial activation, vessel wall damage, or increased maternal pressure in the intervillous space (see chapters 5, 6, and 8) (26). Chronic hypoxia itself can affect umbilical venous return via constriction of umbilical-hepatic venous anastomosis (78). This causes decreased hepatic blood flow and increased flow through the ductus venosis to the systemic circulation. Reduced liver perfusion may then decrease insulin-like growth factor-I (IGF-I) production leading to a compensatory inhibition of fetal growth (fetal growth restriction).

Maternal Arterial Perfusion/Placental Lobule

The maternal blood supply to the intervillous space is provided by the 80 to 100 spiral arteries that perforate the basal plate. In normal pregnancies, most of these arteries are remodeled to provide low resistance to uterine blood flow. Nevertheless, further accommodation is required in late pregnancy to supply the rapidly growing fetus. This is provided by an increase in the maternal cardiac output and a two-fold increase in the luminal diameter of the main uterine arteries (46). These additional modifications result in a doubling of uterine blood flow between 20 and 38 weeks' gestation. Nevertheless, overall uterine blood flow per gram of fetal tissue still decreases by 81 percent over this period. This decrease is compensated for by continuing distal villogenesis and increased efficiency of mature terminal villi (increased syncytial knots, formation of vasculosyncytial membranes, and decreased villous connective tissue).

The physiologic unit of maternal perfusion is the placental lobule (84). Anchoring villi and their associated distal branching villi constitute the periphery of the lobule. The area overlying the opening of each spiral artery is the center. A single villous tree may contribute to several placental lobules. Blood from the spiral artery is propelled toward the roof of the intervillous space, displacing villi from the periphery of the lobule and creating spaces known as lucencies or cavities. Blood flow is arrested at the fibrin-covered undersurface of the chorionic plate and flows back down around major stem villi in the upper half of the placenta where little gas extraction occurs. The still-oxygenated blood then slowly percolates through the maze of branching distal villi in the lower two thirds of the placenta, where the majority of gas exchange occurs. Poorly developed (hypoplastic) distal villous trees not only extract less oxygen based on their decreased absorptive surface, but also fail to retard lobular blood flow, leading to a decreased duration of exposure to oxygenated maternal blood.

Maternal Venous Drainage/Marginal Sinus

Maternal blood exits the placenta via uterine veins, which travel obliquely or parallel to the basal plate and bear no fixed relationship to the arterial lobule. Because the majority of blood flow enters the placenta in its central portion (inner two thirds), venous drainage is enhanced in the periphery (outer one third). Obstruction to venous drainage increases intervillous pressure and leads to decreased fetal placental blood flow due to villous compression or rupture of marginal veins, resulting in premature uteroplacental separation (see chapter 6). Causes of elevated venous pressure include altered placental geometry following the rupture of membranes, distorted uterine anatomy secondary to leiomyomas or cervical dilatation, and increased maternal venous pressure related to cardiac insufficiency or obstruction to the inferior vena cava by pressure from the gravid uterus.

Umbilical Cord Dynamics

Fetal vessels in the umbilical cord are surrounded by Wharton's jelly, a hydrated hyaluronic acid–rich gel with thixotropic properties that normally allows it to resist extremely high pressures (58). This normally protective function can be compromised by fetal volume depletion and the subsequent loss of hydration of the gel (decreased Wharton's jelly), chronic unremitting pressure, or excessive torsion (11,19,47,50).

Most umbilical cords are twisted and the majority have a left helix (twists from upper left to lower right) for reasons that are unclear, but might involve the direction of intestinal looping as it leaves the body stalk and returns to the fetal abdomen (48). Twisting results in the formation of a spiraled vascular sheath provided by the thick-walled umbilical arteries surrounding the thin-walled umbilical vein. The degree of twisting is most pronounced near the fetal cord insertion (8). Both decreases and increases in twisting (measurable by the umbilical coiling index) are associated with increased perinatal morbidity: the former as a reflection of decreased fetal movement and the latter because of a propensity for cord occlusion as described above (76).

Umbilical cord length is determined by tension, which is a function of fetal activity and the amount of space for movement in the amnionic cavity (see chapter 8, Cord Length) (56). Excessively long umbilical cords, generally caused by looping around body parts, have higher intrinsic resistance due to their length (3). Intrinsic resistance can be aggravated by the external pressure exerted by the cord loops themselves.

Membranes and Labor

The membranous chorion and amnion are avascular and free floating prior to fusion with the opposite wall of the uterus at 17 to 20 weeks. Fusion juxtaposes the metabolically active amnion and chorion with vascularized decidua and adjacent uterine smooth muscle.

Time does not permit a detailed consideration of the still poorly understood mechanisms of both premature and normal labor. However, it is generally acknowledged that local increases in cortisol and prostaglandins lead to a cascade of events that trigger labor and allow coordinated uterine contractions. The chorion laevae trophoblast appears to play a pivotal negative role in preventing the premature onset of labor by expressing high levels of prostaglandin dehydrogenase, which inactivates prostaglandins. This tonic inhibition can be overcome by several mechanisms. Normal (physiologic) labor is believed to be triggered by increases in corticotropin-releasing hormone and cortisol, which lead to induction of prostaglandin synthase activity, inhibition of prostaglandin dehydrogenase, and a consequent increase in active prostaglandins (1,18,55,68). Local prostaglandin production stimulates cortisol levels by inducing 11 beta-hydroxysteroid dehydrogenase (HDS) 1 enzyme activity, which converts inactive cortisone to cortisol in the chorionic trophoblast.

Three pathologic mechanisms trigger labor: chronic hypoxia, infection, and physical disruption of the chorion laevae trophoblast (49, 82). Hypoxia is thought to increase the production of chorionic corticotropin-releasing hormone (17). Infection (chorioamnionitis) can both decrease prostaglandin dehydrogenase in chorion laevae trophoblast and lead to the elaboration of cytokines, which can activate the labor cascade. Physical disruptions, such as rupture of membranes, retroplacental hemorrhage, cervical dilatation, and "membrane stripping," may separate the myometrium from the tonic inhibition usually exerted by chorion laevae trophoblast.

Syncytiotrophoblast and Maternal Physiology

The syncytiotrophoblast, in addition to its roles in transport and protection, also functions as a transplanted fetal endocrine organ in the maternal circulation (reviewed in reference 66). Hormones such as human chorionic gonadotropin (HCG), human placental lactogen (HPL), and human growth hormone (HGH) usurp the normal pituitary regulation of luteinizing hormone (LH) and growth hormone (GH). Other pregnancy-specific proteins modulate coagulation, vasodilation, bioavailability of maternal hormones, and a panoply of other maternal physiologic processes in ways that facilitate growth and development of the fetus (9). Regulation of syncytiotrophoblast hormone secretion is passive, depending only on total placental mass and fetal genetic background (32).

This evolutionary mode of regulation allows well-developed, well-nourished infants to make a positive contribution to their own well being in utero. Conversely, abnormal fetuses often have small placentas that are deficient in syncytiotrophoblast protein synthesis, which can contribute to pregnancy loss. Adding another layer of complexity, specific alleles favor the production of high levels of syncytiotrophoblast proteins, promoting the transmission of paternally derived genes into the next generation. In support of this goal, some placental proteins have evolved mechanisms ensuring expression from the paternal allele only (genomic imprinting) (85). Overexpression of these alleles in androgenetic conceptuses, such as complete and partial moles, may explain some of the unregulated trophoblast cell growth seen in these premalignant conditions.

REFERENCES

1. Alfaidy N, Xiong ZG, Myatt L, Lye SJ, MacDonald JF, Challis JR. Prostaglandin F2alpha potentiates cortisol production by stimulating 11beta-hydroxysteroid dehydrogenase 1: a novel feedback loop that may contribute to human labor. J Clin Endocrinol Metab 2001;86:5585–92.
2. Ashkar AA, Di Santo JP, Croy BA. Interferon gamma contributes to initiation of uterine vascular modification, decidual integrity, and uterine natural killer cell maturation during normal murine pregnancy. J Exp Med 2000;192:259–70.
3. Baergen RN, Malicki D, Behling C, Benirschke K. Morbidity, mortality, and placental pathology in excessively long umbilical cords: retrospective study. Pediatr Dev Pathol 2001;4:144–53.
4. Benirschke K, Kaufmann P. Pathology of the human placenta, 4th ed. New York, NY: Springer; 2000.
5. Bianchi DW, Wilkins-Haug LE, Enders AC, Hay ED. Origin of extraembryonic mesoderm in experimental animals: relevance to chorionic mosaicism in humans. Am J Med Genet 1993;46:542–50.
6. Blankenship TN, Enders AC, King BF. Trophoblastic invasion and modification of uterine veins during placental development in macaques. Cell Tissue Res 1993;274:135–44.
7. Blankenship TN, King BF. Developmental changes in the cell columns and trophoblastic shell of the macaque placenta: an immunohistochemical study localizing type IV collagen, laminin, fibronectin and cytokeratins. Cell Tissue Res 1993;274:457–66.
8. Blickstein I, Varon Y, Varon E. Implications of differences in coiling indices at different segments of the umbilical cord. Gynecol Obstet Invest 2001;52:203–6.
9. Bohn H, Winckler W, Grundmann U. Immunochemically detected placental proteins and their biological functions. Arch Gynecol Obstet 1991;249:107–18.
10. Boyd JD, Hamilton WJ. The human placenta. Cambridge: Heffer; 1970.
11. Bruch JF, Sibony O, Benali K, Challier JC, Blot P, Nessmann C. Computerized microscope morphometry of umbilical vessels from pregnancies with intrauterine growth retardation and abnormal umbilical artery Doppler. Hum Pathol 1997;28:1139–45.
12. Caniggia I, Grisaru-Gravnosky S, Kuliszewsky M, Post M, Lye SJ. Inhibition of TGF-beta 3 restores the invasive capability of extravillous trophoblasts in preeclamptic pregnancies. J Clin Invest 1999;103:1641–50.
13. Caniggia I, Mostachfi H, Winter J, et al. Hypoxia-inducible factor-1 mediates the biological effects of oxygen on human trophoblast differentiation through TGFbeta(3). J Clin Invest 2000;105:577–87.
14. Carson DD, Bagchi I, Dey SK, et al. Embryo implantation. Dev Biol 2000;223:217–37.
15. Carter AM. When is the placental circulation established in man? Placenta 1997;18:83–7.
16. Castellucci M, Scheper M, Scheffen I, Celona A, Kaufmann P. The development of the human placental villous tree. Anat Embryol 1990;181:117–28.
17. Challis JR, Matthews SG, Van Meir C, Ramirez MM. Current topic: the placental corticotrophin-releasing hormone-adrenocorticotrophin axis. Placenta 1995;16:481–502.
18. Cheung PY, Walton JC, Tai HH, Riley SC, Challis JR. Immunocytochemical distribution and localization of 15-hydroxyprostaglandin dehydrogenase in human fetal membranes, decidua, and placenta. Am J Obstet Gynecol 1990;163(5 Pt 1):1445–9.
19. Collins JH. Nuchal cord type A and type B. Am J Obstet Gynecol 1997;177:94.
20. Craven CM, Chedwick LR, Ward K. Placental basal plate formation is associated with fibrin deposition in decidual veins at sites of trophoblast cell invasion. Am J Obstet Gynecol 2002;186:291–6.
21. Craven CM, Morgan T, Ward K. Decidual spiral artery remodelling begins before cellular interaction with cytotrophoblasts. Placenta 1998;19:241–52.
22. Craven CM, Zhao L, Ward K. Lateral placental growth occurs by trophoblast cell invasion of decidual veins. Placenta 2000;21:160–9.
23. Cross JC, Werb Z, Fisher SJ. Implantation and the placenta: key pieces of the development puzzle. Science 1994;266:1508–18.
24. Damsky CH, Fitzgerald ML, Fisher SJ. Distribution patterns of extracellular matrix components and adhesion receptors are intricately modulated during first trimester cytotrophoblast differentiation along the invasive pathway, in vivo. J Clin Invest 1992;89:210–22.
25. Demir R, Kaufmann P, Castellucci M, Erbengi T, Kotowski A. Fetal vasculogenesis and angiogenesis in human placental villi. Acta Anat 1989;136:190–203.
26. DeSa DJ. Rupture of fetal vessels on placental surface. Arch Dis Child 1971;46:495–501.
27. Feinberg RF, Kliman HJ, Lockwood CJ. Is oncofetal fibronectin a trophoblast glue for human implantation? Am J Pathol 1991;138:537–43.
28. Fox H. The villous cytotrophoblast as an index of placental ischaemia. J Obstet Gynaecol Br Commonw 1964;71:885–93.

29. Fujimoto T, Parry S, Urbanek M, et al. A single nucleotide polymorphism in the matrix metalloproteinase-1 (MMP-1) promoter influences amnion cell MMP-1 expression and risk for preterm premature rupture of the fetal membranes. J Biol Chem 2002;277:6296–302.
30. Goldenberg R, Hauth J, Andrews W. Intrauterine infection and preterm delivery. N Engl J Med 2000;342:1500–7.
31. Gurtner GC, Davis V, Li H, McCoy MJ, Sharpe A, Cybulsky MI. Targeted disruption of the murine VCAM1 gene: essential role of VCAM-1 in chorioallantoic fusion and placentation. Genes Dev 1995;9:1–14.
32. Haig D. Genetic conflicts in human pregnancy. Q Rev Biol 1993;68:495–532.
33. Harris BA. Peripheral placental separation: a review. Obstet Gynecol Surv 1988;43:577–81.
34. Hecher K, Campbell S, Doyle P, Harrington K, Nicolaides K. Assessment of fetal compromise by Doppler ultrasound investigation of the fetal circulation. Arterial, intracardiac, and venous blood flow velocity studies. Circulation 1995;91:129–38.
35. Hemberger M, Cross JC. Genes governing placental development. Trends Endocrinol Metab 2001;12:162–8.
36. Hertig A. Human trophoblast. Springfield, IL: Thomas; 1968.
37. Hoeldtke NJ, Napolitano PG, Moore KH, Calhoun BC, Hume RF Jr. Fetoplacental vascular tone during fetal circuit acidosis and acidosis with hypoxia in the ex vivo perfused human placental cotyledon. Am J Obstet Gynecol 1997;177:1088–92.
38. Huppertz B, Kingdom J, Caniggia I, et al. Hypoxia favours necrotic versus apoptotic shedding of placental syncytiotrophoblast into the maternal circulation. Placenta 2003;24:181–90.
39. Jaffe R, Jauniaux E, Hustin J. Maternal circulation in the first trimester human placenta: myth or reality. Am J Obstet Gynecol 1997;176:695–705.
40. Jauniaux E, Watson AL, Hempstock J, Bao YP, Skepper JN, Burton GJ. Onset of maternal arterial blood flow and placental oxidative stress. A possible factor in human early pregnancy failure. Am J Pathol 2000;157:2111–22.
41. Jazayeri A, Politz L, Tsibris JC, Queen T, Spellacy WN. Fetal erythropoietin levels in pregnancies complicated by meconium passage: does meconium suggest fetal hypoxia? Am J Obstet Gynecol 2000;183:188–90.
42. Karimu AL, Burton GJ. Human term placental capillary endothelial cell specialization: a morphometric study. Placenta 1995;16:93–9.
43. Kaufmann P, Kingdom JC. Development of the vascular system in the placenta. In: Risau W, Rubanyi GM, eds. Morphogenesis of endothelium. Amsterdam: Harwood Academic; 2000.
44. Keep D, Zaragoza M, Hassold T, Redline RW. Very early complete hydatidiform mole. Hum Pathol 1996;27:708–13.
45. Kingdom J. Adriana and Luisa Castellucci Award Lecture 1997. Placental pathology in obstetrics: adaptation or failure of the villous tree? Placenta 1998;19:347–51.
46. Konje JC, Kaufmann P, Bell SC, Taylor DJ. A longitudinal study of quantitative uterine blood flow with the use of color power angiography in appropriate for gestational age pregnancies. Am J Obstet Gynecol 2001;185:608–13.
47. Labarrere C, Sebastiani M, Siminovich M, et al. Absence of Wharton's jelly around the umbilical cord; an unusual cause of perinatal mortality. Placenta 1985;6:555–9.
48. Lacro RV, Jones KL, Benirschke K. The umbilical cord twist: origin, direction, and relevance. Am J Obstet Gynecol 1987;157(4 Pt 1):833–8.
49. Lockwood CJ. Recent advances in elucidating the pathogenesis of preterm delivery, the detection of patients at risk, and preventative therapies. Curr Opin Obstet Gynecol 1994;6:7–18.
50. Machin GA, Ackerman J, Gilbert-Barness E. Abnormal umbilical cord coiling is associated with adverse perinatal outcomes. Pediatr Dev Pathol 2000;3:462–71.
51. MacLennan AH, Sharp F, Shaw-Dunn J. The ultrastructure of human trophoblast in spontaneous and induced hypoxia using a system of organ culture. A comparison and ultrastructural changes in pre-eclampsia and placental insufficiency. J Obstet Gynaecol Br Commonw 1972;79:113–21.
52. Makikallio K, Vuolteenaho O, Jouppila P, Rasanen J. Association of severe placental insufficiency and systemic venous pressure rise in the fetus with increased neonatal cardiac troponin T levels. Am J Obstet Gynecol 2000;183:726–31.
53. Mayhew TM. Villous trophoblast of human placenta: a coherent view of its turnover, repair and contributions to villous development and maturation. Histol Histopathol 2001;16:1213–24.
54. Mayhew TM, Barker BL. Villous trophoblast: morphometric perspectives on growth, differentiation, turnover and deposition of fibrin-type fibrinoid during gestation. Placenta 2001;22:628–38.
55. McLean M, Bisits A, Davies J, Woods R, Lowry P, Smith R. A placental clock controlling the length of human pregnancy. Nat Med 1995;1:460–3.
56. Moessinger AC, Blanc WA, Merone PA, Polsen DC. Umbilical cord length as an index of fetal activity: experimental study and clinical implications. Pediatr Res 1982;16:109–12.
57. Myatt L. Control of vascular resistance in the human placenta. Placenta 1992;13:329–41.

58. Nanaev AK, Kohnen G, Milovanov AP, Domogatsky SP, Kaufmann P. Stromal differentiation and architecture of the human umbilical cord. Placenta 1997;18:53–64.
59. Nanaev AK, Kosanke G, Kemp B, Frank HG, Huppertz B, Kaufmann P. The human placenta is encircled by a ring of smooth muscle cells. Placenta 2000;21:122–5.
60. Nelson DM, Crouch EC, Curran EM, Farmer DR. Trophoblast interaction with fibrin matrix. Epithelialization of perivillous fibrin deposits as a mechanism for villous repair in the human placenta. Am J Pathol 1990;136:855–65.
61. Ogino S, Redline RW. Villous capillary lesions of the placenta: distinctions between chorangioma, chorangiomatosis, and chorangiosis. Hum Pathol 2000;31:945–54.
62. O'Rahilly R, Muller F. Developmental stages in human embryos. Washington D.C.: Carnegie Institute of Washington; 1987.
63. Pijnenborg R, Bland JM, Robertson WB, Dixon G, Brosens I. The pattern of interstitial trophoblastic invasion of the myometrium in early human pregnancy. Placenta 1981;2:303–16.
64. Raio L, Ghezzi F, di Naro E, et al. In-utero characterization of the blood flow in the Hyrtl anastomosis. Placenta 2001;22:597–601.
65. Ramsey EM, Donner MW. Placental vasculature and circulation. Stuttgart: Thieme; 1980.
66. Redline RW. The placenta. In: Stefaneanu L, DSasano H, Kovacs K, eds. Molecular and cellular endocrine pathology. London, UK: Arnold; 2000:335–52.
67. Redline RW, Wilson-Costello D. Chronic peripheral separation of placenta. The significance of diffuse chorioamnionic hemosiderosis. Am J Clin Pathol 1999;111:804–10.
68. Riley SC, Walton JC, Herlick JM, Challis JR. The localization and distribution of corticotropin-releasing hormone in the human placenta and fetal membranes throughout gestation. J Clin Endocrinol Metab 1991;72:1001–7.
69. Robinson HN, Anhalt GJ, Patel HP, Takahashi Y, Labib RS, Diaz LA. Pemphigus and pemphigoid antigens are expressed in human amnion epithelium. J Invest Dermatol 1984;83:234–7.
70. Robson SC, Ball E, Lyall F, Simpson H, Ayis S, Bulmer JN. Endovascular trophoblast invasion and spiral artery transformation: the "two wave" theory revisited. Placenta 2001;22:A25.
71. Rockelein G, Kobras G, Becker V. Physiological and pathological morphology of the umbilical and placental circulation. Pathol Res Pract 1990;186:187–96.
72. Roth NS, ... AK. The role of placental trophoblast in the pathophysiology of the antiphospholipid antibody syndrome. Am J Reprod Immunol 1998;39(2):125–36.
73. Roth I, Fisher SJ. IL-10 is an autocrine inhibitor of human placental cytotrophoblast MMP-9 production and invasion. Dev Biol 1999;205:194–204.
74. Sepulveda W, Shennan AH, Peek MJ. Reverse end-diastolic flow in the middle cerebral artery: an agonal pattern in the human fetus. Am J Obstet Gynecol 1996;174:1645–7.
75. Simpson RA, Mayhew TM, Barnes PR. From 13 weeks to term, the trophoblast of human placenta grows by the continuous recruitment of new proliferative units: a study of nuclear number using the disector. Placenta 1992;13:501–12.
76. Strong TH Jr., Jarles DL, Vega JS, Feldman DB. The umbilical coiling index. Am J Obstet Gynecol 1994;170(Pt 1):29–32.
77. Tanaka S, Kunath T, Hadjantonakis AK, Nagy A, Rossant J. Promotion of trophoblast stem cell proliferation by FGF4. Science 1998;282:2072–5.
78. Tchirikov M, Kertschanska S, Schroder HJ. Obstruction of ductus venosus stimulates cell proliferation in organs of fetal sheep. Placenta 2001;22:24–31.
79. Todros T, Sciarrone A, Piccoli E, Guiot C, Kaufmann P, Kingdom J. Umbilical Doppler waveforms and placental villous angiogenesis in pregnancies complicated by fetal growth restriction. Obstet Gynecol 1999;93:499–503.
80. Tominaga T, Page EW. Accommodation of the human placenta to hypoxia. Am J Obstet Gynecol 1966;94:679–91.
81. Trudinger BJ, Giles WB, Cook CM. Uteroplacental blood flow velocity-time waveforms in normal and complicated pregnancy. Br J Obstet Gynaecol 1985;92:30–6.
82. van Meir CA, Matthews SG, Keirse MJ, Ramirez MM, Bocking A, Challis JR. 15-hydroxyprostaglandin dehydrogenase: implications in preterm labor with and without ascending infection. J Clin Endocrinol Metab 1997;82:969–76.
83. Veille JC, Kanaan C. Duplex Doppler ultrasonographic evaluation of the fetal renal artery in normal and abnormal fetuses. Am J Obstet Gynecol 1989;161(Pt 1):1502–7.
84. Wigglesworth JS. Vascular organization of the human placenta. Nature 1967;216:1120–1.
85. Wilkins JF, Haig D. Genomic imprinting of two antagonistic loci. Proc R Soc Lond B Biol Sci 2001;268:1861–7.
86. Zhou Y, Fisher SJ, Janatpour M, et al. Human cytotrophoblasts adopt a vascular phenotype as they differentiate. A strategy for successful endovascular invasion? J Clin Invest 1997;99:2139–51.

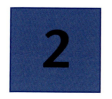

2 BASIC PATHWAYS OF PRENATAL AND PERIPARTUM INJURY: A PATHOGENIC APPROACH TO PLACENTAL INTERPRETATION

INTRODUCTION

The underlying basis of prenatal and peripartum injury is poorly understood, but recent advances in molecular genetics, embryonic development, and vascular biology have set the stage for dramatic advances over the next few years. In the broadest sense, all prenatal and peripartum injury can be explained by some combination of three basic mechanisms: 1) genetic causes of abnormal structure, such as karyotypic abnormalities, single gene defects, polygenic disease, or other genetic abnormalities (peroxisomal and mitochondrial disorders, imprinting disorders); 2) developmental abnormalities affecting fetoplacental reserve, such as an inadequate maternal supply line, nutritional deficiencies, or abnormalities in the maternal immune response to pregnancy; and 3) stochastic (random) events causing specific damage, such as exposure to teratogens, infection, vascular accidents, or membrane rupture. A specific listing of some of the clinical risk factors for injury is provided in Table 2-1.

Placental pathologists play a critical role in explaining prenatal and peripartum injury by revealing morphologic findings that both support and extend the clinical findings. To be useful, a pathology consultation needs to consider three questions, each of which is considered in greater detail in the remainder of this chapter: 1) What are the primary outcomes to be explained? From the standpoint of prenatal and peripartum injury, three perinatal outcomes stand out: preterm delivery, fetal growth restriction, and hypoxic ischemic injury; 2) What are the placental lesions and where do they exert their influence? Lesions can be categorized into groups indicating maternal (preplacental), fetal (postplacental), or intrinsic (placental) disease processes (Table 2-2); 3) What are the pathways of injury? How can underlying risk factors, specific events of the pregnancy as provided by (or elicited from) the clinician, and the nature, magnitude, and timing of the placental lesions be integrated to provide a plausible explanation of injury and adverse outcome?

PRIMARY ADVERSE OUTCOMES OF PRENATAL AND PERIPARTUM INJURY

To understand prenatal and peripartum injury it is important to first place the type of injury in a specific category. The category should be easily recognized, clearly defined, and clinically relevant. Preterm delivery, fetal growth restriction, and hypoxic-ischemic injury are the

Table 2-1

IMPORTANT RISK FACTORS FOR PRENATAL AND PERIPARTUM INJURY

Demographic	Maternal age Interval between pregnancies First pregnancy Poor obstetric history
Nutritional	Weight gain: excessive or inadequate Hyperemesis/ketosis Vitamin or mineral deficiency Protein calorie: malnutrition
Teratogenic	Smoking Environmental toxins Drugs: illicit or prescribed Trauma: iatrogenic or other Microorganisms
Maternal Disease	Diabetes mellitus Hypertension/renal disease Thyroid disease Autoimmune disease Thrombophilia
Fetal Abnormalities	Abnormal karyotype: fetal or placental Single gene defects Polygenic disorders Congenital malformations
Random (Stochastic) Events	Uteroplacental separation Fetomaternal hemorrhage Umbilical cord occlusion Membrane rupture

Table 2-2
CATEGORIES OF PLACENTAL LESIONS

Preplacental (Maternal)

Vascular obstruction	Increased syncytial knots
	Villous infarcts
Vascular disruption	Abruptio placenta (arterial)
	Marginal abruption (venous)
Developmental	Superficial implantation site
	Decidual arteriopathy
Inflammatory	Acute chorioamnionitis (maternal response)
	Subclinical endometritis
	Chronic villitis (VUE)[a]
Other	Massive perivillous fibrinoid deposition ("maternal floor infarction")

Placental

Fetal vascular obstruction	Fetal thrombotic vasculopathy
	Hemorrhagic endovasculitis
Fetal vascular disruption	Ruptured fetal vessel
	Intervillous thrombi (fetomaternal hemorrhage)
Developmental	Distal villous hypoplasia
	Distal villous immaturity
	Villous capillary lesions
	Mesenchymal dysplasia

Postplacental (Fetal)

	Meconium-associated vascular necrosis
	Acute chorioamnionitis (fetal vasculitis)
	Increased NRBC
	Cord occlusion
	Congenital infection
	Hydrops fetalis
	Genetic/chromosomal abnormality

[a]VUE = villitis of unknown etiology; NRBC = nucleated red blood cells.

primary outcomes that account for the majority of morbidity and mortality in the third trimester. Intrauterine fetal demise is sometimes considered separately, but is too broad and heterogeneous to treat as a single entity. Fetuses at the most severe end of the spectrum of each of the other three categories may all die in utero. In order to provide clinically useful information, pathologists should have a thorough understanding of the definition, differential diagnosis, and potential complications associated with each of the primary adverse outcomes.

Preterm Delivery

Prematurity is commonly defined as birth at less than 37 weeks after the last menstrual period (LMP). Gestational age, as determined from the LMP, may sometimes be modified by uterine size in early pregnancy, ultrasound in the first and second trimesters, or newborn examination to yield a more accurate estimate (15). Neonatologists often subdivide premature infants by birth weight into a low birth weight group weighing between 1,550 and 2,499 g and a very low birth weight group weighing less than 1,500 g. With the dramatic increase in the survival of very small infants, a third category of extremely low birth weight infants weighing less than 1,000 g has also been recognized (6). Obstetricians more commonly categorize preterm deliveries based on the presenting symptom, premature onset of labor or premature rupture of membranes, and separate both from indicated premature births due to maternal disease (31,46). Distinctions between the first two categories have little direct relevance for pathologists, but placentas from the third group are notable for having a high incidence of associated maternal vascular lesions.

Maternal (preplacental) risk factors for preterm delivery can be separated into five groups: demographic factors (maternal age less than 20 years, previous preterm birth, short interpregnancy interval); psychosocial factors (poor prenatal care, inadequate nutrition, low socioeconomic index, psychosocial stress); constitutional factors (low prepregnancy weight, poor pregnancy weight gain, short cervix as determined by antenatal ultrasound); teratogen exposure (cocaine, smoking); and infections (bacterial vaginosis, sexually transmitted disease, urinary tract infections) (7,24,28,30,45,60,61). All indicate a threatening environment not fully supportive of fetal development and maternal well being. In an evolutionary sense, preterm labor can almost be considered an adaptive response for both mother and fetus. The fetus is benefitted by delivery prior to substantial injury while the mother is allowed to recover from nutritional, infectious, and other pregnancy-related threats to her general and reproductive health.

Evolution may select for mechanisms that promote the expulsion of abnormal fetuses. Such fetal (postplacental) abnormalities as congenital infection, malformations, chromosomal abnormalities, and genetic defects often lead to preterm delivery for reasons that are poorly understood but may include abnormal hormonal function or the elaboration of inflammatory cytokines.

Placental lesions associated with preterm labor generally affect the membranous amniochorion where the corticosteroid-modulated prostaglandin cascade that regulates labor is centered. Acute chorioamnionitis, maternal underperfusion, chronic deciduitis, and marginal separation with retroplacental hemorrhage can all actively modulate this pathway by mechanisms that include the release of cytokines, regulatory neuropeptides, and other mediators (40,59). Many underlying causes of preterm labor and delivery have as a final common pathway inappropriate access of pathogenic microorganisms to the contents of the uterus resulting in placental chorioamnionitis (see chapter 5, Acute Chorioamnionitis). It would be a mistake, however, to assume that infection is the primary event in all such cases (23).

Mortality in the preterm infant usually follows delivery, but intrauterine fetal death sometimes occurs. Acute chorioamnionitis, by itself, is not usually a direct cause of fetal death. Associated conditions, such as abruption, fetal vascular thrombosis associated with inflammation, or fetal sepsis documented by culture of a highly pathogenic organism with a significant fetal inflammatory response, are exceptions. The most important complications of prematurity leading to significant early morbidity are central nervous system lesions (interventricular hemorrhage and white matter damage), chronic lung disease, and necrotizing enterocolitis (29,51,62). Long-term complications include cerebral palsy, developmental delay, restrictions in the activities of daily living, and visual impairment (26,47).

Fetal Growth Restriction

The expected weight for gestational age is usually obtained from one of several standardized charts derived from populations of varying socioeconomic, racial, and geographic origins (2,19,71). However, the use of any arbitrary cutoff to define fetal growth restriction (FGR) necessarily includes some infants below the threshold who have reached their biologic maximum growth potential and excludes other infants above the threshold who have a growth potential that has not been realized due to in utero factors. For this reason, some authors have proposed that each infant's specific demographic factors and growth trajectory be used to define FGR (70). By these criteria, some infants falling below the 10th percentile would be considered normal while others above the 10th percentile would have FGR. Unfortunately, the data needed for individualized assessment are often not available, particularly to the pathologist. A practical approach is to consider any infant born at less than the 3rd percentile for gestational age as almost certainly having FGR and infants weighing less than 2.5 kg at term as having a high likelihood of FGR. Infants can be both premature and have FGR. In fact, recent serial ultrasound studies suggest that a large percentage of infants who are born prematurely are growth restricted compared to infants born at term (36,72).

Maternal (preplacental) causes of FGR can be separated into three groups. First, are conditions associated with a small constant impairment in fetal growth, including short stature, weight less than 100 lbs, poor pregnancy weight gain, smoking, and uterine structural abnormalities (13,33). Infants from these mothers usually have borderline FGR and a good prognosis. Second are conditions associated with decreased maternal perfusion, such as preeclampsia and the preeclampsia-like syndromes associated with underlying thrombophilia and renovascular disease (16,32,73). Lastly are conditions associated with an intrinsically poor maternal adaptation to pregnancy, such as failure to expand intravascular volume, autoimmunity, and global reproductive failure (infertility, repetitive spontaneous abortion, prior FGR, or prior fetal death) (8,10,14, 21,53). Poor adaptation to pregnancy in some cases may be the result of maternofetal immunologic incompatibility or dysregulated interactions between placental growth factors and maternal growth factor receptors (3,27,39,68). This latter group is as yet poorly understood.

Fetal (postplacental) causes of FGR include a variety of genetic and chromosomal disorders. One specific chromosomal disorder that may be under-recognized is confined placental mosaicism. In this condition the placental karyotype is abnormal, often trisomic, while the fetal karyotype is diploid (58). FGR is particularly common when the diploid fetal karyotype contains chromosomes entirely derived from one parent (uniparental disomy). The clinical consequences of uniparental disomy are believed to be related to genomic imprinting, an epigenetic phenomenon in which a subset of genes is only expressed from alleles inherited from either the mother or the father, but not both.

Placental lesions associated with FGR often directly affect substrate delivery and include chronic peripheral separation ("chronic abruption"), chronic villitis, fetal thrombotic vasculopathy, chronic histiocytic intervillositis, and massive perivillous fibrinoid deposition ("maternal floor infarction") (10,55,56). Developmental abnormalities, such as single umbilical artery, placenta previa, large chorangioma, and abnormal placental shape, are less consistently associated with FGR. No typical histologic features associated with confined placental mosaicism have yet been described.

Severe FGR may culminate in fetal death, usually after a period of progressive circulatory collapse as is sometimes documented by antenatal pulsed flow Doppler testing (17,38). Liveborn infants with FGR are at early risk for thrombocytopenia, neutropenia, hypocalcemia, and hyperglycemia. They have an increased risk for failure to thrive and learning disabilities in later childhood (9,64). Emerging data suggest that infants with FGR may also have a substantially increased risk for cardiovascular and renal diseases in adulthood (11).

Hypoxic-Ischemic Injury

Injuries attributed to decreased oxygen tension (hypoxia), decreased blood flow (ischemia), or both are most common in term infants. An important component in the current conception of hypoxic-ischemic injury is that although hypoxia/ischemia may be the proximate cause of injury, the underlying threshold for injury can vary significantly from case to case. In many cases, the magnitude of the insult required to produce injury may be very low. Potential modulators of this threshold include an inherited predisposition to ischemic neuronal injury, maternal endocrine-metabolic status (particularly thyroid status), and underlying preexisting placental pathology.

Clinically significant hypoxia/ischemia, sometimes called "birth asphyxia," may be defined in several ways. Obstetricians generally use blood gas data obtained at or before the time of birth. Any pH less than 7.2 is abnormal, but an umbilical artery base deficit of more than 12 mmol/L (generally, but not always, accompanied by a pH of less than 7.0) is the most commonly accepted definition (18,41). Another less specific criterion is low Apgar score. Although designed only to identify infants needing resuscitation, an Apgar score of less than 6 at 5 minutes is used by some as a surrogate marker for hypoxia/ischemia (69). On the other hand, neonatologists and neurologists make the diagnosis of hypoxia/ischemia by its effects on the neonate (37). Hypoxic-ischemic encephalopathy (or more properly, neonatal encephalopathy) is defined by specific neurologic criteria, generally including seizures in the first 24 hours of life, and is often accompanied by coexisting cardiac, hepatic, metabolic, and renal abnormalities (44). Perinatal physiologists distinguish four subcategories of hypoxic-ischemic injury: near total anoxia, subtotal hypoxia with acidosis, gradually progressive hypoxia without acidosis, and hypoxia complicated by anoxia and acidosis (48). The presence of repetitive hypoxic insults was later added as a fifth subcategory (66). Each pattern is associated with a characteristic anatomic distribution of brain injuries, a description of which is beyond the scope of this chapter. Gestational age also plays a significant role in the anatomic distribution of brain lesions (67).

Maternal (preplacental) factors associated with an increased risk for hypoxic-ischemic injury include maternal thyroid disease; family history of seizures or cerebral palsy; vaginal bleeding in the first, second, or third trimester; and postdates pregnancy (over 42 weeks) (5,50,53). Of particular interest are abnormalities of thyroid function which may exert their effects via direct neurodevelopmental toxicity, a decreased threshold for injury, or associated subclinical autoimmune disease (1,42).

Fetal (postplacental) abnormalities are often overlooked in the differential diagnosis of hypoxic-ischemic injury. Fetal thrombophilia can be a direct cause of brain damage (perinatal stroke) or may aggravate injury following a severe hypoxic-ischemic event (34,35,43,49).

Basic Pathways of Prenatal and Peripartum Injury

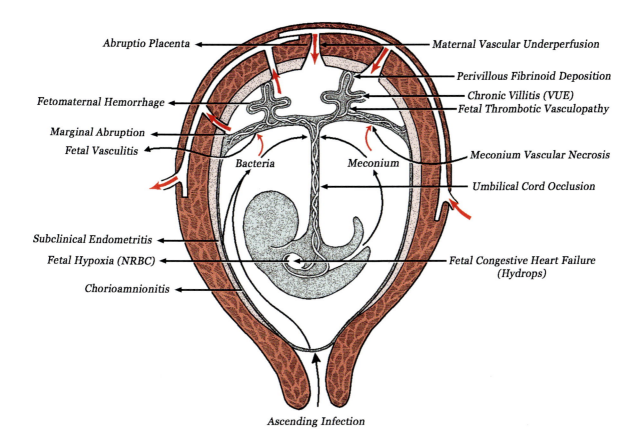

Figure 2-1

ANATOMIC LOCALIZATION OF PLACENTAL LESIONS

The diagram represents a schematic view of the gravid uterus. The fetus and placenta are depicted in blue, the decidualized endometrium in pink, and the uterine myometrium in red. Red arrows illustrate blood flow in and out of the placental intervillous space. Arrows pinpoint the sites of injury for the most common placental disease processes (see Table 2-2 and text). (VUE = villitis of unknown etiology; NRBC = nucleated red blood cells.)

Some fetal genetic diseases can mimic hypoxic-ischemic damage. These include mitochondrial diseases, Rett's syndrome, spinal muscular atrophy, and peroxisomal disorders (58,65).

Placental lesions associated with hypoxic-ischemic damage may be separated into two groups. First are lesions that directly cause circulatory disruption (uteroplacental separation, fetal hemorrhage, umbilical cord compression, placentofetal thromboemboli) and second are lesions identified as risk factors for later neurologic impairment (avascular villi, chorioamnionic hemosiderin deposition, and fetal vascular lesions such as mural thrombosis, necrosis, and severe inflammation) (12,25,53).

Many cases of stillbirth and early neonatal death in the late third trimester are attributable to hypoxia/ischemia. Survivors are at early risk for severe metabolic abnormalities, coagulopathy, and a persistent fetal pattern of circulation associated with severe pulmonary hypertension and refractory neonatal hypoxemia. Long-term complications include cerebral palsy and related static motor disorders, epilepsy, mental retardation, and neurosensory deficits (22). Although most common in term infants, hypoxic-ischemic injury can also complicate either preterm or FGR infants (63).

PLACENTAL LESIONS

A detailed consideration of specific placental lesions, their biologic basis, and their clinical significance may be found in later chapters. An outline of specific lesions by category is provided in Table 2-2 and a schematic diagram depicting their site of action is shown in figure 2-1. The relationship between specific clinical syndromes and placental pathology is discussed in chapter 3. This section provides some perspective on how to think about specific lesions, how to recognize patterns of lesions, and how to put placental pathology into a pathophysiologic context.

Histologic lesions in the placenta require time to develop: generally at least 2 to 4 hours. Sudden dramatic events at the time of delivery such as abruptio placenta, fetal hemorrhage, and cord accidents are apparent only if placental tissue is physically disrupted or accumulations of blood remain adherent to the placenta.

Lesions may be diffuse, multifocal, or isolated. Lesions that are diffusely distributed and recognizable in any random histologic section include acute chorioamnionitis, meconium, increased nucleated red blood cells (NRBC), villous dysmaturity, and chorangiosis. Lesions that are sufficiently multifocal to permit diagnosis in most well-sampled placentas are chronic villitis, avascular villi, and decidual arteriopathy. Isolated lesions include infarcts, intervillous thrombi, ruptured fetal vessels, and placenta accreta. The absence of pathology in a case with poor outcome may warrant reexamination of the gross specimen and submission of additional random sections.

Lesions may either affect fetal well being in direct proportion to their extent and severity, or may serve primarily as indicators of a more profound underlying process affecting the fetoplacental unit. Examples of the former include perivillous fibrin deposition, retroplacental hemorrhage, and chronic villitis. Examples of the latter include increased NRBCs, villous chorangiosis, acute atherosis, avascular villi, decidual plasma cells, and membrane hemosiderin.

Not every placental lesion is associated with a bad outcome. Extensive disease can be compensated for by placental reserve and may be clinically silent. One common example is the isolated marginal villous infarct, which is often not associated with significant morbidity and mortality in an otherwise normal term placenta.

Each anatomic compartment has its own underlying sensitivity to injury. For example, dramatic findings associated with maternal underperfusion seem to have less impact on outcome than more subtle processes affecting large fetal vessels, such as mural inflammation, necrosis, or nonocclusive luminal thrombi (4,54,57).

Placental lesions are often markers for specific genetic, infectious, immunologic, thrombophilic, or vasodestructive processes. Identification of a placental lesion may predict recurrence risk, guide strategies for definitive diagnosis, or suggest options for prevention or therapy.

Subcategorization

Time of Onset/Duration (Stage). Placental lesions can be separated into chronic, subacute, and acute subgroups (53). Chronic lesions begin weeks to months before delivery and include maternal vasculopathy, chronic villitis, fetal thrombotic vasculopathy, chronic abruption, and increased perivillous fibrin deposition (55). Subacute lesions begin within days of delivery and include fetal chorioamnionitis, prolonged meconium exposure, and increased NRBCs. Acute lesions occur within hours of delivery and include abruptio placenta, cord accidents, and fetal hemorrhage. In general, lesions occurring at each time period decrease placental reserve and increase the chance that a subsequent lesion will lead to an adverse outcome (53).

Intensity (Grade) and Character. Another way of subclassifying lesions is by the specific histologic characteristics. For example, intensity (grade), activity (acute superimposed on chronic), subtype (lymphoplasmacytic, histiocytic, granulomatous), and associated findings (increased perivillous fibrin deposition, stem villous vasculitis, avascular villi) are characteristics that are particularly applicable to a description of chronic villitis. While the clinical utility of such distinctions varies from lesion to lesion, these attributes should all be considered in the final interpretation.

Extent of Involvement. Lesions such as chronic villitis, increased perivillous fibrin deposition, retroplacental hemorrhage, avascular villi, and villous infarcts vary considerably in their extent of involvement, which then changes their impact on pregnancy. Also relevant is the status of the uninvolved placental tissue; for example, the significance of 20 percent villous infarction at term may differ in a 600 g placenta with otherwise normal villi and a 280 g placenta with distal villous hypoplasia, increased syncytial knots, and intervillous fibrin-type fibrinoid deposits (intervillous fibrin).

Multiple Findings Suggestive of a Single Underlying Disease Process. It is often useful to gather related findings in a single category. One example is "findings consistent with maternal underperfusion," which may include various combinations of decreased weight, altered villous morphology, intervillous fibrin, decidual vasculopathy, superficial implantation site, decreased Wharton's jelly, and villous infarcts. Grouping of related findings makes sense from two perspectives: it reinforces the validity of the interpretation, and it discourages overestimating the significance of multiple interrelated findings.

Multiple Findings Each Suggestive of a Separate Disease Process. When separate independent processes affect the same placenta, placental reserve is challenged and the capacity for compensatory change to occur is restricted (20,57). This is particularly true when lesions occur in different anatomic compartments or at different stages of gestation. Maternal plus fetal vascular disease or perivillous fibrin deposition plus acute chorioamnionitis may have additive or even synergistic effects on outcome. Alternatively, combinations such as prolonged meconium exposure and intense fetal inflammation acting on the same chorionic vessel may cause greater damage than either one alone.

Physiologic Consequences

The physiologic consequences of a placental lesion, regardless of its cause, are sometimes predicted by its anatomic location and the functional compartments it affects (fig. 2-1). In considering each functional compartment it is important to distinguish primary lesions from compensatory secondary adaptations. Although the analogies are not perfect, comparisons with diseases affecting a more familiar gas exchanging organ, the lung, may be helpful.

Lesions affecting the basal plate and maternal arteries decrease maternal perfusion. These lesions are analogous to airway obstruction and tend to cause both hypoxia and hypercarbia. Possible adaptations include accelerated villous maturation, which augments the efficiency of gas exchange, and increases in maternal blood pressure or cardiac output to increase perfusion.

Lesions affecting the interhemal membrane (terminal villous capillaries, stroma, trophoblast, and adjacent intervillous space), such as perivillous fibrin deposition, chronic villitis, or villous edema, act like interstitial lung disease or acute respiratory distress syndrome to affect diffusion and reduce fetal oxygen tension. Possible adaptations include an increase in the number of villous capillaries (chorangiosis) or in total fetal red blood cell mass (increased NRBCs, polycythemia).

Lesions affecting chorionic and stem villous vessels affect conductance of fetal blood to the interhemal membrane. These lesions, often thrombotic in nature, may be compared to pulmonary thromboembolic disease. They result in a mismatch between the maternal and fetal circulations, significantly reduce the fetal vascular bed, and can lead to hypoxia, circulatory obstruction, and generalized vasomotor instability.

Obstruction of umbilical blood flow, fetal hyperviscosity, and fetal cardiovascular insufficiency can all exert global alterations on placental blood flow. These processes lead to vascular stasis and increased fetal venous pressure, and are analogous to those seen with chronic congestive heart failure. Placental lesions associated with such global decreased perfusion include hemorrhagic endovasculitis and villous hydrops.

PATHWAYS OF INJURY

The pathologist, in conjunction with other health care professionals, including obstetricians, neonatologists, neurologists, and the hospital risk management staff, needs to consider all of the available evidence to identify the primary and secondary factors contributing to a bad outcome and to reconstruct the most plausible sequence of events. This integrated analysis should start with underlying maternal risk factors and the events of early gestation; proceed to consider the influence of placental lesions of varying duration, severity, and number; and take into account intrinsic abnormalities of the fetus. These prenatal events can then be placed in context with clinical findings at delivery and the immediate neonatal period (fig. 2-2). Moving beyond this academic exercise, it is important that the results of such an analysis be promptly transmitted to clinical caregivers and the family in order to fully document, disclose, and understand the past pregnancy and guide the clinical management of future pregnancies.

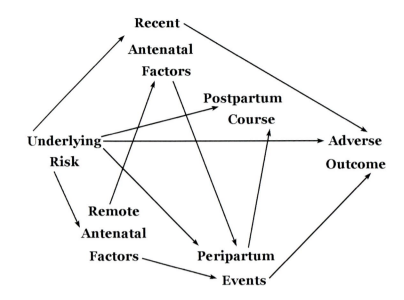

Figure 2-2

DETERMINANTS OF PREGNANCY OUTCOME

Schematic diagram illustrating the potential interplay of underlying risk factors, remote and recent antenatal risk factors, peripartum events, and postpartum course in determining adverse perinatal outcome.

REFERENCES

1. Abramson J, Stagnaro-Green A. Thyroid antibodies and fetal loss: an evolving story. Thyroid 2001;11:57–63.
2. Alexander GR, Himes JH, Kaufman RB, Mor J, Kogan M. A United States national reference for fetal growth. Obstet Gynecol 1996;87:163–8.
3. Allen WR, Skidmore JA, Stewart F, Antczak DF. Effects of fetal genotype and uterine environment on placental development in equids. J Reprod Fertil 1993;98:55–60.
4. Altshuler G, Hyde S. Meconium-induced vasocontraction: a potential cause of cerebral and other fetal hypoperfusion and of poor pregnancy outcome. J Child Neurol 1989;4:137–42.
5. Badawi N, Kurinczuk JJ, Keogh JM, et al. Antepartum risk factors for newborn encephalopathy: the Western Australian case-control study. BMJ 1998;317:1549–53.
6. Bahado-Singh RO, Dashe J, Deren O, Daftary G, Copel JA, Ehrenkranz RA. Prenatal prediction of neonatal outcome in the extremely low-birth-weight infant. Am J Obstet Gynecol 1998;178:462–8.
7. Basso O, Olsen J, Christensen K. Study of environmental, social, and paternal factors in preterm delivery using sibs and half sibs. A population-based study in Denmark. J Epidemiol Community Health 1999;53:20–3.
8. Bendon RW, Hommel AB. Maternal floor infarction in autoimmune disease: two cases. Pediatr Pathol Lab Med 1996;16:293–7.
9. Bos AF, Einspieler C, Prechtl HF. Intrauterine growth retardation, general movements, and neurodevelopmental outcome: a review. Dev Med Child Neurol 2001;43:61–8.
10. Boyd TK, Redline RW. Chronic histiocytic intervillositis: a placental lesion associated with recurrent reproductive loss. Hum Pathol 2000;31:1389–96.
11. Byrne CD, Phillips DI. Fetal origins of adult disease: epidemiology and mechanisms. J Clin Pathol 2000;53:822–8.
12. Cass H, Reilly S, Owen L, et al. Findings from a multidisciplinary clinical case series of females with Rett syndrome. Dev Med Child Neurol 2003;45:325–37.
13. Catalano PM, Thomas AJ, Huston LP, Fung CM. Effect of maternal metabolism on fetal growth and body composition. Diabetes Care 1998;21(Suppl 2):B85–90.
14. Coulam CB, Wagenknecht D, McIntyre JA, Faulk WP, Anneggers JF. Occurrence of other reproductive failures among women with recurrent spontaneous abortion. Am J Reprod Immunol 1991;25:96–8.
15. Cunningham FG, Williams JW. William's obstetrics, 20th ed. Stamford, CT: Appleton & Lange; 1997.
16. Dekker GA, deVries JI, Doclizsch PM, et al. Underlying disorders associated with severe early onset preeclampsia. Am J Obstet Gynecol 1995;173:1042–8.

17. Devoe LD, Gardner P, Dear C, Faircloth D. The significance of increasing umbilical artery systolic-diastolic ratios in third-trimester pregnancy. Obstet Gynecol 1992;80:684–92.
18. Dijxhoorn MJ, Visser GH, Huisjes HJ, Fidler V, Touwen BC. The relation between umbilical pH values and neonatal neurological morbidity in full term appropriate-for-dates infants. Early Hum Dev 1985;11:33–42.
19. Dombrowski MP, Wolfe HM, Brans YW, Saleh AA, Sokol RJ. Neonatal morphometry. Relation to obstetric, pediatric, and menstrual estimates of gestational age. Am J Dis Child 1992;146:852–6.
20. Driscoll S. Autopsy following stillbirth: a challenge neglected. In: Ryder O, Byrd M, eds. One medicine. Berlin: Springer-Verlag; 1984:20–31.
21. Duvekot JJ, Cheriex EC, Pieters FA, Menheere PP, Schouten HJ, Peeters LL. Maternal volume homeostasis in early pregnancy in relation to fetal growth restriction. Obstet Gynecol 1995;85:361–7.
22. Gaffney G, Flavell V, Johnson A, Squier M, Sellers S. Cerebral palsy and neonatal encephalopathy. Arch Dis Child 1994;70:F195–200.
23. Goldenberg RL, Hauth JC, Andrews WW. Intrauterine infection and preterm delivery. N Engl J Med 2000;342:1500–7.
24. Goldenberg RL, Tamura T, Neggers Y, et al. The effect of zinc supplementation on pregnancy outcome. JAMA 1995;274:463–8.
25. Grafe MR. The correlation of prenatal brain damage with placental pathology. N Neuropathol Exp Neurol 1994;53:407–15.
26. Hack M, Taylor HG, Klein N, Mercuri-Minich N. Functional limitations and special health care needs of 10- to 14-year-old children weighing less than 750 grams at birth. Pediatrics 2000;106:554–60.
27. Haig D. Genetic conflicts in human pregnancy. Q Rev Biol 1993;68:495–532.
28. Iams JD, Goldenberg RL, Meis PJ, et al. The length of the cervix and the risk of spontaneous premature delivery. National Institute of Child Health and Human Development Maternal Fetal Medicine Unit Network. N Engl J Med 1996;334:567–72.
29. Jobe AH, Ikegami M. Mechanisms initiating lung injury in the preterm. Early Hum Dev 1998;53:81–94.
30. Khoshnood B, Lee KS, Wall S, Hsieh HL, Mittendorf R. Short interpregnancy intervals and the risk of adverse birth outcomes among five racial/ethnic groups in the United States. Am J Epidemiol 1998;148:798–805.
31. Kimberlin DF, Hauth JC, Owen J, et al. Indicated versus spontaneous preterm delivery: an evaluation of neonatal morbidity among infants weighing </=1000 grams at birth. Am J Obstet Gynecol 1999;180:683–9.
32. Kliman HJ. Uteroplacental blood flow. The story of decidualization, menstruation, and trophoblast invasion. Am J Pathol 2000;157:1759–68.
33. Kramer MS. Intrauterine growth and gestational duration determinants. Pediatrics 1987;80:502–11.
34. Kraus FT. Cerebral palsy and thrombi in placental vessels of the fetus: insights from litigation. Hum Pathol 1997;28:246–8.
35. Kraus FT, Acheen VI. Fetal thrombotic vasculopathy in the placenta: cerebral thrombi and infarcts, coagulopathies, and cerebral palsy. Hum Pathol 1999;30:759–69.
36. Lackman F, Capewell V, Richardson B, daSilva O, Gagnon R. The risks of spontaneous preterm delivery and perinatal mortality in relation to size at birth according to fetal versus neonatal growth standards. Am J Obstet Gynecol 2001;184:946–53.
37. Leviton A, Nelson KB. Problems with definitions and classifications of newborn encephalopathy. Pediatr Neurol 1992;8:85–90.
38. Ley D, Marsal K. Doppler velocimetry in cerebral vessels of small for gestational age infants. Early Hum Dev 1992;31:171–80.
39. Lie RT, Rasmussen S, Brunborg H, Gjessing HK, Lie-Nielsen E, Irgens LM. Fetal and maternal contributions to risk of pre-eclampsia: population based study. BMJ 1998;316:1343–7.
40. Lockwood CJ. Predicting premature delivery—no easy task. N Engl J Med 2002;346:282–4.
41. Low JA. Intrapartum fetal asphyxia: definition, diagnosis, and classification. Am J Obstet Gynecol 1997;176:957–9.
42. Lucas A, Morley R, Fewtrell MS. Low triiodothyronine concentration in preterm infants and subsequent intelligence quotient (IQ) at 8 year follow up. BMJ 1996;312:1132–3.
43. Lynch JK, Hirtz DG, DeVeber G, Nelson KB. Report of the National Institute of Neurological Disorders and Stroke Workshop on perinatal and childhood stroke. Pediatrics 2002;109:116–23.
44. Martin-Ancel A, Garcia-Alix A, Gaya F, Cabanas F, Burgueros M, Quero J. Multiple organ involvement in perinatal asphyxia. J Pediatr 1995;127:786–93.
45. Meis PJ, Goldenberg RL, Mercer B, et al. The preterm prediction study: significance of vaginal infections. Am J Obstet Gynecol 1995;173:1231–5.
46. Mercer BM, Goldenberg RL, Meis PJ, et al. The Preterm Prediction Study: prediction of preterm premature rupture of membranes through clinical findings and ancillary testing. The National Institute of Child Health and Human Development Maternal-Fetal Medicine Units Network. Am J Obstet Gynecol 2000;183:738–45.

47. Murphy DJ, Hope PL, Johnson A. Neonatal risk factors for cerebral palsy in very preterm babies: case-control study. BMJ 1997;314:404–8.
48. Myers RE. Four patterns of perinatal brain damage and their conditions of occurrence in primates. Adv Neurol 1975;10:223–34.
49. Nelson KB, Dambrosia JM, Grether JK, Phillips TM. Neonatal cytokines and coagulation factors in children with cerebral palsy. Arch Neurol 1998;44:665–75.
50. Nelson KB, Ellenberg JH. Obstetric complications as risk factors for cerebral palsy or seizure disorders. JAMA 1984;251:1843–8.
51. Paneth N, Rudelli R, Kazam E, Monte W. Brain damage in the preterm infant. London: MacKeith Press; 1994:171–85.
52. Redline RW, Abramowsky CR. Clinical and pathologic aspects of recurrent placental villitis. Hum Pathol 1985;16:727–31.
53. Redline RW, O'Riordan MA. Placental lesions associated with cerebral palsy and neurologic impairment following term birth. Arch Pathol Lab Med 2000;124:1785–91.
54. Redline RW, Pappin A. Fetal thrombotic vasculopathy: the clinical significance of extensive avascular villi. Hum Pathol 1995;26:80–5.
55. Redline RW, Patterson P. Patterns of placental injury. Correlations with gestational age, placental weight, and clinical diagnosis. Arch Pathol Lab Med 1994;118:698–701.
56. Redline RW, Wilson-Costello D. Chronic peripheral separation of placenta. The significance of diffuse chorioamnionic hemosiderosis. Am J Clin Pathol 1999;111:804–10.
57. Redline RW, Wilson-Costello D, Borawski E, Fanaroff AA, Hack M. Placental lesions associated with neurologic impairment and cerebral palsy in very low birth weight infants. Arch Pathol Lab Med 1998;122:1091–8.
58. Robinson WP, Barrett IJ, Bernard L, et al. Meiotic origin of trisomy in confined placental mosaicism is correlated with presence of fetal uniparental disomy, high levels of trisomy in trophoblast, and increased risk of fetal intrauterine growth restriction. Am J Hum Genet 1997;60:917–27.
59. Romero R, Sepulveda W, Baumann P, et al. The preterm labor syndrome: biochemical, cytologic, immunologic, pathologic, microbiologic, and clinical evidence that preterm labor is a heterogeneous disease [Abstract]. Am J Obstet Gynecol 1993;168:288.
60. Schieve LA, Cogswell ME, Scanlon KS, et al. Prepregnancy body mass index and pregnancy weight gain: associations with preterm delivery. The NMIHS Collaborative Study Group. Obstet Gynecol 2000;96:194–200.
61. Scholl TO. High third-trimester ferritin concentration: associations with very preterm delivery, infection, and maternal nutritional status. Obstet Gynecol 1998;92:161–6.
62. Sonntag J, Grimmer I, Scholz T, Metze B, Wit J, Obladen M. Growth and neurodevelopmental outcome of very low birthweight infants with necrotizing enterocolitis. Acta Paediatr 2000;89:528–32.
63. Soothill PW, Nicolaides KH, Campbell S. Prenatal asphyxia, hyperlacticaemia, hypoglycaemia, and erythroblastosis in growth retarded fetuses. Br Med J 1987;294:1051–3.
64. Soothill PW. Diagnosis of intrauterine growth retardation and its fetal and perinatal consequences. Acta Paediatr Suppl 1994;399:55–8, discussion 59.
65. Sue CM, Bruno C, Andreu AL, et al. Infantile encephalopathy associated with the MELAS A3243G mutation. J Pediatr 1999;134:696–700.
66. Tan S, Zhou F, Nielson VG, Wang ZW, Gladson CL, Parks DA. Increased injury following intermittent fetal hypoxia-reoxygenation is associated with increased free radical production in fetal rabbit brain. J Neuropathol Exp Neurol 1999;58:972–81.
67. Towbin A. Brain damage in the newborn and its neurologic sequels. Danvers, MA: PRM Publishing; 1998.
68. Trupin LS, Simon LP, Eskenazi B. Change in paternity: a risk factor for preeclampsia in multiparas. Epidemiology 1996;7:240–4.
69. Use and abuse of the Apgar Score. Committee on Fetus and Newborn, American Academy of Pediatrics and Committee on Obstetric Practice, American College of Obstetricians and Gynecologists. Pediatrics 1996;98:141–2.
70. Wilcox MA, Johnson IR, Maynard PV, Smith SJ, Chilvers CE. The individualised birthweight ratio: a more logical outcome measure of pregnancy than birthweight alone. Br J Obstet Gynaecol 1993;100:342–7.
71. Yudkin PL, Aboualfa M, Eyre JA, Redman CW, Wilkinson AR. New birthweight and head circumference centiles for gestational ages 24 to 42 weeks. Early Hum Dev 1987;15:45–52.
72. Zeitlin J, Ancel PY, Saurel-Cubizolles MJ, Papiernik E. The relationship between intrauterine growth restriction and preterm delivery: an empirical approach using data from a European case-control study. Br J Obstet Gynaecol 2000;107:750–8.
73. Zhang J, Zeisler J, Hatch MC, Berkowitz G. Epidemiology of pregnancy-induced hypertension. Epidemiol Rev 1997;19:218–32.

3 CLINICAL SYNDROMES AND THEIR PATHOLOGIC CORRELATES IN THE PLACENTA

The information that accompanies a placenta submitted for pathologic evaluation is necessarily limited, but should include at least the most probable diagnostic considerations, specifically related to the mother or newborn, and ideally to both. These data are necessary for the conduct of an informed examination. A pathology report that is not responsive to the questions raised by the clinical problems is not useful. Clinical data are usually transmitted to the pathologist by an abbreviation code (see chapter 13, Table 13-2), which can be very helpful when mounted in a convenient spot, adjacent to both the dissecting bench and the microscope.

The question in the mind of the pathologist is "given a specific clinical problem, what should I look for, both grossly and microscopically?" The placenta uniquely relates to two very different individuals, a context unlike any other organ. The nature of the pathologic lesion potentially responsible for the different clinical problems of the two patients connected to a placenta is not obvious. This chapter is intended as a guide to the sections of this atlas that describe the placental pathology of the lesions responsible for most of the common clinical problems.

The following categories are separated according to the conventional clinical context of mother and fetus. We emphasize that placental lesions may put both mother and fetus at risk for injury. A responsive report necessarily considers both individuals and must communicate to both obstetricians and pediatricians.

CLINICAL DIAGNOSES BASED PRIMARILY ON MATERNAL HISTORY OR MATERNAL EXAMINATION

Pregnancy-Induced Hypertension, Preeclampsia, and Eclampsia

Pregnancy-induced hypertension (PIH) implies that the blood pressure of a pregnant woman with previously normal blood pressure rises to 140/90 mm Hg or greater after 20 weeks' gestation, on at least two occasions, separated by at least 6 hours.

Preeclampsia means PIH plus proteinuria (1+ or greater on a random urine dipstick confirmed by a timed 24-hour collection containing 300 mg protein or greater). Generalized edema is common, but is no longer a specific criterion. Severe preeclampsia implies the addition of one or more of the following: blood pressure over 160 mm Hg systolic or 110 mm Hg diastolic; proteinuria greater than 5 g per 24 hours, or 3+ or greater on two random dipstick evaluations at least 4 hours apart; headache; visual disturbances; epigastric or right upper quadrant pain; oliguria; thrombocytopenia; liver enzyme elevation; fetal growth restriction; and pulmonary edema. Eclampsia is preeclampsia with maternal seizures. The *HELLP syndrome* is a form of severe preeclampsia with a specific triad of additional findings: maternal red blood cell hemolysis, elevated liver enzymes, and low platelet count.

Two different types of placental change occur in preeclampsia and eclampsia. The first and most common is a small placenta, often delivered prematurely. Multiple infarcts and decidual vasculopathy, especially acute atherosis, are usually present (see chapter 6), and in severe cases the villi are small and slender, a pattern called *accelerated maturation,* or *distal villous hypoplasia* (see chapter 4). The second type is a large placenta with abundant, immature villous cytotrophoblast, which may occur in women with diabetes mellitus, multifetal gestations, and hydropic placentas, especially those with hydatidiform moles. Preeclampsia occurs only in the presence of trophoblast; a fetus need not be present. Treatment may improve symptoms, but the condition itself can be eliminated only by delivery of the placenta.

Despite extensive study for many years, the etiology of these conditions is unknown. Failure of adaptive vascular remodeling of spiral arteries may be the result of inappropriate immune reactions between the invading placental site trophoblast and maternal leukocytes (24). Placental ischemia and diffuse maternal endothelial injury, possibly related to oxidative stress and other inflammatory effects of blood-borne fragments of syncytiotrophoblast, all seem to be important (23,84,91,95). There appears to be a genetic predisposition, transmitted by both maternal and paternal routes (58). Among possible causes, upregulation of a gene expressing soluble fms-like tyrosine kinase 1, which reduces the amount of endothelial-stabilizing factors, has been implicated (71).

Acute Fatty Liver of Pregnancy

This specific form of maternal hepatic failure occurs in about 1 in 10,000 pregnancies, usually in the clinical context of the HELLP syndrome. Women with acute fatty liver of pregnancy (AFLP) present in the third trimester with jaundice, epigastric pain, nausea, vomiting, profound hypoglycemia, and encephalopathy. Liver biopsies show centrilobular steatosis and necrosis. Fulminant hepatic failure, coagulopathy, bleeding, and maternal death occur if delivery is not performed, and fetal mortality is also high. An inherited long-chain 3-hydroxyacyl-CoA dehydrogenase (LCHAD) deficiency in the fetus, associated with a mutant *E474Q* gene, is one very important cause of this syndrome (48,106). A much smaller proportion of women with the HELLP syndrome have the same basic genetic abnormality.

The newborn is at risk for sudden hypoglycemia, cardiomyopathy, hepatic steatosis, and sudden death. Screening of both parents and the cord blood for the *E474Q* mutation, and appropriate postnatal molecular testing of the newborn, may be lifesaving. The placental pathology in one case was a maternal (placental) floor infarct (70), but in most instances, placental studies have not been recorded.

Essential Hypertension

Placental lesions from women with preexisting hypertension not complicated by superimposed preeclampsia have received little attention. Jones and Fox (49) found that some ischemic changes in placental villi were qualitatively similar, but less pronounced, than those they had previously found in preeclamptic women (50). Placental weight may be normal or even increased, possibly due to increased maternal perfusion pressure, but more likely a consequence of associated maternal obesity or glucose intolerance. Hyperplastic arteriosclerotic changes may occur in the walls of intramyometrial vessels sufficient to produce placental ischemia, but portions of spiral arteries in the decidua basalis undergo the usual physiologic change. Vessels in the decidua capsularis may also show physiologic change. Acute atherosis, typical in preeclampsia, does not occur in uncomplicated chronic hypertension.

Maternal Thrombophilia (Including Maternal Deep Vein Thromboses, Pulmonary Infarcts, Cerebral Vascular Accidents)

The risk of maternal thrombotic disease is eight times greater in pregnant women with inherited coagulopathies than in pregnant women in general (65). Acquired thrombophilic states, especially the presence of antiphospholipid antibodies, promote intraplacental clotting, apparently by interfering with the normal antithrombotic annexin V phospholipid-binding protein (86). A history of previous thrombotic episodes is significant in pregnancy, even if laboratory testing has not identified a cause. The most common inherited coagulopathies are the *G1691A* mutation in the factor V gene (factor V Leiden), the *G20210A* mutation in the prothrombin gene, and the *C677T* mutation in the methylene tetrahydrofolate reductase gene (111). Less common are deficiencies in antithrombin III, protein S, and protein C. Diabetes mellitus is commonly associated with a hypercoagulable state (105).

The maternal risk is mainly venous thromboembolism, but arterial thrombosis also occurs (38,99). There is a strong association with severe preeclampsia (2). Adverse pregnancy outcomes occurred in 54 percent of women with thrombophilia, and placental thrombotic lesions of all kinds are common (2,80). The fetus of a mother with thrombophilia is at risk for intrauterine growth restriction and stillbirth (28,38,68,80). Of a group of 22 infants with prenatal or perinatal stroke, 14 had coagulation abnormalities and 6 had family histories suggesting thrombosis (37). In another study of 24 infants with perinatal infarcts, 10 had thrombophilias, and neurodevelopmental disabilities were more prevalent in those with thrombophilia (74). Treatment of thrombophilic women after repeated pregnancy losses (three or more) with low molecular weight heparin may improve future pregnancy outcomes (12,80).

Placental lesions associated with maternal thrombophilias include fetal thrombotic vasculopathy, abruption, infarcts, and hematomas (5,56,69).

Diabetes Mellitus

Diabetes in pregnancy is separated into two distinct groups: women with preexisting diabetes, usually type I, and women developing glucose intolerance during pregnancy who have an increased risk for developing type II diabetes in later life. The age of onset, duration of disease, and presence of vascular complications in type I diabetes vary considerably, and may affect perinatal outcome directly. Good metabolic control throughout pregnancy (as compared with poor control) influences perinatal morbidity and mortality in all types of diabetic pregnancy.

The gross and microscopic histopathology of the placenta varies considerably, but there is no direct relationship with any of these diabetic clinical variations. The extensive review of Haust (45) covers placental as well as fetal and neonatal pathology in great detail. In about half of diabetic pregnancies, the size, weight, and gross and microscopic appearance of the placenta are normal. There are no specific gross or microscopic changes. However, those placentas that are abnormal have a common constellation of features: they are larger, thicker, more friable, and heavier than normal placentas of the same gestational age, and the umbilical cord is often conspicuously thicker. A single umbilical artery is more common (3 to 5 percent) than in the general population (about 1 percent) (45).

The histologic appearance of the placenta may also be normal, but some abnormalities are distinctive when present. Villi commonly appear immature, with mild stromal edema, enlarged villous diameters, and an increase in the prominence of cytotrophoblast cells (see chapter 4, Distal Villous Immaturity). Cytotrophoblast proliferation with mitoses may occur, possibly as a response to syncytiotrophoblast necrosis (51). Decidual vasculopathy may also be present. The stem vessel and villous changes of fetal thrombotic vasculopathy (32) and chorangiosis (3) are common, as might be expected in view of the thrombophilia associated with diabetes (15). Fetal and neonatal thrombi are disproportionately more frequent in maternal diabetes (81). In the presence of maternal vascular disease, renal disease, or concurrent preeclampsia, the placenta may be smaller, with infarcts and accelerated maturation. Even ideal levels of control of diabetic hyperglycemia do not appear to improve or affect placental morphology to any significant degree (61).

Maternal Anemias

There are no specific histologic abnormalities due to acquired, mostly nutritional, maternal anemias. A recent study has shown that placentas from anemic patients are more deeply implanted (the placental site trophoblast invades more deeply) than normal placentas (52). This is exactly opposite of placental changes in preeclampsia. Preterm birth is more common. Placentas have been described both as larger than normal (36) or smaller (92), with a significant reduction in villous volume.

In maternal sickle cell anemia placental infarcts are common (see chapter 6). The infarcts have no unique features apart from the presence of sickled erythrocytes. Both the placenta and the newborn are usually small for gestational age. Villous hydrops, as noted by Shanklin (101), may result from associated nutritional problems, although there is no consensus on this. Abruption may occur. Uncomplicated sickle cell trait is unlikely to cause gross placental lesions, but the maternal red blood cells often sickle after formalin fixation. Rarely, prenatal sickling may occur in the intervillous space after severe maternal hypoxia.

The pathology of the placenta and fetus in maternal homozygous alpha- and beta-thalassemias differ. Homozygosity for abnormal alpha-globin chains directly blocks formation of fetal hemoglobin, resulting in severe fetal anemia. Both the fetus and placenta are severely hydropic, and fetal death occurs in utero or soon after birth (47). In contrast, the placenta and fetus in homozygous beta-thalassemia

(thalassemia major, or Cooley's anemia) are normal at birth but the infant soon becomes severely anemic as the protective hemoglobin F declines. Pregnancy only occurs rarely in women with thalassemia major and then only in those with disease of mild or intermediate severity (98).

Recurrent Spontaneous Abortion (Recurrent Pregnancy Loss, Habitual Abortion)

The clinical diagnosis of recurrent spontaneous abortion is usually based on the occurrence of three or more consecutive spontaneous abortions. The probability that a recognizable underlying pathologic basis for this sequence can be demonstrated is small, but the identifiable causes are potentially significant. They include maternal thrombophilias, especially syndromes related to autoimmune antibodies; anatomic problems, such as incompetent cervix or leiomyomas; and maternal endocrinopathies, mainly poorly controlled diabetes mellitus. Parental chromosomal anomalies account for less than 5 percent of cases.

The first and easiest, but too often neglected, diagnostic step is to reexamine together all of the pathologic material from the previous pregnancies. Such placental lesions as maternal floor infarct, massive perivillous fibrin deposition, and extensive chronic villitis may cause repeated miscarriage, often in the third trimester. Early gestational pathology in a subgroup of these patients can be abnormal, showing the above lesions plus other distinctive lesions including chronic histiocytic intervillositis (massive chronic intervillositis), lymphoplasmacytic deciduitis, and chronic decidual perivasculitis (90). Although uncommon, these diagnoses are significant, because fetal difficulties are typically sudden and unexpected. Serial nonstress tests and ultrasound studies, with a goal of delivery as soon as maturity is reached, may be life-saving (see chapters 5 and 6, figs. 5-42, 5-55, 6-30–6-40).

PRIMARILY FETAL CONDITIONS

Clinical Chorioamnionitis (Versus Histologic Chorioamnionitis)

From the point of view of an obstetrician, the occurrence of maternal fever suggests the possibility of intrauterine infection. The obstetrician may reasonably make a clinical diagnosis of chorioamnionitis on this basis. However, pathologic confirmation of chorioamnionitis in the placenta occurs in only 60 percent of such cases (103). Maternal fever often is unrelated to the infection; for example, maternal fever occurs more commonly in patients with epidural anesthesia in comparison with other anesthetics, independent of infection. Symptomatic intrauterine maternal infections are more usually the result of an endometritis (deciduitis), which can be, but often is not, associated with chorioamnionitis. The unfortunate misnomer "maternal chorioamnionitis" tends to appear in this context. Chorioamnionitis is a *fetal* disease—mothers don't have chorioamnionitis. Unfortunately, there are many other potential causes of maternal fever, and even worse, severe chorioamnionitis with fetal injury frequently occurs without maternal fever. Maternal leukocytosis, uterine tenderness, and purulent-appearing vaginal discharge are nonspecific clinical findings suggestive of chorioamnionitis, but they are unreliable indicators in comparison with histologic chorioamnionitis, demonstrated by placental examination. Other measures of fetal infection, such as increased cord blood interleukin-6 levels, are much better predictors of fetal morbidity than the clinical symptoms of the mother (104).

The adverse implications of fetal and neonatal injury correlate well with the histopathologic demonstration of chorioamnionitis in the placenta, and poorly, if at all, with "clinical" chorioamnionitis (1,22,29,113). Although clinical diagnoses based on maternal signs and symptoms help in patient management, the important distinction between a definite intrauterine fetal infection (histologic chorioamnionitis) and a possible intrauterine infection (clinical chorioamnionitis) is blurred. As an unfortunate result of this ambiguity, the importance of placental examination and the appreciation of significant clinical correlations of amnionic fluid infection have been obscured. For instance, recognition of the importance of chorioamnionitis as a major risk factor in the pathogenesis of cerebral palsy was delayed for approximately one century.

The important pathologic features of chorioamnionitis and other placental infections are described in chapter 5.

Preterm Birth, Preterm Labor, Premature Rupture of Membranes

Term births are those that occur after 37 weeks' gestation. It is generally accepted that the fetus should mature by 260 days (37 weeks) after implantation, after which labor may safely begin within the next 2 to 3 weeks, followed by delivery some few to several hours later.

Preterm births, those occurring before 37 weeks, are the most significant cause of neonatal morbidity and mortality. The most severe sequelae (neonatal death and cerebral palsy) among newborn survivors occur to those born before 34 weeks. The most common causes of preterm birth are preterm premature rupture of the membranes, spontaneous preterm labor, and a medically indicated premature delivery (e.g., a cesarean section) initiated because of deterioration of fetal well-being.

Based upon placental evaluations, preterm premature rupture of the membranes (PPROM) occurs mainly in the context of infection (chorioamnionitis) and vascular thrombotic or bleeding problems (6). Spontaneous preterm labor should be distinguished from PPROM because the clinical associations are different. These include severe maternal illnesses, uteroplacental underperfusion, uterine fundal and cervical abnormalities, and fetal anomalies. Chorioamnionitis may present as spontaneous preterm labor, with membranes still intact. The most common reasons for a mandated preterm delivery are severe maternal hypertension, the more severe classes of diabetes mellitus, placental abruption, and abnormalities of fetal growth.

Post-term Pregnancy

The definition of prolonged, or post-term, pregnancy proposed by the World Health Organization (114) is 42 completed weeks (294 days) or more following the onset of the last menses. There is a marked increase in perinatal mortality in pregnancies of 43 and 44 weeks. A combination of progressive oligohydramnios and meconium release appears to lead to cord compression and risk of pulmonary failure, possibly due to aspiration of viscous meconium. The postmature newborn, well illustrated by Clifford (13), has a characteristic thin body, with slender elongated limbs; dried, wrinkled, often meconium-tinged skin; long fingernails; and an apprehensive or worried expression. The postmature placenta has no distinctive or definitive abnormalities (11,31,60). Malformations, especially anencephaly and adrenal hypoplasia, may result in postmaturity due to hormonal imbalances caused by poor pituitary function (66).

Intrapartum Electronic Fetal Monitoring: Nonreassuring Fetal Heart Rate, Bradycardia, Decelerations

Based upon an assumption that most neonatal injury occurs during labor, electronic fetal monitoring became widely employed in the past 40 years. The frequency of cesarean section has increased five-fold, but the prevalence of cerebral palsy is essentially unchanged. Some recent studies of the prenatal experiences of injured neonates now lead to a consensus that no more than 10 percent of prenatal injuries occur during labor (7,9). An exposure to some of the terminology is useful in understanding the clinical data often submitted with the placenta.

Fetal well-being is commonly evaluated during labor with an electronic fetal heart rate monitoring system (cardiotocogram). This provides a continuous tracing of the fetal heart rate, in a manner comparable to a fetal electrocardiogram. The tracing can be matched to other events, such as uterine contractions or some form of fetal stimulation. Certain heart rate abnormalities that are regarded as potentially threatening frequently lead to cesarean section. While both the newborn and the placenta may be normal, the chance of significant placental abnormalities is increased when the fetal heart rate is abnormal (88). These circumstances commonly are an indication for placental examination, but they are not specific for any one problem or group of problems.

Patterns of concern in the heart rate tracing include decelerations (of cardiac contraction rate) and baseline abnormalities. Early decelerations, coincident with uterine contractions, are believed to relate to head compression and are considered benign. Late decelerations, which are delayed relative to uterine contractions, may signify acidosis. Variable decelerations, which have an irregular shape and an inconsistent relationship to uterine contractions, are believed to be caused by cord compression in some cases.

Baseline abnormalities include a decrease in heart rate variability (decreased beat-to-beat variation), absence of accelerations in response to fetal movement, and most ominously with respect to possible central nervous system (CNS) injury, an oscillating sinusoidal rhythm with no response to uterine contractions. Bradycardia below a rate of 110 may be of concern, especially if prolonged.

It is important for pathologists to realize that the interpretation of these tracings is not an exact science. In one multicenter study, 17 experts were asked to review 50 tracings on two occasions, 1 month apart (54). About 20 percent changed their interpretations, and 25 percent could not agree with their colleagues.

Fetal Growth Restriction, Intrauterine Growth Restriction, and the Small for Gestational Age Newborn

Infants born with a weight below 2,500 g are classified as low birthweight. Many low birthweight babies are normal and healthy but small, because of constitutional factors such as parental size or ethnicity. Infants whose birthweight lies below an expected percentile (which may be arbitrarily put at the 3rd, 5th, or 10th percentile) for gestational age may be classified as small for gestational age (SGA), and qualify as intrauterine growth restricted (IUGR) babies. The fetal death rate increases by a factor of eight as the birthweight falls from the 10th to the 3rd percentile. For those below the 3rd percentile, the death rate is nearly 20 times the average population (63,73). In addition to fetal demise, the prevalence of such adverse clinical markers as seizures in the first day of life, need for intubation at birth, sepsis, "birth asphyxia," hypothermia, hypoglycemia, and meconium aspiration are all increased. The medical problems of the survivors persist into adulthood, and include hypertension, coronary artery disease, and noninsulin-dependent diabetes mellitus (79).

The standard method of prenatal diagnosis is by measurements obtained by ultrasound studies, including (at least) fetal abdominal circumference, head circumference, biparietal diameter, and femur length (93), which are converted to fetal weight estimates. The amniotic fluid volume is also estimated. When the foregoing are abnormal, Doppler studies of blood flow through the fetal vessels in the umbilical cord, middle cerebral artery, or other sites may be obtained.

Fetal growth restriction (FGR) is said to be symmetric when the fetal head and abdominal measurements are decreased proportionately, and asymmetric when a greater decrease in the abdominal organs has occurred. The clinical and pathologic significance of this distinction is uncertain, but asymmetric SGA infants are at increased risk for intrapartum and neonatal complications, even after exclusion of infants with anomalies (20). Poor blood flow in the umbilical vessels, as determined by Doppler velocimetry, is a common feature which may begin early and persist for weeks until delivery (94).

Maternal factors associated with FGR are poor (starvation level) nutrition, hypertension, preeclampsia, chronic renal disease, tobacco and other drug abuse, and a poor obstetric history in general. Fetal factors include chromosomal anomalies, congenital malformations, and multiple gestations (63). Placental lesions associated with FGR include: 1) the vascular lesions that affect uteroplacental blood flow (maternal vasculopathy, chronic abruption); 2) lesions that reduce placental-fetal blood flow (fetal thrombotic vasculopathy, large chorangiomas); and 3) lesions that increase the diffusion distance at the interhemal membrane (villitis of unknown etiology, maternal floor infarct, developmental disorders) as described in chapters 4, 5, and 6 (96).

It should be clear to a pathologist who examines a placenta designated as "IUGR" that the newborn is probably in trouble, that the medical team requesting the pathologic studies already has a sophisticated concept about the newborn and its placenta, and that a detailed explanation of the pathology should ordinarily be possible and will be expected.

Cerebral Palsy. This neurologic disability is characterized by nonprogressive motor abnormalities of early onset, involving one or more limbs, with muscular spasticity or paralysis. The diagnosis is usually not apparent until about 6 months of age.

(*Historical Note:* W. J. Little, a distinguished orthopedic surgeon, describing his experience with 47 neurologically disabled children to the Obstetrical Society of London in 1861, attributed their spastic rigidity to "asphyxia neonatorum," an injury caused by anoxia ("failure of decarbonization of the blood") during parturition (64). It was a significant insight, but not based on the obstetrical observations of Dr Little. Little was not an obstetrician and had not been connected with the deliveries of the affected children. Sigmund Freud, well known as a neurologist, concluded in 1897 that diplegic forms of cerebral palsy, especially, originated long before birth in intrauterine life (14). His more scientific, pathology-based monograph (33) received little attention in the 20th century, and "Little's disease" thereafter came to be regarded as the result of obstetrical misfortune during labor and delivery, and often in more recent years as the result of obstetrical mismanagement. The failure to follow up on Freud's observations delayed the search for the real causes of cerebral palsy for nearly 100 years.)

Intrauterine infections associated with bacterial growth in the amnionic fluid are the most common placental lesions associated with cerebral palsy in term and premature infants (39,77,100). About half of all cases of cerebral palsy occur in infants of normal birth weight, born at term, and the prevalence has not changed despite extensive intrapartum monitoring (76). The significant placental pathology is acute chorioamnionitis, especially when associated with funisitis and inflammation of surface fetal vessels (87,89,116). Experimental studies of injury to the brain in this context suggest that injury to the white matter in chorioamnionitis may be an indirect effect of bacterial toxins (43) and is associated with the production of inflammatory cytokines (34,115). Even cortical polymicrogyria, a lesion more commonly regarded as a malformation, may be an indirect result of chorioamnionitis (110). Preterm infection consistently leads to preterm birth, itself an additional strong determinant of cerebral palsy. Cognitive limitations also occur in the context of preterm intrauterine infection (19).

Thrombotic events (5,55), especially in the fetal circulation (fetal thrombotic vasculopathy) (56,108), represent the second main etiologic category for cerebral palsy. A high proportion of neonates with cerebral infarcts (68 percent) have genetically determined coagulopathies (41). Other significant thrombotic or vaso-occlusive events in the placentas of surviving infants include extensive infarction, massive perivillous fibrin deposits, placental floor infarct, and massive chronic villitis. Cerebral palsy in a twin is usually the result of intrauterine fetal death of the co-twin (40).

Cytomegalic inclusion virus and toxoplasmosis are important, but less common, causes of neurologic injury. Neurodevelopmental delay and severe respiratory failure in the newborn are associated with Coxsackie virus infection (30). Prematurity is also a significant risk factor; maternal hypothyroidism and hypothyroxinemia in prematurity also may have adverse effects on prenatal neurologic development (42, 62). Both the severity and the cumulative number of placental lesions directly increase the risk for CNS lesions at birth (112).

Antepartum risk factors for newborn encephalopathy are far more common than intrapartum factors (7,8). Acute placental abruption and some instances of cord compression can cause intrapartum anoxia severe enough to produce bilateral cerebral injury, just as Little believed, but only about 6 to 10 percent of cases can be attributed to this type of acute event (8,78). In such cases of true intrapartum hypoxia, the survivors may be born limp, acidotic, and unable to breathe spontaneously, and have neonatal seizures; they also usually have evidence of multiorgan injury, such as renal failure, pulmonary insufficiency, bowel necrosis, or cardiac injury in the immediate postpartum period. An international cerebral palsy task force has published a consensus statement defining the criteria for establishing a causal relationship between intrapartum events and cerebral palsy (Table 3-1) (67).

Typical cerebral white matter lesions (leukomalacia) occur prenatally in cases of severe nonimmune fetal hydrops (59). Genetically determined forms of cerebral palsy may account for 1 or 2 percent of cases, and probably are somewhat more common in consanguineous families (72). Rett's syndrome, a progressive neurologic disorder caused by a *MECP2* gene mutation (117), occurs only in women. The clinical features may resemble, but need to be distinguished from, cerebral palsy.

Germinal Matrix Hemorrhage (GMH) and Intraventricular Hemorrhage (IVH). The germinal matrix is a zone of immature neural growth that lies just beneath the ependyma of

Table 3-1

CRITERIA TO DEFINE AN ACUTE INTRAPARTUM HYPOXIC EVENT[a]

Essential Criteria

Evidence of metabolic acidosis in intrapartum fetal, umbilical arterial, cord, or very early neonatal blood samples. pH < 7.0 and base deficits >12 mmol/L

Early onset of severe or moderate neonatal encephalopathy in infants > 34 weeks' gestation

Cerebral palsy is of the spastic quadriplegic or dyskinetic type

Criteria that Together Suggest an Intrapartum Timing but by Themselves are Nonspecific

A sentinel (signal) hypoxic event occurring immediately before or during labor

A sudden, rapid and sustained deterioration of the fetal heart rate pattern, usually following the hypoxic sentinel event where the pattern was previously normal

Apgar scores of 0-6 for longer than 5 minutes

Early evidence of multisystem involvement

Early imaging evidence of acute cerebral abnormality

[a]Table 1 from MacLennan A. A template for defining a causal relationship between acute intrapartum events and cerebral palsy: international concensus statement. BMJ 1999;319:1054–9.

the lateral ventricles. This region is characterized by numerous, very delicate, thin-walled capillary spaces that are especially susceptible to injury, resulting in hemorrhages. Premature infants are especially susceptible to GMH, especially during the 24th to 26th week. This anatomic region matures and disappears by the 35th week and is no longer disproportionately susceptible to injury. First-degree GMHs are small and confined to the germinal matrix area, second-degree lesions bulge into the ventricular lumen, and third-degree lesions indicate blood or clot in the ventricles (IVH). The most common placental lesions associated with GMH are those listed under cerebral palsy, occurring in association with prematurity.

Periventricular Leukomalacia (PVL). PVL is diagnosed by ultrasound, computed tomography (CT), or magnetic resonance imaging (MRI) techniques applied to the brain of surviving newborns, or by postmortem examination of the brains of premature infants who die in the perinatal or neonatal period. The periventricular "watershed" zone between the lenticulostriate arteries and the deep penetrating branches of the middle cerebral arteries becomes at first necrotic, followed over a period of days and weeks by gliosis and cyst formation in the cerebral white matter.

The most common placental lesions are those listed under cerebral palsy, in association with prematurity. In a series of 1,439 preterm infants delivered before 34 weeks, 34 were found to have PVL (57). In this study, the placental lesions included circulatory problems (abruption, infarcts, ischemic villi) and chorioamnionitis.

Hypoxic-Ischemic Encephalopathy (HIE). This is an imprecise clinical diagnostic term that indicates the observation of apparent neonatal neurologic abnormalities, such as low Apgar scores, poor respiratory function, abnormal reflexes, and neonatal seizures. The hypoxia and ischemia are commonly assumed but infrequently demonstrated. The term *neonatal encephalopathy* is now preferred because of the frequent ambiguity regarding causation. The most common placental lesions are those listed under cerebral palsy.

Perinatal or Intrapartum Asphyxia. This is an imprecise clinical diagnostic term that indicates an observation of one or more of the following: low Apgar scores, abnormal muscle tone (a limp, "floppy" neonate), need for resuscitation, neonatal seizures, neonatal acidosis, and reduced oxygenation of the cord blood. An obstetrician may base the diagnosis on fetal heart rate decelerations, low fetal scalp or umbilical cord pH, and thick meconium, while the pediatrician may focus on low Apgar scores, delayed spontaneous breathing, and early neurologic deficits. Of these, only the neurologic abnormality has a reasonable association with cerebral palsy, and even that is a poor predictor. None of these observations is specific for an asphyxiated state (76). The expression "hypoxia/asphyxia" seems to imply that some initiating event comparable to suffocation or drowning has definitely caused hypoxia. This may be true in instances of abruption, fetomaternal hemorrhage, or cord compression, but it is an erroneous assumption in most cases, which are initiated by sepsis or thrombosis (78). All too often the only basis for reporting that "intrauterine hypoxia/birth asphyxia" actually occurred is a clinical impression which led to the recording of an ICD-9 code of 768 in the mother's chart (27).

The most common placental lesions associated with hypoxia or asphyxia are those listed above under cerebral palsy. It is important to recognize that a hypoxic event sufficient to cause neonatal encephalopathy also causes objective evidence of injury to other organ systems (44). Another significant feature of fetal hypoxia is the presence of many nucleated red blood cells in the fetal circulation. This form of reactive erythroblastosis is not specific for hypoxia: it is associated with chorioamnionitis, and also with the many conditions that cause fetal or placental hydrops (see chapter 10). This important subject requires the detailed analysis that follows.

Erythroblastosis: Nucleated Red Blood Cells in the Fetal Circulation of the Placenta

Nucleated red blood cells (NRBC) are rarely identifiable in the fetal blood when histologic sections of the fetal blood vessels in a normal placenta are examined. Differential counts of fetal or neonatal blood in the third trimester average about 500 to 1,000 NRBC/mm^3, or 1 to 10 NRBC/100 WBC (white blood cells) (46). The finding of more than an occasional NRBC in histologic sections of a placenta suggests that important clinical and pathologic lesions may be present. A semiquantitative evaluation is recommended, and has been applied in practice (87). The feasibility of using histologic sections to quantify NRBC counts with an accuracy comparable to actual blood counts has been investigated (17) and deserves further study. Fetal lymphocyte counts also rise (82), but this relationship has been less comprehensively studied.

There are numerous causes of erythroblastosis, as listed in Hermansen's review (46). Acute hypoxia (as in acute abruption), chronic hypoxia (large or numerous infarcts, severe preeclampsia), and maternal diabetes mellitus are probably the most common. Other causes are fetal anemia, chorioamnionitis and many other infections, and intrauterine growth restriction. In our experience, fetal thrombotic vasculopathy is commonly associated with increased NRBC counts, especially when the lesions are extensive or acute.

The time required to produce an NRBC elevation is not established. This issue is frequently raised in litigated cases if the timing of an injury is in dispute. Benirschke (10) reported a newborn with a NRBC response within 1 hour of an acute fetal hemorrhage caused by placental vessel injury during instrumentation with a monitoring device. The applicability of this observation to NRBC elevations from other more chronic causes is questionable. Phelan et al. (82) concluded that NRBC counts are higher and hypoxic events of longer duration in cases associated with brain injury. In many instances of obvious chronic or progressive placental lesions (severe preeclampsia, growth restriction, fetal thrombotic vasculopathy), the NRBC rise is more directly related to the incremental stress of labor. When sequential counts are available, the evidence of a rise or fall in NRBC counts may assist in estimating the onset of the rise, but not necessarily the timing of, a silent injury hours or days before.

Fetal or Neonatal Thrombocytopenias

The clinical problem associated with thrombocytopenia is fetal or neonatal bleeding. The most serious complication is prenatal intracranial hemorrhage, as a result of prenatal thrombocytopenia in the neonate. The most common causes are maternal immune thrombocytopenia and fetomaternal alloimmunization to paternally-derived platelet antigens inherited by the fetus. Maternal IgG antibodies pass through the placental barrier into the fetal circulation, resulting in the destruction of fetal platelets (97). This occurs in 1 in 500 to 1,000 deliveries. No specific or distinctive lesions in the placenta have been identified in cases the authors have examined or in most of the reported cases. The placenta described by de Tar et al. (26) had typical features of fetal thrombotic vasculopathy and extensive chronic villitis, possibly related to human leukocyte antigen (HLA) alloimmunization in the same patient.

Severe but transient neonatal thrombocytopenia may be associated with maternal antiplatelet autoimmunity, even without overt maternal thrombocytopenia (107). Ultrasound and Doppler monitoring of fetuses at risk for intracranial hemorrhage may detect indicators of a worsening prognosis before an intracranial hemorrhage occurs, allowing for intrauterine intervention (25). Neonatal thrombocytopenia may also occur in association with large placental hemangiomas (see chapter 11), with any form of disseminated intravascular coagulation in the fetus or newborn, and in some cases of preeclampsia.

Meconium-Stained Amnionic Fluid and the Meconium Aspiration Syndrome

Meconium is present in the amnionic fluid of about 14 percent of deliveries. It has long been a reputed but inconsistent indicator of postnatal morbidity or mortality. It has been implicated as a basic initiating factor in the meconium aspiration syndrome (35), and a role in causing fetal hypoxia by stimulating umbilical vessel constriction has been proposed (4,75). However, most newborns with meconium-stained amnionic fluid seem to have a more basic underlying problem, such as intrauterine infection (16,83), acute or chronic hypoxia, or acidosis, suggesting that the meconium is either an accessory factor (85) or even an epiphenomenon, rather than a primary etiologic factor (35). The placenta should be carefully examined for other significant lesions before assuming that the meconium itself is a major or initiating factor in a prenatal or perinatal injury (53,109).

The placental pathologic features associated with meconium staining are presented in chapter 7.

Abnormal Amnionic Fluid Volume

The presence of an excess of amnionic fluid is called *hydramnios* or *polyhydramnios*. A diminished amount is called *oligohydramnios*. A quantification technique based upon the addition of multiple ultrasound measurements, called the amnionic fluid index, is commonly used. An index below 5 cm is abnormally low (oligohydramnios) and an index of 24 cm or more indicates hydramnios.

In a consecutive series of 672 pregnancies complicated by hydramnios, 77 (11 percent) of the fetuses had significant abnormalities, mainly malformations (21). The most common anomalies were anencephaly, spina bifida, esophageal atresia, nonimmune hydrops, and various abnormal karyotypes (18). The recipient twin affected by the twin-twin transfusion syndrome commonly has hydramnios.

The most common cause of oligohydramnios is leakage of amnionic fluid caused by premature membrane rupture. Oligohydramnios also occurs in nearly all cases of bilateral renal agenesis and fetal urinary tract obstruction. Other associations include various other fetal malformations, abnormal karyotypes, growth restriction, post-term pregnancies, preeclampsia, maternal hypertension, and the donor twin in the twin-twin transfusion syndrome. Some instances of chronic partial placental abruption may cause oligohydramnios (102). The umbilical cord is subject to compression, especially with severe oligohydramnios, and pulmonary hypoplasia is common. Simple compression of fetal parts may cause a variety of skeletal deformities, such as clubfoot (102).

REFERENCES

1. Alexander JM, McIntire DM, Leveno KJ. Chorioamnionitis and the prognosis for term infants. Obstet Gynecol 1999;94:274–8.
2. Alfirevic Z, Roberts D, Martlew V. How strong is the association between maternal thrombophilia and adverse pregnancy outcome? A systematic review. Eur J Obstet Gynecol Reprod Biol 2002;101:6–14.
3. Altshuler G. Chorangiosis. An important placental sign of neonatal morbidity and mortality. Arch Pathol Lab Med 1984;108:71–4.
4. Altshuler G, Hyde S. Meconium-induced vasocontraction: a potential cause of cerebral and other fetal hypoperfusion and of poor pregnancy outcome. J Child Neurol 1989;4:137–42.
5. Arias F, Romero R, Joist H, Kraus FT. Thrombophilia: a mechanism of disease in women with adverse pregnancy outcome and thrombotic lesions in the placenta. J Matern Fetal Med 1998;7:277–86.
6. Arias F, Victoria A, Cho K, Kraus FT. Placental histology and clinical characteristics of patients with preterm premature rupture of membranes. Obstet Gynecol 1997;89:265–71.

7. Badawi N, Kurinczuk JJ, Keogh JM, et al. Antepartum risk factors for newborn encephalopathy: the Western Australian case-control study. BMJ 1998;317:1549–53.
8. Badawi N, Kurinczuk JJ, Keogh JM, et al. Intrapartum risk factors for newborn encephalopathy: the Western Australian case-control study. BMJ 1998;317:1554–8.
9. Bakketeig LS. Only a minor part of cerebral palsy cases begin in labour. But still room for controversial childbirth issues in court. BMJ 1999;319:1016–7.
10. Benirschke K. Placental pathology questions to the perinatologist. J Perinatol 1994;14:371–5.
11. Benirschke K, Kaufmann P. Pathology of the human placenta, 4th ed. New York: Springer; 2000:443–54.
12. Brenner B, Hoffman R, Blumenfeld Z, Weiner Z, Younis JS. Gestational outcome in thrombophilic women with recurrent pregnancy loss treated by enoxaparin. Thromb Haemost 2000;83:693–7.
13. Clifford SH. Postmaturity with placental dysfunction. Clinical syndromes and pathologic findings. J Pediatr 1954;44:1–13.
14. Collier JS. The pathogenesis of cerebral diplegia. Proc R Soc Med 1924;17 (Section of Neurology):1–11.
15. Colwell JA, Jokl R. Vascular thrombosis in diabetes. In: Porte D, Sherwin RS, eds. Ellenberg and Rifkin's diabetes mellitus, 5th ed. Stamford, Conn: Appleton & Lange; 1997:207–16.
16. Coughtry H, Jeffery HE, Henderson-Smart DJ, Storey B, Poulos V. Possible causes linking asphyxia, thick meconium, and respiratory distress. Aust N Z J Obstet Gynaecol 1991;31:97–102.
17. Curtin WM, Shehata BM, Khuder SA, Robinson HR, Brost BC. The feasibility of using histologic placental sections to predict newborn nucleated red blood cell counts. Obstet Gynecol 2002;110:305–10.
18. Damato N, Filly RA, Goldstein RB, et al. Frequency of fetal anomalies in sonographically detected polyhydramnios. J Ultrasound Med 1993;12:11–5.
19. Dammann O, Kuban K, Leviton A. Perinatal infection, fetal inflammatory response, white matter damage, and cognitive limitations in children born preterm. Ment Retard Dev Disabil Res Rev 2002;8:46–50.
20. Dashe JS, McIntire DD, Lucas MJ, Leveno KJ. Effects of symmetric and asymmetric fetal growth on pregnancy outcomes. Obstet Gynecol 2000;96:321–7.
21. Dashe JS, McIntire DD, Ramus RM, Santos-Ramos R, Twickler DM. Hydramnios: anomaly prevalence and sonographic detection. Obstet Gynecol 2002;100:134–9.
22. DeFelice C, Toti P, Laurini RN, et al. Early neonatal brain injury in histologic chorioamnionitis. J Pediatr 2001;138:101–4.
23. Dekker GA, Sibai BM. Etiology and pathogenesis of preeclampsia: current concepts. Am J Obstet Gynecol 1998;179:1359–75.
24. Dekker GA, Sibai BM. The immunology of preeclampsia. Semin Perinatol 1999;23:24–33.
25. DeSpirlet M, Goffenet F, Philippe HJ, Bailly M, Couderc S, Nisand I. Prenatal diagnosis of a subdural hematoma associated with reverse flow in the middle cerebral artery: case report and literature review. Ultrasound Obstet Gynecol 2000;16:72–76.
26. de Tar MW, Klohe E, Grosset A, Rau T. Neonatal alloimmune thrombocytopenia with HLA alloimmunization: case report with immunohematologic and placental findings. Pediatr Devel Pathol 2002;5:200–5.
27. Dite GS, Bell R, Reddihough DS, Bessell C, Brennecke S, Sheedy M. Antenatal and perinatal antecedents of moderate and severe spastic cerebral palsy. Aust N Z J Obstet Gynaecol 1998;38:377–83.
28. Dizon-Townson DS, Meline L, Nelson L, Varner M, Ward K. Fetal carriers of the factor V Leiden mutation are prone to miscarriage and placental infarction. Am J Obstet Gynecol 1997;177:402–5.
29. Elimian A, Verma U, Beneck D, Cipriano R, Visintainer P, Tejani N. Histologic chorioamnionitis, antenatal steroids, and perinatal outcomes. Obstet Gynecol 2000;96:333–6.
30. Euscher E, Davis J, Holzman I, Nuovo GJ. Coxsackie virus infection of the placenta associated with neurodevelopmental delays in the newborn. Obstet Gynecol 2001;98:1019–26.
31. Fox H. Pathology of the placenta, 2nd ed. Philadelphia: Saunders; 1997.
32. Fox H. Thrombosis of the foetal stem arteries in the human placenta. J Obstet Gynaecol Br Commonw 1966;73:961–5.
33. Freud S. Die infantile cerebrallahmung. Wien: Alfred Holder; 1897.
34. Gaudet LM, Smith GN. Cerebral palsy and chorioamnionitis: the inflammatory cytokine link. Obstet Gynecol Surv 2001;56:433–6.
35. Ghidini A, Spong CY. Severe meconium aspiration syndrome is not caused by aspiration of meconium. Am J Obstet Gynecol 2001;185:931–8.
36. Godfrey KM, Redman CW, Barker DJ, Osmund C. The effect of maternal anaemia and iron deficiency on the ratio of fetal weight to placental weight. Brit J Obstet Gynaecol 1991;98:886–91.

37. Golomb MR, MacGregor DL, Domi T, et al. Presumed pre- or perinatal arterial ischemic stroke: risk factors and outcomes. Ann Neurol 2001; 50:163–8.
38. Greer IA. Thrombosis in pregnancy: maternal and fetal issues. Lancet 1999;353:1258–65.
39. Grether JK, Nelson KB. Maternal infection and cerebral palsy in infants of normal birth weight. JAMA 1997;278:207–11.
40. Grether JK, Nelson KB, Cumminns SK. Twinning and cerebral palsy: experience in four northern California counties, births 1983 through 1985. Pediatrics 1993;92:854–8.
41. Gunther G, Junker R, Strater R, et al. Symptomatic ischemic stroke in full term neonates: role of acquired and genetic prothrombotic risk factors. Stroke 2000;31:2437–41.
42. Haddow JE, Palomaki GE, Allan WC, et al. Maternal thyroid deficiency during pregnancy and subsequent neuropsychological development of the child. N Engl J Med 1999;341:549–55.
43. Hagberg H, Peebles D, Mallard C. Models of white matter injury: comparison of infectious, hypoxic-ischemic, and excitotoxic insults. Ment Retard Dev Disabil Res Rev 2002;8:30–8.
44. Hankins GD, Koen S, Gei AF, Lopez SM, Van Hook JW, Anderson GD. Neonatal organ system injury in acute birth asphyxia sufficient to result in neonatal encephalopathy. Obstet Gynecol 2002;99:688–91.
45. Haust MD. Maternal diabetes mellitus-effects on the fetus and placenta. In: Naeye RL, Kissane JM, Kaufman N, eds. Perinatal diseases. Baltimore: Williams & Wilkins; 1981:201–85.
46. Hermansen MC. Nucleated red blood cells in the fetus and newborn. Arch Dis Child Fetal Neonatal Ed 2001;84:F211–5.
47. Hsia YE. Detection and prevention of important alpha-thalassemia variants. Semin Perinatol 1991;15:35–41.
48. Ibdah JA, Bennett MJ, Rinaldo P, et al. A fetal fatty acid oxydation disorder as a cause of liver disease in pregnant women. N Eng J Med 1999;340:1723–31.
49. Jones CJ, Fox H. An ultrastructural and ultrahistochemical study of the human placenta in maternal essential hypertension. Placenta 1981;2:193–204.
50. Jones CJ, Fox H. An ultrastructural and ultrahistochemical study of the human placenta in maternal pre-eclampsia. Placenta 1980;1:61–76.
51. Jones CJ, Fox H. An ultrastructural and ultrahistochemical study of the placenta of the diabetic woman. J Pathol 1976;119:91–9.
52. Kadyrov M, Black S, Kaufmann P, Huppertz B. Preeclampsia and maternal anaemia display reduced apoptosis and opposite invasive phenotypes of extravillous trophoblast. Placenta 2003;24:540–38.
53. Kaspar HG, Abu-Musa A, Hannoun A, et al. The placenta in meconium staining: lesions and early neonatal outcome. Clin Exp Obstet Gynecol 2000;27:63–6.
54. Keith RD, Beckley S, Garibaldi JM, Westgate JA, Ifeachor EC, Greene KR. A multicentre comparative study of 17 experts and an intelligent computer system for managing labour using the cardiotocogram. Br J Obstet Gynaecol 1995;102:688–700.
55. Kraus FT. Placental thrombi and related problems. Semin Diag Pathol 1993;10:275–83.
56. Kraus FT, Acheen VI. Fetal thrombotic vasculopathy in the placenta: cerebral thrombi and infarcts, coagulopathies, and cerebral palsy. Hum Pathol 1999;30:759–69.
57. Kumazaki K, Nakayama M, Sumida Y, et al. Placental features in preterm infants with periventricular leukomalacia. Pediatrics 2002;109:650–5.
58. Lachmeijer AM, Dekker GA, Pals G, Aarnoudse JG, ten Kate LP, Arngrimsson R. Searching for preeclampsia genes: the current position. Eur J Obstet Gynecol Reprod Biol 2002;105:94–113.
59. Larroche JC, Aubry MC, Narcy F. Intrauterine brain damage in nonimmune hydrops fetalis. Biol Neonate 1992;61:273–80.
60. Larsen LG, Clausen HV, Anderson B, Graem N. A steriologic study of postmature placentas fixed by dual perfusion. Am J Obstet Gynecol 1995;172:500–7.
61. Laurini RN, Visser GH, Ballegooie E, Schoots CJ. Morphological findings in placentae of insulin-dependent diabetic patients treated with continuous subcutaneous insulin infusion (CSII). Placenta 1987;8:153–65.
62. Leviton A, Paneth N, Reuss L, et al. Hypothyroxinemia of prematurity and the risk of cerebral white matter damage. J Pediatr 1999;134:706–11.
63. Lin CC, Santolaya-Forgas J. Current concepts of fetal growth restriction: Part 1. Causes, classification, and pathophysiology. Obstet Gynecol 1998;92:1044–55.
64. Little WJ. On the influence of abnormal parturition, difficult labour, premature birth, and asphyxia neonatorum on the mental and physical condition of the child, especially in relation to deformities. Clin Orthop 1966;46:7–22.
65. Lockwood CJ. Heritable coagulopathies in pregnancy. Obstet Gynecol Surv 1999;54:754–65.
66. MacDonald PC, Siiteri PK. Origin of estrogen in women pregnant with an anencephalic fetus. J Clin Invest 1965;44:465–74.

67. MacLennan A. A template for defining a causal relationship between acute intrapartum events and cerebral palsy: international concensus statement. BMJ 1999;319:1054–9.
68. Many A, Elad R, Yaron Y, Eldor A, Lessing JB, Kupferminc M. Third trimester unexplained intrauterine fetal death is associated with inherited thrombophilia. Obstet Gynecol 2002;99:684–7.
69. Many A, Schreiber L, Rosner S, Lessing JB, Eldor A, Kupferminc M. Pathologic features of the placenta in women with severe pregnancy complications and thrombophilia. Obstet Gynecol 2001;98:1041–4.
70. Matern D, Shehata BM, Shekhawat P, Strauss AW, Bennett MJ, Rinaldo P. Placental floor infarction complicating the pregnancy of a fetus with long-chain 3-hydroxyacyl-CoA dehydrogenase (LCHAD) deficiency. Mol Genet Metab 2001;72:265–8.
71. Maynard S, Min JY, Merchan J, et al. Excess placental soluble fms-like tyrosine kinase 1 (sFlt1) may contribute to endothelial dysfunction, hypertension, and proteinuria in preeclampsia. J Clin Invest 2003;111:649–58.
72. McHale DP, Mitchell S, Bundey S, et al. A gene for autosomal recessive symmetrical spastic cerebral palsy maps to chromosome 2q24-25. Am J Hum Genet 1999;64:526–32.
73. McIntire DD, Bloom SL, Casey BM, Leveno KJ. Birth weight in relation to morbidity and mortality among newborn infants. N Engl J Med 1999;340:1234–8.
74. Mercuri E, Cowan F, Gupte G, et al. Prothrombotic disorders and abnormal neurodevelopmental outcome in infants with neonatal cerebral infarction. Pediatrics 2001;107:1400–4.
75. Naeye RL. Can meconium in the amnionic fluid injure the fetal brain? Obstet Gynecol 1995;86:720–4.
76. Nelson KB. The epidemiology of cerebral palsy in term infants. Ment Retard Dev Disabil Res Rev 2002;8:146–50.
77. Nelson KB, Dambrosia JM, Grether JK, Phillips TM. Neonatal cytokines and coagulation factors in children with cerebral palsy. Ann Neurol 1998;44:665–75.
78. Nelson KB, Grether JK. Causes of cerebral palsy. Curr Opin Pediatr 1999;11:487–91.
79. Newham J. Consequences of fetal growth restriction. Curr Opin Obstet Gynecol 1998;10:145–9.
80. Ogueh O, Chen MF, Spurli G, Benjamin A. Outcome of pregnancy in women with hereditary thrombophilia. Int J Gynecol Obstet 2001;74:247–53.
81. Oppenheimer EH, Esterly JR. Thrombosis in the newborn: comparison between infants of diabetic and nondiabetic mothers. J Pediatr 1965;67:549–56.
82. Phelan JP, Korst LM, Ahn MO, Martin GI. Neonatal nucleated red blood cell and lymphocyte counts in fetal brain injury. Obstet Gynecol 1998;91:485–9.
83. Piper JM, Newton ER, Berkus MD, Peairs WA. Meconium: a marker for peripartum infection. Obstet Gynecol 1998;91:741–745.
84. Pipkin FB. Risk factors for preeclampsia. N Engl J Med 2001;344:924–6.
85. Ramin KD, Leveno KJ, Kelly MA, Carmody TJ. Amnionic fluid meconium: a fetal environmental hazard. Obstet Gynecol 1996;87:181–4.
86. Rand JH, Wu XX, Andree HA, et al. Pregnancy loss in the antiphospholipid-antibody syndrome—a possible thrombogenic mechanism. N Engl J Med 1997;337:154–60.
87. Redline RW, O'Riordan MA. Placental lesions associated with cerebral palsy and neurologic impairment following term birth. Arch Pathol Lab Med 2000;124:1785–91.
88. Redline RW, Patterson P. Patterns of placental injury: correlation with gestational age, placental weight, and clinical diagnosis. Arch Pathol Lab Med 1994;118:698–701.
89. Redline RW, Wilson-Costello D, Borawski E, Fanaroff AA, Hack M. Placental lesions associated with neurologic impairment and cerebral palsy in very low-birth weight infants. Arch Pathol Lab Med 1998;122:1091–8.
90. Redline RW, Zaragoza M, Hassold T. Prevalence of developmental and inflammatory lesions in nonmolar first-trimester spontaneous abortions. Hum Pathol 1999;30:93–100.
91. Redman CW, Sargent IL. Placental debris, oxidative stress, and pre-eclampsia. Placenta 2000;21:597–602.
92. Reshetnikova OS, Burton GJ, Teleshova OV. Placental histomorphometry and morphologic diffusing capacity of the villous membrane in pregnancies complicated by iron-deficiency anemia. Am J Obstet Gynecol 1995;173:724–7.
93. Resnik R. Intrauterine growth restriction. Obstet Gynecol 2002;99:490–6.
94. Rigano S, Bozzo M, Ferrazzi E, Belloti M, Battaglia FC, Galan HL. Early and persistent reduction in umbilical vein flow in the growth restricted fetus: a longitudinal study. Am J Obstet Gynecol 2001;185:834–8.
95. Roberts JM, Hubel CA. Is oxidative stress the link in the two-stage model of pre-eclampsia? Lancet 1999;354:788–9.

96. Salafia CM, Pezzullo JC, Minior VK, Divon MY. Placental pathology of absent and reversed end-diastolic flow in growth-restricted fetuses. Obstet Gynecol 1997;90:830–6.
97. Savoia HF, Brennecke SP, Burrows RF, et al. Investigation and management of fetomaternal alloimmune thrombocytopenia. Aust N Z J Obstet Gynaecol 2000;40:176–9.
98. Savonara-Ventura C, Bonello F. Beta thalassemia syndromes and pregnancy. Obstet Gynecol Surv 1994;49:129–37.
99. Seligsohn U, Lubetsky A. Genetic susceptibility to venous thrombosis. N Engl J Med 2001;344:1222–31.
100. Shalak LF, Perlman JM. Infection markers and early signs of neonatal encephalopathy in the term infant. Ment Retard Dev Disabil Res Rev 2002;8:14–9.
101. Shanklin DR. Clinicopathologic correlates in placentas from women with sickle cell disease (abstract). Am J Pathol 1976;82:5a.
102. Shenker L, Reed KL, Anderson CF, Borjon JA. Significance of oligohydramnios complicating pregnancy. Am J Obstet Gynecol 1991;164:1597–600.
103. Smulian JC, Shen-Schwartz S, Vintzileos AM, Lake MF, Ananth CV. Clinical chorioamnionitis and histologic placental inflammation. Obstet Gynecol 1999;94:1000–5.
104. Smulian JC, Vintzileos AM, Lai YL, Santiago J, Shen-Schwartz S, Campbell WA. Maternal chorioamnionitis and umbilical vein interleukin-6 levels for identifying early neonatal sepsis. J Matern Fetal Med 1999;8:88–94.
105. Sowers JR, Lester MA. Diabetes and cardiovascular disease. Diabetes Care 1999;22(Supp 3):c14–20.
106. Strauss AW, Bennett MJ, Rinaldo P, et al. Inherited long chain 3-hydroxyacyl-CoA dehydrogenase deficiency and a fetal-maternal interaction cause maternal liver disease and other pregnancy complications. Sem Perinatol 1999;23:100–12.
107. Tchernia G, Morel-Kopp MC, Yvart J, Kaplan C. Neonatal thrombocytopenia and hidden maternal autoimmunity. Brit J Haematol 1993;84:457–63.
108. Thorarensen O, Ryan S, Hunter J, Younkin DP. Factor V Leiden 19 mutations: an unrecognized cause of hemiplegic cerebral palsy, neonatal stroke, and placental thrombosis. Ann Neurol 1997;42:372–5.
109. Thureen PJ, Hall DM, Hoffenberg A, Tyson RW. Fatal meconium aspiration in spite of appropriate perinatal airway management: pulmonary and placental evidence of prenatal disease. Am J Obstet Gynecol 1997;176:967–75.
110. Toti P, DeFelice C, Palmeri LD, Villanova M, Martin JJ, Buoncore G. Inflammatory pathogenesis of cortical polymicrogyria: an autopsy study. Pediatr Res 1998;44:291–6.
111. Unfried G, Griesmacher A, Weismuller W, Nagele F, Huber JC, Tempfer CB. The C677T polymorphism of the methylene tetrahydrofolate reductase gene and idiopathic recurrent miscarriage. Obstet Gynecol 2002;99:614–9.
112. Viscardi RM, Sun CC. Placental lesion multiplicity: risk factor for IUGR and neonatal cranial ultrasound abnormalities. Early Hum Devel 2001;62:1–10.
113. Williams MC, O'Brien WF, Nelson RN, Spellacy WN. Histologic chorioamnionitis is associated with fetal growth restriction, in term and preterm infants. Am J Obstet Gynecol 2000;183:1094–9.
114. World Health Organization (WHO). Recommended definition terminology and format for statistical tables related to the perinatal period and rise of a new certification for cause of perinatal deaths. Acta Obstet Gynecol Scand 1977;56:247–53.
115. Yanowitz TD, Jordan JA, Gilmour CH, et al. Hemodynamic disturbances in premature infants born after chorioamnionitis: association with cord blood cytokine concentrations. Pediatr Res 2002;51:310–6.
116. Yoon BH, Romero R, Park JS, Kim CJ, Choi JH, Han TR. Fetal exposure to an intra-amniotic inflammation and the development of cerebral palsy at the age of three years. Am J Obstet Gynecol 2000;182:675–81.
117. Zoghbi HY. Introduction: Rett syndrome. Ment Retard Dev Disabil Res Rev 2002;8:59–60.

4 DISORDERS OF PLACENTAL DEVELOPMENT

INTRODUCTION

Formation of the placental disc and its adnexa (umbilical cord and membranes) follows a developmental program with shared general features but many minor variations that are highly species specific (12,71). In humans, implantation generally occurs in the body of the uterus and extends through the endometrial decidua into the tissues and vessels of the inner myometrium. Membranes form by secondary atrophy of the initially spherical chorionic sac and are continuous with the margin of the definitive discoid placenta. The fetal vascular supply is gathered in an umbilical cord that inserts centrally into the placental disc at its original site of implantation.

Disorders of placental development occur by several mechanisms. Primary abnormalities in placental gene expression can alter development, irrespective of the surrounding maternal environment (cell autonomous). Developmental abnormalities may arise because of an abnormal maternal environment or disordered interactions between the fetal genetic program and the environment (conditionally specified). Alternatively, an initially normal developmental sequence can be interrupted by discrete events that damage the developing placenta, leading to alterations in structure. These same mechanisms have been invoked for birth defects in the fetus and have been termed malformation, deformation, and disruption, respectively. Important determinants of placental structure, as discussed below, include genetic and chromosomal abnormalities, anatomic defects at the initial site of implantation, local oxygen supply, and the metabolic status of the mother. Major causes of disruption are hemorrhage, thrombosis, infection, and substance abuse.

DISORDERS OF MEMBRANE DEVELOPMENT

Placenta Membranacea

Definition. Placenta membranacea is a failure of normal placental membrane formation leading to a gestational sac almost completely surrounded by vascularized chorionic villi.

Incidence and Etiology. This extremely rare anomaly is poorly understood (2). Regression of villi in the membranous portion of the placenta normally occurs between 10 and 14 weeks, coincident with degenerative changes caused by oxidative damage in peripheral portions of the placenta (37). This may provide a mechanistic explanation for previous suggestions that placenta membranacea may be related to poor blood supply to the decidual basalis and overvascularization of the decidua capsularis (34). Failure of regression could also be genetic and related to abnormal expression of critical fetoplacental or uterine genes. The lack of a clearcut recurrence risk argues against the latter, although there is one anecdotal report of recurrence in the second generation (daughter of an affected mother) (8). Some have proposed that diffuse endometrial hypoplasia may be a causative factor. Placenta membranacea is the normal condition in marine mammals, some domestic animals, and a few lower primates.

Clinical Features. Premature separation, placenta previa, and either maternal hemorrhage or gravid hysterectomy, due to retained placenta, are reported complications. Life-threatening fetal hemorrhage may occur at the time of membrane rupture.

Gross and Microscopic Findings. In most reported cases, there is a small patch of clear membranous tissue at one aspect of the sac (fig. 4-1). The placenta tends to be abnormally thin and the maternal surface is often disrupted due to placenta accreta. Areas of potential fetal hemorrhage should be carefully evaluated at gross examination in cases with a poor pregnancy outcome. Histologic examination of areas of possible accreta or fetal hemorrhage is indicated.

Circumvallation/Circummargination

Definition. Circumvallation is the complete or partial insertion of the fetal membranes in the placental disc away from the peripheral

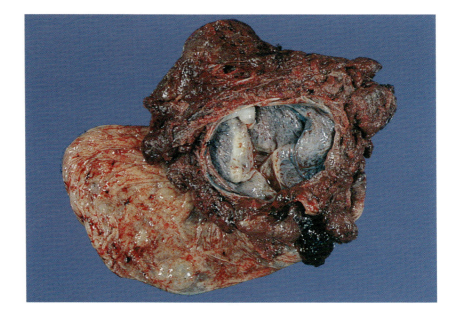

Figure 4-1

PLACENTA MEMBRANACEA

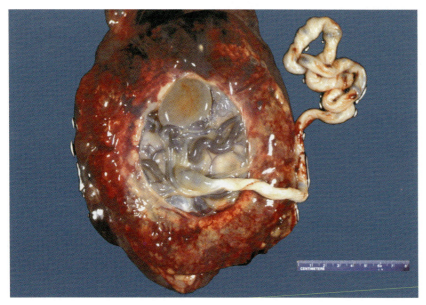

Figure 4-2

CIRCUMVALLATE PLACENTA

margin, with or without a distinct ridge of degenerating blood clot (fig. 4-2). Occasionally, circumvallate placentas have an inner concentric ridge but the membranes are secondarily attached such that they appear to arise from the periphery. The term circummarginate refers to cases without the ridge and should probably be abandoned for the sake of clarity.

Incidence and Etiology. This relatively common abnormality occurs in 1 to 7 percent of placentas (26). The preponderance of opinion is that most cases are due to marginal venous hemorrhage ("marginal abruption"), which pushes or folds the membranes, and sometimes the entire peripheral placenta, inward over the chorionic plate (9,64,79). In most cases, this sequence represents a disruption related to increased maternal venous pressure or changes in the intrauterine geometry that accompany rupture of membranes (60). Other explanations include abnormally deep implantation and premature fixation of the disc-membrane boundary (premature formation of the "closure ring"), with subsequent placental growth (94). Even in

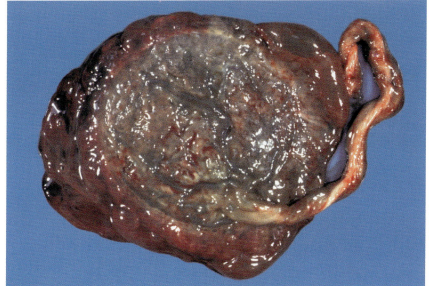

Figure 4-3
CIRCUMVALLATE PLACENTA
Green discoloration in circumvallate placenta is due to chronic hemorrhage.

these latter scenarios, it is likely that hemorrhage is either a secondary event leading to the final lesion or a cause of the premature closure ring.

Clinical Features. Circumvallate placentas are often associated with recurrent vaginal bleeding in all trimesters (see chapter 6, Retroplacental Hematomas, Marginal Hematomas, and Placenta Abruption) (98). In the most severe cases, features of the chronic abruption-oligohydramnios sequence, including decreased amnionic fluid, leakage of clear fluid, and premature delivery, are seen (22). Term infants with evidence of circumvallation or chronic marginal hemorrhage may have mild intrauterine growth restriction (IUGR) and have an increased risk of long-term neurologic impairment (76). Placentas with chronic marginal hemorrhages are also at increased risk for later abruptio placenta (23). Clinical sequelae seem to parallel the amount of associated hemorrhage and cases with mild or focal circumvallation, without evidence of substantial hemorrhage, are often without clinical consequences.

Gross Findings. Placentas tend to be somewhat small for gestational age and often have areas of larger, degenerating, brownish blood clots (see chapter 6, fig. 6-29). Areas of more recent, dark red marginal hemorrhage are also common. If blood has gained entry to the amniotic fluid, green discoloration of the fetal surface secondary to biliverdin staining may be seen (fig. 4-3). In terms of the circumvallate insertion itself, the percentage of the circumference affected should be recorded and a representative section through the insertion area submitted for microscopic examination.

Microscopic Findings. Marginal sections show foci of old decidual hemorrhage either separating amniochorion from marginal villi or lying within redundant folds of membrane, and/or peripheral placenta on the surface of the chorionic plate (fig. 4-4). Local hemosiderin deposition is the rule and in severe cases diffuse chorioamnionic hemosiderosis affects the entire placenta (figs. 4-5, 4-6).

DISORDERS OF UTERINE IMPLANTATION

Placenta Previa

Definition. Placenta previa is defined as placental implantation in the lower uterine segment with some tissue near or overlying the uterine cervical os. Central placenta previa is a placenta whose implantation is centered over the os; complete placenta previa occurs when one edge completely covers the os; and partial placenta previa is a placenta whose edge lies within 2 cm of the os.

Incidence. Complete or partial placenta previa is seen in approximately 0.3 to 0.5 percent of deliveries (16).

Etiology. The trophectoderm of the early blastocyst and the endometrial epithelium have no intrinsic affinity for one another. Implantation

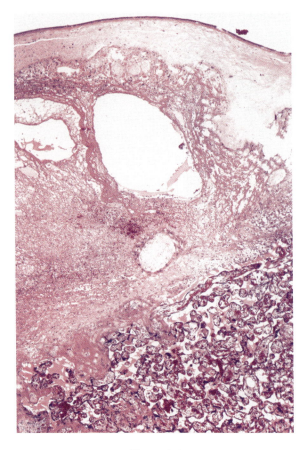

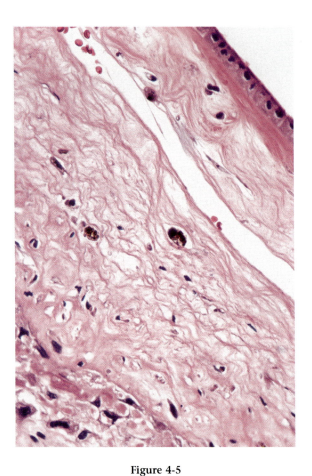

Figure 4-4

CIRCUMVALLATE PLACENTA

A large aggregate of old clotted blood and fibrin elevates the membranes away from the marginal insertion site (to the left of field). Placental margin is at the left. Villi are pressed downward to the lower right.

Figure 4-5

MEMBRANE HEMOSIDERIN

Golden brown refractile pigment is seen with the chorionic fibrous connective tissue (hematoxylin and eosin stain).

Figure 4-6

MEMBRANE HEMOSIDERIN

Numerous nests of blue pigment throughout the amniochorionic connective tissue represent diffuse uptake of degenerating blood products from the amnionic fluid (iron stain).

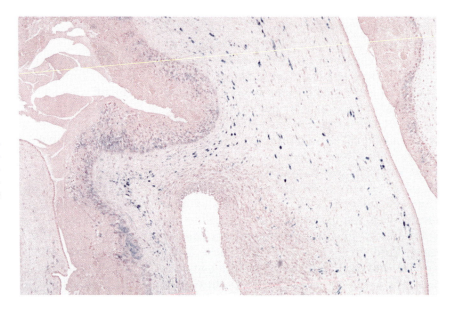

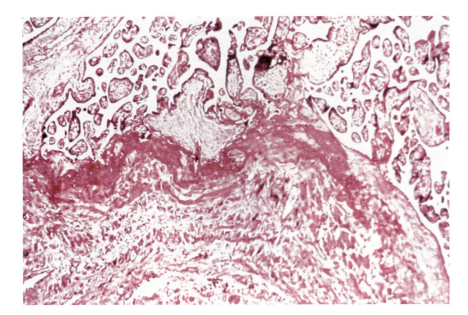

Figure 4-7

PLACENTA ACCRETA

Anchoring villi implant directly on the uterine smooth muscle, without intervening decidual cells.

generally occurs in the uterine fundus and is coordinated by factors secreted from the mature blastocyst, which act on appropriately primed mullerian epithelium. The epithelium is thereby induced to express the appropriate adhesion molecules and trigger a specific sequence of events in the underlying endometrial stroma (69). On the other hand, trophectoderm rapidly attaches to and invades surfaces coated with extracellular matrix without additional signals.

Epithelial alterations that expose or change the composition of the extracellular matrix might be expected to increase the chance of low implantation. This is born out by clinical associations with previous curettage, prior cesarean section, and multiple vaginal deliveries. Other conditions predisposing to low implantation are anatomic abnormalities of the fundus, such as large leiomyomas and uterine malformations.

Clinical Features. Placental migration toward sites of greater blood supply (discussed below) often leads to resolution of cases of placenta previa diagnosed by early ultrasound (16). A positive sonographic diagnosis at 20 to 25 weeks' gestation is associated with only a 3 percent prevalence of placenta previa at delivery, compared to a 24 percent incidence following diagnosis at 30 to 35 weeks. Placenta previa often results in premature separation of the placenta, leading to profuse vaginal bleeding, premature labor, or both. Rapid evaluation by ultrasound and prompt cesarean section are necessary to prevent the risk of life-threatening fetal exsanguination related to tearing of the placental parenchyma overlying the cervical os.

Gross and Microscopic Findings. Placenta previa is often accompanied by a marginal retroplacental hematoma. In placentas delivered vaginally with complete membranes, a diagnosis of partial placenta previa may be suspected when the point of membrane rupture is at the disc margin. Disruption of the maternal surface due to placenta accreta is common. There are no specific histologic features associated with placenta previa.

Placenta Accreta, Increta, Percreta

Definition. In these conditions, anchoring villi implant on uterine smooth muscle without intervening decidua (fig. 4-7). Accreta is limited to superficial myometrium; increta extends into the myometrium; and percreta extends to or through the uterine serosa (fig. 4-8).

Incidence. The incidence of placenta accreta is dependent on the definition of cases and the diligence of histologic examination; it varies from 1 in 540 to 70,000 deliveries (16). One review notes a 10-fold increase over the past 10 years and cites a current incidence of 1 in 2,500 deliveries (1).

Etiology. Matrix molecules, local growth factors, and large granular leukocytes present in decidualized endometrium are believed to play

Placental Pathology

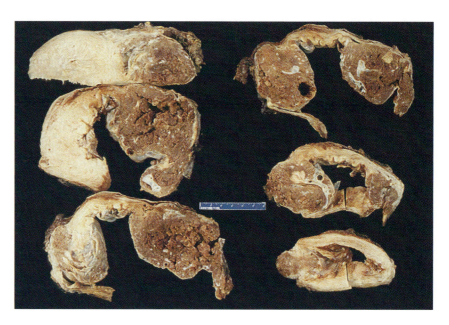

Figure 4-8

PLACENTA PERCRETA

Multiple cross sections of a gravid hysterectomy specimen show placenta growing through the uterine wall.

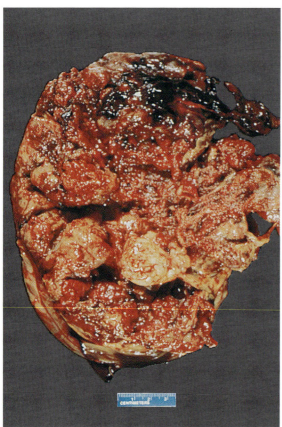

Figure 4-9

FRAGMENTED MATERNAL SURFACE WITH EMBEDDED LEIOMYOMA

See chapter 11, Intraplacental Leiomyoma, for discussion.

a role in regulating trophoblast invasiveness and the formation of a normal basal plate (72,73). Accreta is thought to be the consequence of placental implantation in a region of absent or abnormal decidualized endometrium. Predisposing conditions include maternal age greater than 35 years, previous uterine instrumentation (abortion, dilation and curettage [D&C], cesarean section), congenital or acquired uterine structural defects (uterine septa, leiomyomas, Asherman's syndrome), and ectopic implantation (placenta previa, cornual pregnancy).

Clinical Features. Antepartum complications of placenta accreta include recurrent vaginal spotting, overt hemorrhage, and uterine rupture. Hemorrhage is often due to coexisting placenta previa. Uterine rupture is usually confined to cases of percreta, particularly when associated with a previous cesarean section scar. Postpartum complications include early or delayed postpartum hemorrhage, which may necessitate gravid hysterectomy in some cases; endomyometritis, particularly in cases with chorioamnionitis; and the development of a hyalinized placental polyp when adherent placental fragments are retained for a prolonged period of time.

Gross and Microscopic Findings. In cases of placenta accreta, the maternal surface is generally disrupted and often incomplete. On rare occasions, an adherent leiomyoma may be delivered with the placenta (fig. 4-9). Histologically, the basal plate often shows a diffuse increase in matrix-type fibrinoid. Focal absence of decidua is the critical diagnostic feature. The common misperception that well-vascularized villi must directly abut large fragments of smooth muscle is probably responsible for the opinion that microscopic evaluation of the delivered placenta for signs of accreta is unrewarding. The authors' experience has been quite the contrary. Most cases of suspected accreta show smooth muscle cells in near proximity to an anchoring villus (generally lacking fetal capillaries), with only fibrin or intermediate trophoblast intervening. This diagnostic feature is usually seen with routine sampling (three full-thickness sections, with one or more taken directly adjacent to the disrupted maternal surface) and is not present in normal placentas. The presence of occasional smooth muscle cells in a basal plate containing decidua is a normal finding following vaginal birth after a cesarean section (VBAC) (36). The recognition of placenta accreta in postpartum curettings is important in the differential diagnosis of postpartum hemorrhage and may sometimes require immunostains for keratin and muscle-specific actin to delineate the true relationship between villi and myometrium.

Superficial Implantation

Definition. A deficiency of interstitial and endovascular intermediate trophoblast in the decidua basalis and basal plate arteries of the delivered placenta is termed a superficial implantation.

Incidence. Superficial implantation is the underlying anatomic abnormality in preeclampsia, which affects 2.6 percent of all pregnancies and is more common in nulliparous (4- to 5-fold) than multiparous women (87,101). Other related disorders associated with superficial implantation include fetal growth restriction (FGR), maternal thrombophilia, and abruptio placenta (20,49,96).

Etiology. The placenta is anchored to the uterus by the intermediate trophoblast, which differentiates from the cytotrophoblast covering the undersurface of the anchoring villi (see chapter 1, fig. 1-15). Proliferative immature intermediate trophoblast directly adjacent to the anchoring villi give rise to infiltrative mature intermediate trophoblast cells at deeper levels of the endometrium. Intermediate trophoblast finally coalesce as placenta site giant cells at the deepest point of invasion in the inner third of the myometrium (see fig. 1-16). Endovascular trophoblast cells are derived from the early cytotrophoblast shell. They block the lumens of basal arteries in early pregnancy and later invade the arterial wall down to the level of the inner third of the myometrium (see figs. 1-26, 1-28, and 1-29).

Brosens (10) first described superficial implantation in 1972 after a systematic study of gravid hysterectomy specimens from preeclamptic and normal patients. His observation was that trophoblast in preeclamptic placentas was restricted to the endometrium, never reaching the myometrium. This association was strengthened by several large patient series using placental bed biopsies taken at the time of cesarean section (84). Fisher (103) later reported that the trophoblast in preeclamptic placentas lacked the specific integrin adhesion molecules required for uterine invasion. Subsequent work suggested that this integrin defect was part of a generalized failure of intermediate trophoblast maturation (55).

One important regulator of trophoblast maturation is decreased oxygen tension, which acts directly on trophoblast regulatory genes via a hypoxia response element in the upstream regulatory regions of the genes (11). Local hypoxia during early gestation may be the critical factor leading to superficial implantation in susceptible patients. A potential cause of early local hypoxia is hypertrophic narrowing of endometrial arterioles. Such hypertrophy is increased in patients with the angiotensinogen Thr235 variant (61), a known predisposing factor for preeclampsia (see chapter 6, fig. 6-3). However, simple hypoxia is unlikely to be the whole story since maternal anemia in humans and chronic constriction of the aorta in rhesus monkeys are both associated with excessively deep placental implantation (45,102).

The association of preeclampsia with first pregnancies and autoimmune disease suggests a pathogenic immunologic factor. Supporting this hypothesis are data showing that cytokines can regulate trophoblast invasion and endometrial arteriolar caliber in humans and experimental animals (73). Altered human leukocyte antigen (HLA) expression on trophoblast does not appear to be a factor (17). The mechanism of disordered implantation in patients with underlying thrombophilia is unclear, but could potentially involve either early thrombosis in the endometrial vascular bed or the direct actions of thrombin itself, which is a known regulator of vascular remodeling at other sites (30).

Clinical Features. Superficial implantation is associated with changes related to maternal underperfusion of the intervillous space, including FGR and preterm delivery (see also chapter 3, Preeclampsia). It is not yet clear whether all preeclamptic placentas are superficially implanted. Currently, patients with preeclampsia are separated into two distinct subgroups: those with small placentas showing evidence of significant maternal underperfusion and those with large placentas containing excessive amounts of trophoblast. Conditions associated with preeclampsia and trophoblast excess include diabetes, multiple pregnancy, hydrops fetalis, and gestational trophoblastic disease. The final common pathway leading to clinical disease that links these two disparate subgroups of patients may be the excessive release of trophoblast breakdown products, such as oxidized serum proteins or other specific ligands (soluble vascular endothelial growth factor [VEGF receptor]-1) into the maternal circulation (58,81).

Gross and Microscopic Findings. Superficially implanted placentas are often small for gestational age, but otherwise show no gross abnormalities. Upon microscopic examination, the best evidence of superficial implantation is the finding of muscularized basal plate arteries underlying the inner two thirds of the placental disc (fig. 4-10). The walls of the arteries at this location should contain only trophoblast and fibrinoid matrix (fig. 4-11). Acute atherosis, a characteristic finding in preeclampsia (see chapter 6), is usually seen in the small arteries of the placental membranes. However, since atherosis affects only muscularized arteries, its presence in the basal plate is also diagnostic of superficial implantation (see chapter 6, fig. 6-1).

Two other typical findings in superficial implantation are numerous placental site giant cells within the basal plate, surrounded by loose decidual tissue lacking intermediate trophoblast (fig. 4-12, left), and sheets of cohesive immature intermediate trophoblast in close proximity to anchoring villi in the basal plate (7,55,56,77). Immature intermediate trophoblast may show

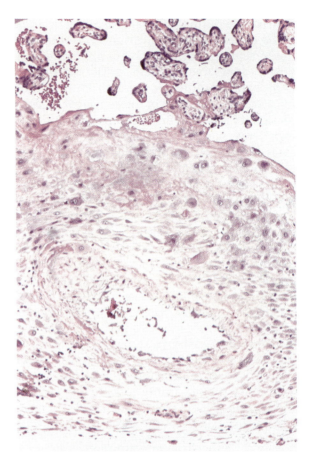

Figure 4-10

PERSISTENT SMOOTH MUSCLE IN WALL OF BASAL PLATE ARTERY

areas of cytoplasmic clearing and cystic degeneration similar to that seen in the chorion laevae in some cases (fig. 4-12, right). These changes are sensitive but not specific and should not be the sole basis for making a diagnosis of a preeclampsia-like syndrome in the absence of other supporting findings.

DISORDERS OF PLACENTAL MIGRATION

Shape Abnormalities

Definition. An *accessory lobe* occurs when the placental parenchyma is completely separated from the main placental disc by surrounding membranes, with bridging fetal blood vessels (fig. 4-13). *Multilobation* represents membranous indentations of the placental disc measuring greater than 50 percent of the disc diameter,

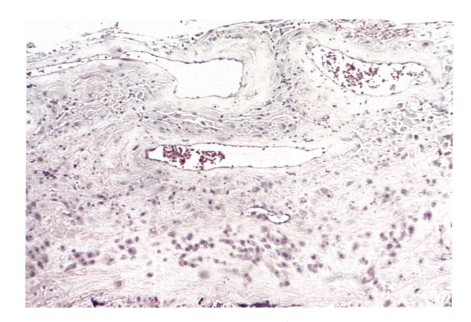

Figure 4-11

NORMAL BASAL PLATE ARTERY

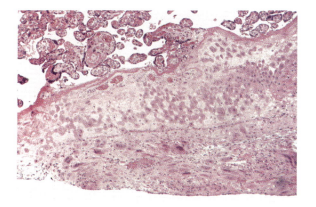 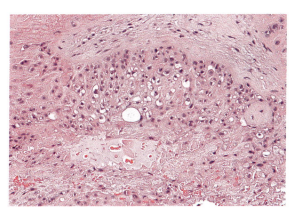

Figure 4-12

SUPERFICIAL IMPLANTATION SITE

Left: Abundant trophoblast giant cells in loose decidual tissue, basal plate.
Right: Immature intermediate trophoblast with cytoplasmic vacuolation and cystic degeneration below an anchoring villus in the basal plate (multiparous patient with preeclampsia and severe intrauterine growth restriction at 37 weeks).

with or without bridging vessels (fig. 4-14). *Atrophy* is a greater than 50 percent reduction in placental thickness occupying more than 10 percent of the total placental disc surface area (fig. 4-15).

Incidence. Accessory lobes (also known as *succenturiate lobes*) are found in 3 to 6 percent of placentas (8,26). Incidence figures for multilobation and atrophy are not available.

Etiology. Accessory lobes are a normal component of placentation in some primates (63). Shape abnormalities in humans are generally considered to reflect atrophy and differential growth of the developing placenta in response to local reduction of uterine perfusion. Causes of decreased uterine blood supply include leiomyomas, uterine septa, previous curettage or cesarean section, and implantation in anatomic regions such as the lower uterine segment, uterine cornua, and cervical os.

Clinical Features. Aside from serving as markers for possible underlying uterine pathology, shape abnormalities are of little clinical significance. Placenta accreta and placenta previa

Placental Pathology

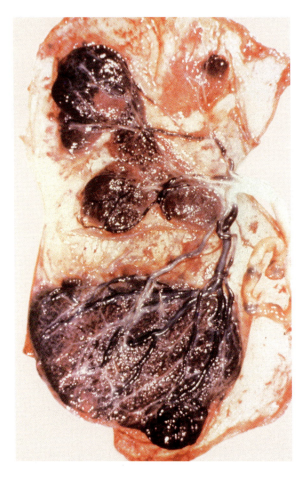

Figure 4-13
ACCESSORY LOBES

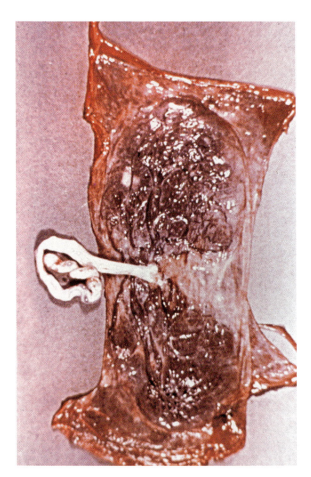

Figure 4-14
MULTILOBATION

Figure 4-15
MARGINAL ATROPHY

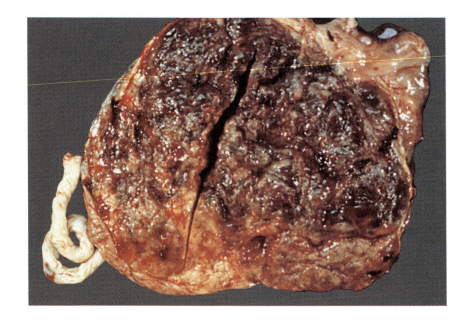

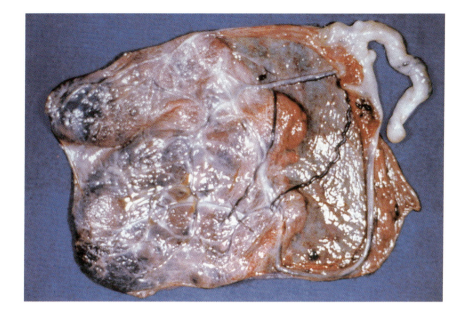

Figure 4-16

MEMBRANOUS INSERTION OF UMBILICAL CORD

are both commonly associated with abnormal shape. The most important clinical risk with these lesions is that fetal blood vessels connecting various portions of these placentas can be severed at the time of membrane rupture or during the second stage of labor.

Gross and Microscopic Findings. Shape abnormalities can occur in a myriad of permutations and combinations, which should be described using the above definitions. Fetal blood vessels in the exposed membranes require careful inspection for tears, which are accompanied by extravasated blood, and thrombi, which are particularly frequent in cases of acute chorioamnionitis. The normally abrupt transition between the disc and membranes is often blurred in placentas with shape abnormalities. Atrophic or membranous marginal tissue usually contains chorionic villi and a collapsed intervillous space, with fibrin-type fibrinoid surrounding the stem villi and bridging the chorionic and basal plates.

Peripheral Cord Insertion

Definition. *Membranous (velamentous) insertion* occurs when the umbilical cord terminates because of a loss of Wharton's jelly and decussation of the umbilical vessels in the placental membranes (fig. 4-16). *Marginal insertion* is the insertion of the umbilical cord at the placental margin (fig. 4-17). In *peripheral insertion*, the umbilical cord inserts eccentrically into the placental disc (fig. 4-18). In one study, peripheral insertion was defined as a distance from the cord insertion to the margin of the placenta that is less than 10 percent of the average of the two orthogonal disc diameters (78). When one or more major chorionic vessels traverse the adjacent membranes, it is termed *aberrant membrane vessel* (fig. 4-17).

Incidence. Membranous cord insertion occurs in 1.3 to 1.6 percent of gestations and marginal insertion in 6 to 9 percent (8,26). Peripheral cord insertion is common in twin pregnancies (22 percent) and especially in monochorionic twins (36 percent) (78).

Etiology. Under normal circumstances, with symmetric placental growth and normal membrane formation, the umbilical cord will be at the exact center of the placental disc. Asymmetry of the uterine vascular supply in singletons or competition for the uterine vascular supply in twins can result in eccentric lateral growth, causing the initial implantation site to become incorporated into the placental membranes later in gestation. This concept of placental migration was coined *trophotropism* many years ago and has been documented by serial sonographic studies (8,16).

Clinical Features. There is a slightly increased incidence of FGR and secondary involution of one of the umbilical arteries (single

Placental Pathology

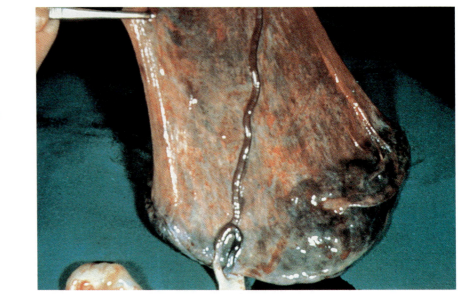

Figure 4-17

MARGINAL INSERTION OF UMBILICAL CORD WITH ABERRANT MEMBRANE VESSEL

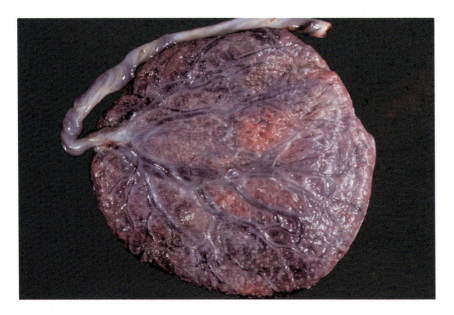

Figure 4-18

PERIPHERAL CORD INSERTION

umbilical artery) in patients with placentas with peripheral cord insertion (53). Twins, both monochorionic and dichorionic, with peripheral cord insertion are more likely to show discordant growth and FGR (70). The major risk of peripheral cord insertion is rupture of membranous vessels at the time of membrane rupture or during the second stage of labor (ruptured vasa previa). Twisting of umbilical vessels at the peripheral insertion site can lead to progressive variable decelerations and fetal acidosis. In extreme cases, vascular occlusion or thrombosis may occur.

Gross and Microscopic Findings. Careful gross examination of membranous vessels to evaluate possible hemorrhage and thrombosis is indicated. Most tears occur after delivery of the fetus and are of no clinical significance. Findings in a depressed neonate that suggest a true ruptured vasa previa are extension of hemorrhage away from the tear site and pressure craters created by extravasated blood (see chapter 8, fig. 8-9). Histologic studies can confirm antenatal hemorrhage by demonstrating hemoglobin breakdown products or recent occlusive thrombi (see also chapter 8, Umbilical Cord Insertion).

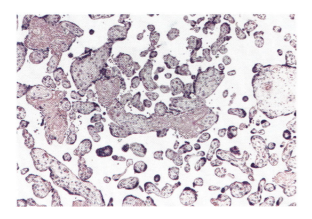 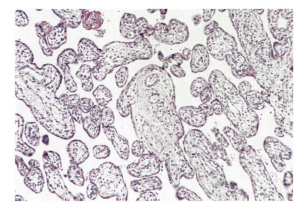

Figure 4-19

DISTAL VILLOUS HYPOPLASIA

Left: Distal villous deficiency, preterm.
Right: Normal preterm placenta.

DISORDERS OF VILLOUS DEVELOPMENT

Distal Villous Hypoplasia with Placental Undergrowth (Peripheral Villous Hypoplasia, "Terminal Villous Deficiency")

Definition. Distal villous hypoplasia is a decreased number of distal villi in the center of the placental lobule. Residual distal villi are thin, nonbranching, poorly vascularized, and may show syncytial knots. Prominent tertiary stem villi at the periphery of the lobule often show increased stromal collagen, muscular hypertrophy of stem villous arterioles, and variable degrees of intervillous fibrin and villous agglutination (fig. 4-19). The term terminal villous deficiency is discouraged since terminal villi are present but abnormal and the process may involve decreased branching of distal stem villi as well as terminal villi. Although formerly combined with increased syncytial, knotting as "accelerated maturation," recent data support separating these two entities (see chapter 6, Decidual Vasculopathy).

Incidence. This pathologic pattern conforms closely to the clinical entity characterized by severe FGR and abnormal pulsed flow Doppler studies which has a prevalence of approximately 10 percent in selected series of high-risk pregnancies (51).

Etiology. Two hypotheses have been invoked regarding the etiology of distal villous hypoplasia. The first is severe uteroplacental underperfusion, leading to fetoplacental underperfusion following fetal circulatory redistribution to the most critical vascular beds. Decreased maternal and fetal placental perfusion in this scenario arrest placental growth and further reduce the fetoplacental vascular bed (92). The second hypothesis is that placental perfusion is decreased due to a primary placental problem, such as an abnormal karyotype or intrinsic arteriolar pathology (hypertrophy or obliteration) (25,33,86). Distal villous hypoplasia could be the final common result of both pathways.

Clinical Features. Although its use for clinical management is controversial, there is little argument that FGR with an abnormal pulsed flow Doppler assessment is associated with increased morbidity and mortality compared to FGR without this abnormality (19). Physiologic studies directly measuring oxygen tension in the intervillous space of patients with abnormal pulsed flow Doppler studies have shown that oxygen tension is actually increased (51). The initial interpretation of this finding challenged the entire concept of decreased uteroplacental perfusion. Upon reflection, a more proper interpretation seems to be that when placentas reach the final stage of distal villous hypoplasia their inability to absorb oxygen outstrips the decrease in oxygen delivery from the maternal circulation. An important consequence of intervillous hyperoxia is that oxygen-free radicals may be toxic for placental development and can further aggravate the placental pathology (39).

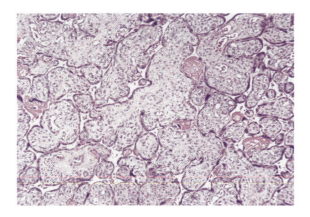
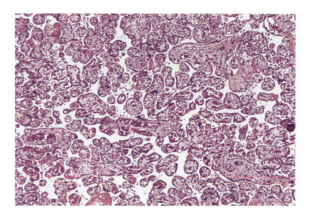

Figure 4-20

DISTAL VILLOUS IMMATURITY

Left: Distal villous immaturity, term.
Right: Normal term placenta.

Gross and Microscopic Findings. Placentas with distal villous hypoplasia are extremely small for gestational age. The fetoplacental weight ratio is generally very high and other manifestations of maternal underperfusion, such as infarction, abruption, and changes consistent with severe oligohydramnios, are common.

Microscopically, the overall ratio between distal villous profiles and tertiary stem villi is markedly decreased. Distal villi in the center of the lobule are sparse. When cut in cross section, they are very small. When cut in longitudinal section, they are long, thin, and unbranched. Tertiary stem villi are fibrotic and contain thickened arterioles that often extend into more distal villi. Secondary changes, such as intervillous fibrin with intermediate trophoblast and villous agglutination, are prominent near tertiary stem villi. Syncytial knotting may be prominent.

Distal Villous Immaturity with Placental Overgrowth ("Delayed Villous Maturation")

Definition. Distal villous immaturity is an increased number of large distal villi with increased capillaries, stromal macrophages, and interstitial fluid uniformly distributed throughout the villous stroma (fig. 4-20).

Incidence. This pattern is most common with gestational diabetes, which complicates approximately 7 percent of pregnancies (52). Not all diabetic pregnancies show these changes. The phenotype may depend on overall glucose control.

Etiology. The etiology of fetoplacental overgrowth in diabetes is maternal hypoglycemia leading to fetal hyperinsulinemia (see chapter 3, Diabetes Mellitus). Insulin binds to placental insulin and insulin-like growth factor (IGF) receptors, stimulating persistent and accelerated fetoplacental growth. Placentas from patients with Beckwith-Wiedemann syndrome (exophthalmos, macroglossia, gigantism) often show similar findings attributable to their known increase in IGF-II expression (91). Morphologically similar changes in nondiabetic placentas are poorly explained but could be due to variations in insulin and IGF availability, which are regulated during pregnancy by intrinsic genetic variations and local IGF binding proteins such as decidual IGF-BP1 and circulating fetal IGF-II receptor (21,31,67).

Clinical Features. Large placentas with distal villous immaturity are most commonly seen with gestational diabetes and type I insulin-dependent diabetes of comparatively recent onset (White class B or C) (88). Patients without overt glucose intolerance in the present pregnancy may be at risk for diabetes in subsequent pregnancies or in later life (28). Infants of diabetic mothers have features that in some ways parallel the changes seen in their placentas (15). They are large for gestational age and have some manifestations of immaturity, such as delayed lung maturation and a mild increase in circulating nucleated red blood cells (NRBC) (100).

Despite a lack of overt abnormalities, these infants are at risk for stillbirth, congenital anomalies, renal vein thrombi, and other adverse outcomes (27,42,68). Postdelivery complications, such as hypoglycemia, hypocalcemia, and transient hypertrophic cardiomyopathy, may occur, particularly if there was poor maternal glucose control (14). Nondiabetic patients with distal villous immaturity and normal fetoplacental growth may be at risk for idiopathic intrauterine fetal distress (IUFD) (90).

Gross and Microscopic Findings. Placentas are usually large for gestational age. Umbilical cords tend to be thick, with abundant Wharton's jelly. Terminal villi are abundant relative to stem villi and have the characteristics listed above. Stem villi have increased connective tissue. Increased capillary vascularity, sometimes reaching the threshold for chorangiosis (see below), is common. Decidual arterioles may show nonspecific mural hypertrophy with large amounts of extracellular matrix (6).

DISORDERS OF FETAL VASCULAR DEVELOPMENT

Chorangioma and Localized Chorangiomatosis

Definition. Chorangioma is an expansile nodular lesion composed of capillary vascular channels, intervening stromal cells, and surrounding trophoblast. It is analogous to hemangiomas at other body sites. Localized chorangiomatosis is a villous stromal process with the same histologic characteristics as chorangioma, but which permeates multiple large stem villi rather than forming a single expansile nodular lesion.

Incidence. Chorangiomas were observed in 0.51 percent of examined placentas over a 10-year period in a recent study by the authors (66). The frequency of localized chorangiomatosis in the same series was 0.32 percent. Both lesions are most common at 32 to 37 weeks, and are increased in placentas from preeclamptic patients and in twin placentas.

Etiology. Chorangioma and localized chorangiomatosis tend to be found under the chorionic plate or at the placental margin, sites of reduced oxygenation. Their rate of coincidence in the same placenta is higher than would be expected based on their incidence in the general population. These factors and the shared association with preeclampsia argue strongly for a common pathogenesis and suggest that decreased oxygen tension may play a role in their development (7). This hypothesis is strengthened by the increased incidence of these entities in populations delivering at high elevations, which has been shown in two independent studies (82, 89). Recurrence in subsequent pregnancies and coexisting hemangiomas in the fetus suggest an underlying predisposition in some patients.

Clinical Features. Small chorangiomas are incidental findings of little clinical significance. Intermediate-sized lesions may be associated with intrauterine growth retardation (62). Large chorangiomas (or extensive chorangiomatosis), often defined as 9 cm or more, are associated with arteriovenous shunting and may cause polyhydramnios, hydrops fetalis, and fetal death (93). Platelet sequestration in the capillary spaces of large chorangiomas or multifocal localized chorangiomatosis can lead to disseminated intravascular coagulation, thrombocytopenia, or a hemorrhagic diathesis in the fetus (see case presented in figure 4-21) (43).

Gross Findings. Chorangiomas may present as single nodules or multinodular masses on the cut surface of the placenta (fig. 4-22). They are firm and homogeneous lesions that rarely contain blood. They are most commonly subchorionic or marginal in location. Localized chorangiomatosis is occasionally apparent upon gross examination (fig. 4-21A).

Microscopic Findings. Chorangiomas have traditionally been separated into angiomatous and cellular subtypes based on the amount of accompanying stroma (figs. 4-23, 4-24). However, this distinction represents two ends of a continuum and has no clinical significance. Two recent reports have emphasized the frequency of associated nonspecific trophoblast hyperplasia in chorangiomas (fig. 4-25) (50,66). Between 50 and 65 percent of the cases showed hyperplasia, which was associated with an increase in MIB-1 staining. This finding may be related to excessive amounts of growth factors. Trophoblast hyperplasia in chorangiomas may account for several case reports of so-called chorangiocarcinoma (40,95), a lesion not yet fully accepted in the pathology literature. Localized chorangiomatosis has an identical histology, but conforms

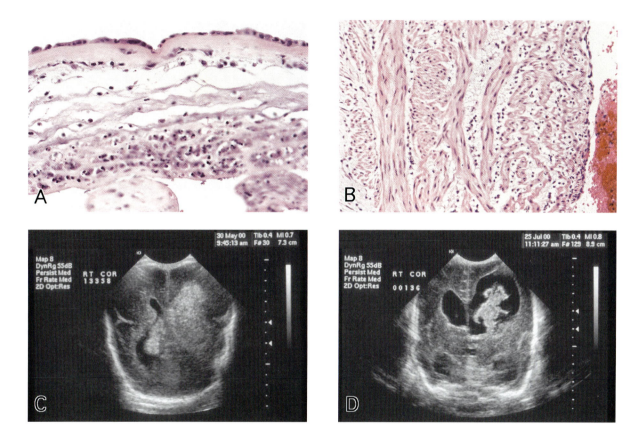

Figure 5-1

ACUTE CHORIOAMNIONITIS, *BACTEROIDES* SP

A 35-year-old woman (G1 P0) delivered at 25 4/7 weeks, 14 days after premature rupture of the membranes.

A: Maternal neutrophilic infiltrate in the membranous amniochorion.

B: Fetal neutrophilic infiltrate in the umbilical vein.

C: Ultrasound on day 2 after birth shows bilateral intraventricular hemorrhage (left, grade 4 with adjacent periventricular leukomalacia; right, grade 1 with ventricular dilatation).

D: Ultrasound on day 29 after birth shows a porencephalic cyst (left) and ventricular dilatation (right). A ventriculoperitoneal shunt was inserted on day 49.

system has recently been proposed by a subcommittee of the Society for Pediatric Pathology-Perinatal Section (95).

Maternal Inflammatory Response. The stage (duration) of the maternal inflammatory response follows a stereotyped sequence as outlined below. Later-stage infections (stages 2 and 3) are associated with increased neonatal morbidity and mortality (45,128).

In stage 1 (early), *acute subchorionitis and/or acute chorionitis* (figs. 5-4, 5-5), maternal neutrophils are in the subchorionic fibrin and/or membranes at the junction between the decidua and chorioamnion. In stage 2 (intermediate), *acute chorioamnionitis* (figs. 5-3, 5-6), maternal neutrophils are in the connective tissues of the chorionic plate and membranous chorioamnion. Stage 3 (late), *necrotizing chorioamnionitis* (fig. 5-7), is characterized by hypereosinophilia of the amnion basement membrane, karyorrhexis of neutrophils, necrosis, and sloughage of amnionic epithelial cells.

The grade (intensity) of the maternal inflammatory response is variable and difficult to quantitate. One definition of severe maternal inflammation is more than 30 neutrophils per high-power field in the chorionic plate (fig. 5-8) (74). This definition has not been predictive of such clinical outcomes as sepsis, chronic lung disease, and cerebral palsy (59,98,101,102). A second histologic feature found in severe (grade 2) maternal inflammation, chorionic microabscess

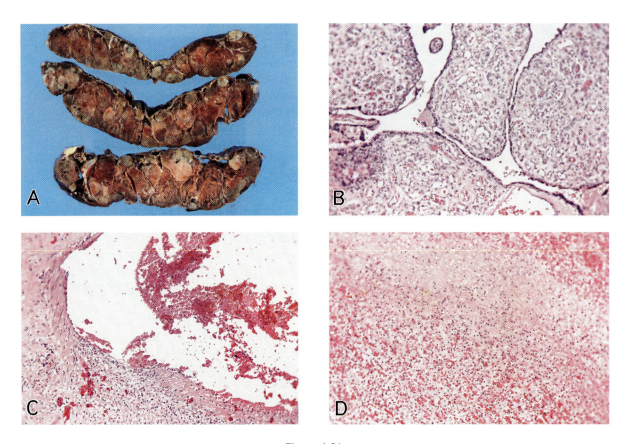

Figure 4-21

LOCALIZED CHORANGIOMATOSIS, MULTIFOCAL

Hydropic newborn was delivered at 39 weeks' gestation with severe congestive heart failure, cardiomegaly, grade I intraventricular hemorrhage, and thrombocytopenia. All resolved with treatment over a period of 9 days.

A: Diffuse nodularity is the result of massive involvement by localized angiomatous lesions of varying sizes, estimated to involve 90 percent of this 684-g placenta.

B: Angiomatous areas vary from expanded villi with stromal replacement in a trophoblastic envelope to masses over 1 cm in diameter.

C: This large stem vessel contained a mural thrombus (attachment site at lower right).

D: Infarcted angiomatous nodule associated with thrombosis.

to the outline of affected stem villi (fig. 4-21B). It does not extend into distal villi (terminal and tertiary stem villi). Chorangioma and localized chorangiomatosis may be distinguished from villous chorangiosis (see below) by the presence of surrounding perivascular cells and a background of increased stromal collagenization and cellularity, leading to increased spacing of the capillary vascular channels (see also chapter 11, Hemangioma [Chorangioma]).

Villous Chorangiosis (Hypercapillarization)

Definition. Villous chorangiosis occurs if more than 10 terminal villi show 10 or more capillaries in several areas of the placenta (3).

Incidence. Chorangiosis was found in 7 percent of placentas in a recent study, which agrees with most other series in the literature (66). The lesion is predominantly seen in term placentas. Chorangiosis is commonly associated with distal villous immaturity (diabetic pregnancies, Beckwith-Wiedemann syndrome). It may be prominent in some cases of chronic villitis, fetal thrombotic vasculopathy, and mild maternal vascular underperfusion. It is increased in placentas delivered at higher elevations (89).

Etiology. Terminal villogenesis is thought to occur by a process of capillary growth and coiling that is followed by surrounding stromal outgrowth (13,18). In chorangiosis these processes

Disorders of Placental Development

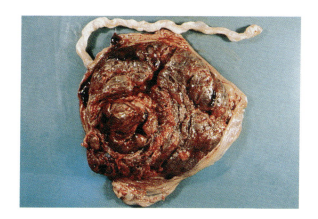
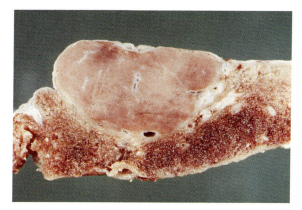

Figure 4-22

CHORANGIOMA

Left: Large nodular mass protrudes through the basal plate.
Right: Large solid lesion arising in a typical location just below the chorionic plate.

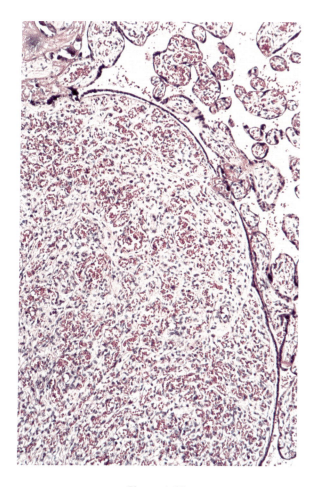

Figure 4-23

CHORANGIOMA, CAPILLARY TYPE

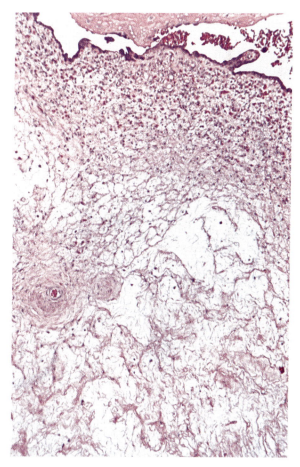

Figure 4-24

CHORANGIOMA, CELLULAR TYPE

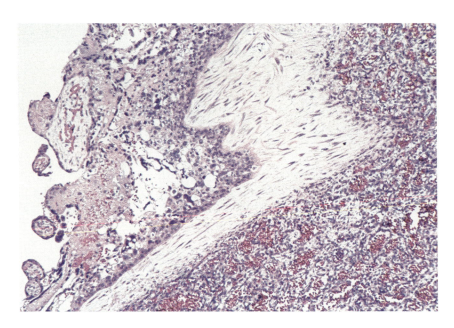

Figure 4-25

NONSPECIFIC TROPHOBLAST HYPERPLASIA IN CHORANGIOMA

may be uncoupled, leading to hypercapillarization, perhaps as an adaptive mechanism to increase gas exchange. Excessive local growth factors (such as trophoblast-derived VEGF), cytokines, and increased capillary pressure have been suggested as possible contributing factors.

Clinical Features. Maternal diabetes and placental overgrowth syndromes (Beckwith-Wiedemann and Smith-Golabi-Behmel) are accepted causes of chorangiosis. Associations with twin gestation and chronic hypoxia are more controversial (44,63,70). While frequent in selected cases with abnormal outcomes, chorangiosis has not yet been shown to be an independent risk factor for adverse outcome.

Gross and Microscopic Findings. Placentas with chorangiosis are often large for gestational age. Histologically, chorangiosis is limited to distal villi (terminal villi and the margins of tertiary stem villi). Capillaries in chorangiosis have a thin, well-circumscribed basement membrane and lack the continuous layer of surrounding pericytes seen with chorangioma and chorangiomatosis. The accepted criteria for the diagnosis of chorangiosis is the "rule of tens" described above. In our experience, occasional villi with 15 or more capillaries are always present and make the diagnosis more secure (fig. 4-26) (66).

Care should be exercised in making the diagnosis of chorangiosis in congested placentas. An apparent increase in capillaries limited to peripheral areas of the slide usually relates to compression of tissue in the cassette prior to paraffin embedding and should not be confused with true chorangiosis. Immunostaining for endothelial antigens with CD31 or CD34 reveals substantially more capillaries than are seen by the hematoxylin and eosin (H&E) stain and should not be used to make the diagnosis unless new quantitative definitions are developed.

Diffuse Multifocal Chorangiomatosis

Definition. Diffuse multifocal chorangiomatosis is the presence of foci of excessive capillary growth, with surrounding pericytes and collagen fibrils, affecting scattered secondary and tertiary stem villi throughout the placenta.

Incidence. Diffuse multifocal chorangiomatosis is relatively rare (0.23 percent of all placentas in a recent series) and predominantly seen in the placentas of very low birth weight infants (less than 32 weeks) (66).

Etiology. Associations with preeclampsia, twin gestation, IUGR, congenital malformations, and avascular villi suggest that this process may represent an aberrant response to hypoxia in very immature placentas.

Clinical Features. The clinical significance of this recently defined and relatively uncommon lesion has not been fully defined. Known associations are listed above.

Gross and Microscopic Findings. No specific gross findings are associated with diffuse villous chorangiomatosis. Placental weight is

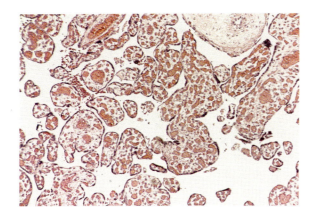 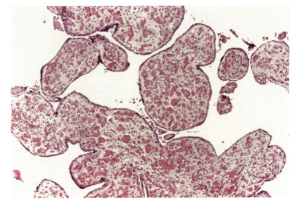

Figure 4-26

VILLOUS CHORANGIOSIS

Left: Numerous villi with greater than 10 capillary profiles.
Right: Isolated larger villi with greater than 15 capillary profiles.

abnormal in over half of cases, but the number of small and large placentas is equivalent (66). Histologic findings as defined above are illustrated in figure 4-27.

GENETIC AND CHROMOSOMAL DISORDERS

Metabolic Storage Diseases

Definition. Placental changes, generally limited to the trophoblast, villous stromal macrophages, and amnionic epithelium, that are secondary to and diagnostic for fetal metabolic storage diseases (figs. 4-28, 4-29).

Incidence and Etiology. Placentas with evidence of storage disease are rare. The incidence and underlying etiologies of the various storage diseases can be obtained from other sources (59). Most are caused by single gene defects transmitted in an autosomal recessive pattern.

Clinical Features. Many metabolic storage diseases are clinically silent or present with nonspecific clinical abnormalities such as hydrops fetalis or isolated organ failure at the time of birth. Placental examination allows for rapid identification and may guide the subsequent diagnostic work-up.

Gross and Microscopic Findings. There are no typical gross findings for placentas showing histologic evidence of storage disease. Histologic examination of the placenta at low-power microscopy often shows an unusually pale staining placental parenchyma (fig. 4-28). At higher

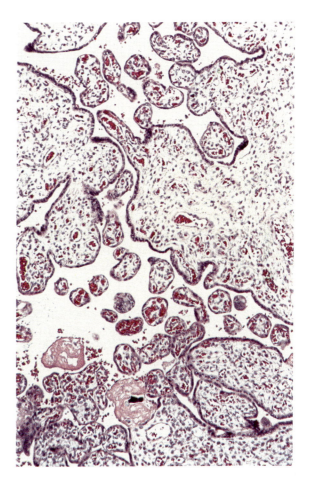

Figure 4-27

DIFFUSE MULTIFOCAL CHORANGIOMATOSIS

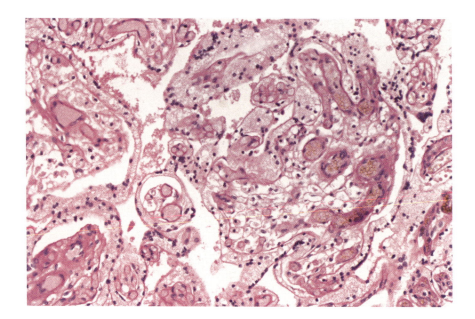

Figure 4-28

I-CELL DISEASE (MUCOLIPIDOSIS II): DIFFUSE VILLOUS VACUOLATION

magnification, this is seen to be due to diffuse vacuolation of the syncytiotrophoblast, villous stromal cells, intermediate trophoblast, and/or amniocytes. In cases affecting the trophoblast, there is an increase in the overall thickness of the syncytiotrophoblast layer and near uniform vacuolation of its cytoplasm (fig. 4-29A). Villous macrophages are usually involved and show an increase in both number and size, with prominent foamy cytoplasm (fig. 4-29B). Changes in the amnionic epithelium and the intermediate trophoblast are more subtle, featuring watery clear cytoplasm (fig. 4-29C,D). Periodic acid-Schiff (PAS) and alcian blue stains have been reported to distinguish between neutral mucins and mucopolysaccharides, which are positive with both stains, and acidic mucopolysaccharides, which are positive for alcian blue alone (83).

Markedly vacuolated syncytiotrophoblast cells are found with galactosialidosis, I-cell disease (mucolipidosis II), GM1 and GM2 gangliosidoses, infantile sialic acid storage disease, sialidosis, cholesterol ester storage disease, and type IV mucopolysaccharidosis. Changes that occur with in beta-glucuronidase deficiency and types I and IVA mucopolysaccharidosis are limited to villous stromal cells. Only amniocytes are affected in types II and IV glycogen storage disease (8,54). Specific placental changes with other genetic diseases are incompletely documented, but additional data are slowly emerging (e.g., placental changes in Bartter's syndrome [24]).

Mesenchymal Dysplasia

Definition. Mesenchymal dysplasia is placental enlargement, with abnormal stem villi showing marked cystic dilatation and vesicle formation, fibroblastic stromal overgrowth, and vascular abnormalities that affect vessels of all sizes.

Incidence. Mesenchymal dysplasia is a recently coined term for a lesion previously reported under a variety of names in case reports and small series (38). The condition is rare, with only 22 published cases. Many additional unpublished cases have been seen by the authors.

Etiology. The underlying cause of placental mesenchymal dysplasia is unknown. Infants in approximately half of the reported cases have anomalies suggestive of Beckwith-Wiedemann syndrome (BWS), such as omphalocele, macroglossia, and visceromegaly. In no case has a diagnostic cytogenetic abnormality associated with BWS been verified. Cases of mesenchymal dysplasia are particularly likely to be associated with fetal omphalocele. Recent data have suggested that patients with BWS and omphalocele are more likely to have genetic abnormalities in the *CDKN1C* gene than at other sites in the 11p15 susceptibility region (57). Another possible etiology for mesenchymal dysplasia is confined placental mosaicism (see below). While all published cases of mesenchymal dysplasia studied by flow cytometry have had diploid DNA content, an anecdotal case (G. Schauer, Ped Path

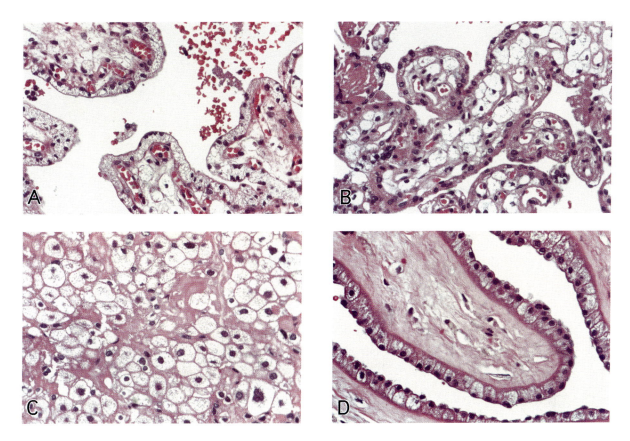

Figure 4-29

GALACTOSIALIDOSIS

A: Syncytiotrophoblast vacuolation.
B: Villous macrophage vacuolation.
C: Intermediate trophoblast vacuolation.
D: Amnionic epithelial vacuolation.

listserver, 5/30/00) has been described with a confined area of tetraploidy. One possible explanation for mesenchymal dysplasia without fetal anomalies is that the 11p15 abnormalities typical of BWS are confined to the placenta. The study of future cases using techniques such as flourescent in situ hybridization and comparative genomic hybridization will be of interest.

Clinical Features. Mesenchymal dysplasia is generally recognized by antenatal ultrasound as a form of partial molar pregnancy. Accompanying preeclampsia is common, probably relating to trophoblast excess. Infants without BWS have no other reported abnormalities.

Gross Findings. Placentas are usually extremely large for gestational age, often exceeding 1,000 g at term. Large stem villi near the chorionic plate are grossly thickened and often show prominent cystic cavitation (fig. 4-30). Elongated, thick-walled, large vessels in primary stem villi and the chorionic plate occasionally protrude extraplacentally into the amnionic cavity or umbilical cord. These large vessels commonly show secondary changes, such as mural hemorrhage, thrombosis, and aneurysmal dilatation.

Microscopic Findings. Enlarged stem villi may show overgrowth of fibroblastic stroma, increased vascularization, or cystic degeneration, without accompanying trophoblast hyperplasia. Many cases show all three features in different areas (fig. 4-31). Smaller stem villous vessels show proliferation, dilatation, abnormal branching, and formation of sinusoids. Associated chorangiomas and areas of localized

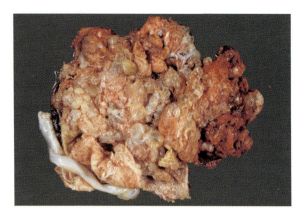 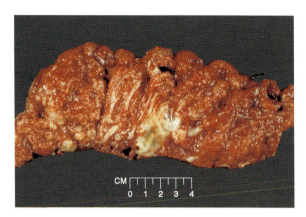

Figure 4-30

MESENCHYMAL DYSPLASIA
Left: Maternal surface
Right: Cut section.

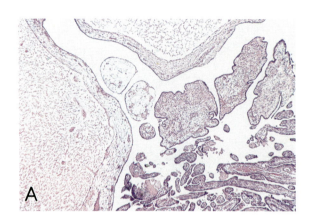 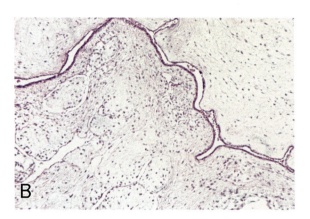

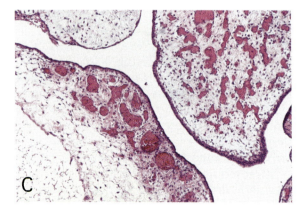

Figure 4-31

MESENCHYMAL DYSPLASIA
A: Hypervascular and hydropic villi.
B: Solid villi.
C: Marked vascular proliferation.

chorangiomatosis are common. Terminal villi are generally normal but can show distal villous immaturity and chorangiosis. While most cases are diffuse, occasional placentas have localized lesions with the same features.

Chromosomal Abnormalities

Definition. The villous morphology is associated with or suggestive of an abnormal karyotype.

Incidence. The incidence of abnormal karyotypes is gestational age–dependent, varying from over 75 percent at 2 weeks of development to 0.59 percent for livebirths in the third trimester. Most chromosomal abnormalities increase with advanced maternal age, as exemplified by the increased incidence of trisomy 21 in women 45 years of age (1 in 30) compared to those 20 years of age (1 in 1,000) (32). Abnormal karyotype limited to the placenta alone (*confined placental mosaicism [CPM]*) is seen in 1 to 3 percent of all first trimester chorionic villus samples (47).

Etiology. The underlying mechanisms leading to chromosomal abnormalities in the fetus are beyond the scope of this chapter. With regard to CPM, most cases detected in the first trimester are apparently normal by term. However, thorough analysis will confirm the presence of at least a minor abnormal cell line in the majority. Mosaicism confined to the placenta may involve the trophoblast, chorionic and villous stroma, or amniocytes in various combinations. Most cases of fetal trisomy 13 and 18 reaching term have at least a subpopulation of nontrisomic villous trophoblast (46). Careful study reveals a minor component of fetal mosaicism in approximately 10 percent of cases of presumed CPM.

CPM arises by two mechanisms: meiotic errors leading to trisomy, with a later loss of one chromosome in the fetus (most common for trisomies 9, 16, 22), and postmeiotic somatic errors occurring in placental tissues after separation from the fetus (most common for trisomies 2, 7, 8, 10, 12) (85). The former may lead to fetuses that carry two copies of the involved chromosome derived from the same parent (uniparental disomy). It is unclear whether uniparental disomy imparts any additional risk above that seen with CPM in the absence of uniparental disomy (99).

Clinical Features. The clinical outcome for constitutional chromosomal anomalies is dependent on the nature of the abnormality. The diagnosis of aneuploid gestations may be facilitated by midtrimester maternal serum testing using various panels of placental hormones (human chorionic gonadotropin [HCG], activin, estriol) and fetal proteins (alpha-fetoprotein) (35). The subgroup of chromosomal abnormalities with over-representation of the paternal genome, molar pregnancies, represents special problems which are beyond the scope of this discussion. Twin pregnancies with one complete hydatidiform mole and late partial hydatidiform moles are occasionally discovered in third trimester placentas and require appropriate clinical follow-up.

CPM has been associated with spontaneous abortion, FGR, and IUFD (41). These complications are more common in cases resulting from meiotic errors and in those with a higher percentage of aneuploid trophoblast. The diagnosis of CPM requires labor intensive specialized techniques such as direct karyotyping, fluorescence in situ hybridization (FISH), and comparative genomic hybridization which are not generally available (5). Accumulating evidence suggests that CPM may be a significant and under-recognized cause of FGR (48).

Gross Findings. Placentas with paternal triploidy (partial mole) and exclusively paternal lineage (complete mole) have grossly recognizable cysts of 2-mm diameter or greater. Cases of CPM involving trisomy 16 have also been reported to have cystic villi (4). Other cases of CPM, especially involving trisomy 9, may be associated with a very small placenta (O. Faye-Peterson, personal communication, 2001).

Microscopic Findings. In addition to cystic villi, some placentas with chromosomal abnormalities may show villous dimorphism (paternal triploidy), nonspecific villous trophoblast hyperplasia (trisomies 7, 15, 21, 22), or other dysmorphic features (trisomies 7, 8, 13, 16, 18, and monosomy X) (74,75,80). These dysmorphic features include an irregular villous outline, villous stromal trophoblast inclusions, stromal karyomegaly, and an abnormal villous capillary vascular pattern (fig. 4-32). Considerable controversy exists as to whether these changes are reliable or useful predictors of aneuploidy (29,65,97). A reasonable approach is to mention these features as being suggestive of a possible chromosomal abnormality when they are unambiguously present, particularly in cases where the karyotype is unavailable. Trophoblast hyperplasia of the magnitude seen in molar pregnancies, but without molar villi (fig. 4-33), is best managed by a single HCG titer at 6 to 8 weeks postpartum to ensure return to baseline. Histologic features attributable to CPM have not been defined (see also chapter 9).

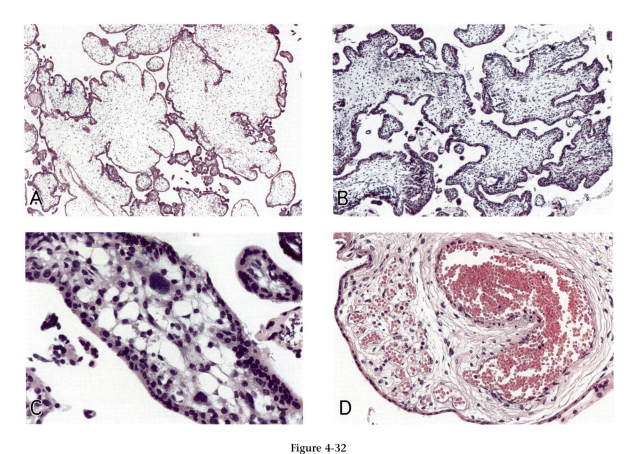

Figure 4-32

DYSMORPHIC VILLI

A: Irregular villous contour.
B: Trophoblast inclusions.
C: Stromal karyomegaly.
D: Aberrant capillary vascular pattern.

Figure 4-33

NONSPECIFIC VILLOUS TROPHOBLAST HYPERPLASIA, TRISOMY 7

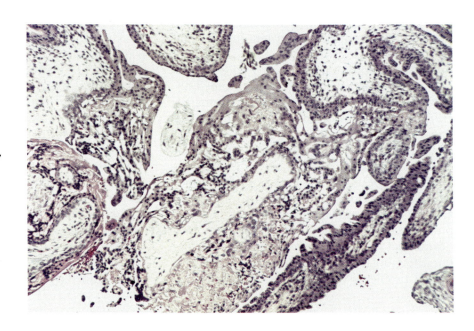

REFERENCES

1. ACOG Committee on Obstetric Practice. ACOG Committee opinion. Number 266, January 2002: placenta accreta. Obstet Gynecol 2002;99:169–70.
2. Ahmed A, Gilbert-Barness E. Placenta membranacea: a developmental anomaly with diverse clinical presentation. Pediatr Dev Pathol 2003;6:201–2.
3. Altshuler G: Chorangiosis. An important placental sign of neonatal morbidity and mortality. Arch Pathol Lab Med 1984;108:71–4.
4. Astner A, Schwinger E, Caliebe A, Jonat W, Gembruch U. Sonographically detected fetal and placental abnormalities associated with trisomy 16 confined to the placenta. A case report and review of the literature. Prenat Diagn 1998;18:1308–15.
5. Barrett IJ, Lomax BL, Loukianova T, Tang SS, Lestou VS, Kalousek DK. Comparative genomic hybridization: a new tool for reproductive pathology. Arch Pathol Lab Med 2001;125:81–4.
6. Barth WH Jr, Genest DR, Riley LE, Frigoletto FD Jr, Benacerraf BR, Greene MF. Uterine arcuate artery Doppler and decidual microvascular pathology in pregnancies complicated by type I diabetes mellitus. Ultrasound Obstet Gynecol 1996;8:98–103.
7. Benirschke K. Recent trends in chorangiomas, especially those of multiple and recurrent chorangiomas. Pediatr Devel Pathol 1999;2:264–9.
8. Benirschke K, Kaufmann P. Pathology of the human placenta, 4th ed. New York: Springer; 2000:778–85.
9. Bey M, Dott A, Miller JM. The sonographic diagnosis of circumvallate placenta. Obstet Gynecol 1991;78:515–7.
10. Brosens IA, Robertson WB, Dixon HG. The role of the spiral arteries in the pathogenesis of preeclampsia. Obstet Gynecol Annu 1972;1:177–91.
11. Caniggia I, Mostachfi H, Winter J, et al. Hypoxia-inducible factor-1 mediates the biological effects of oxygen on human trophoblast differentiation through TGFbeta(3). J Clin Invest 2000;105:577–87.
12. Carter AM. Evolution of the placenta and fetal membranes seen in the light of molecular phylogenetics. Placenta 2001;22:800–7.
13. Castellucci M, Scheper M, Scheffen I, Celona A, Kaufmann P. The development of the human placental villous tree. Anat Embryol 1990;181:117–28.
14. Cooper MJ, Enderlein MA, Tarnoff H, Roge CL. Asymmetric septal hypertrophy in infants of diabetic mothers. Fetal echocardiography and the impact of maternal diabetic control. Am J Dis Child 1992;146:226–9.
15. Cordero L, Treuer SH, Landon MB, Gabbe SG. Management of infants of diabetic mothers. Arch Pediatr Adolesc Med 1998;152:249–54.
16. Cunningham FG, MacDonald P, Gant N, et al. William's obstetrics, 20th ed. Stamford, CT: Appleton & Lange; 1997:765–7.
17. Datema G, van Meir C, Kanhai H, van den Elsen P. Pre-term birth and severe pre-eclampsia are not associated with altered expression of HLA on human trophoblasts. Am J Reprod Immunol 2003;49:193–201.
18. Demir R, Kaufmann P, Castellucci M, Erbengi T, Kotowski A. Fetal vasculogenesis and angiogenesis in human placental villi. Acta Anat 1989;136:190–203.
19. Devoe LD, Gardner P, Dear C, Faircloth D. The significance of increasing umbilical artery systolic-diastolic ratios in 3rd-trimester pregnancy. Obstet Gynecol 1992;80:684–92.
20. Dommisse J, Tiltman AJ. Placental bed biopsies in placental abruption. Br J Obstet Gynaecol 1992;99:651–4.
21. Dunger DB, Ong KK, Huxtable SJ, et al. Association of the INS VNTR with size at birth. ALSPAC Study Team. Avon Longitudinal Study of Pregnancy and Childhood. Nat Genet 1998;19:98–100.
22. Elliott JP, Gilpin B, Strong TH Jr, Finberg HJ. Chronic abruption-oligohydramnios sequence. J Reprod Med 1998;43:418–22.
23. Eriksen G, Wohlert M, Ersbak V, Hvidman L, Hedegaard M, Skajaa K. Placental abruption. A case-control investigation. Br J Obstet Gynaecol 1991;98:448–52.
24. Ernst LM, Parkash V. Placental pathology in fetal Bartter syndrome. Pediatr Dev Pathol 2002;5:76–9.
25. Fok RY, Pavlova Z, Benirschke K, Paul RH, Platt LD. The correlation of arterial lesions with umbilical artery doppler velocimetry in the placentas of small-for-dates pregnancies. Obstet Gynecol 1990;75:578–83.
26. Fox H. Pathology of the placenta, 2nd ed. Major problems in pathology, Vol. 7. London: W.B. Saunders; 1997:54–60.
27. Gabbe SG. Congenital malformations in infants of diabetic mothers. Obstet Gynecol Surv 1977;32:125–32.

28. Gaudier FL, Hauth JC, Poist M, Corbett D, Cliver SP. Recurrence of gestational diabetes-mellitus. Obstet Gynecol 1992;80:755–8.
29. Genest DR, Roberts D, Boyd T, Bieber FR. Fetoplacental histology as a predictor of karyotype: a controlled study of spontaneous first trimester abortions. Hum Pathol 1995;26:201–9.
30. Gibbons GH, Dzau VJ. The emerging concept of vascular remodeling. N Engl J Med 1994;330:1431–8.
31. Gibson JM, Aplin JD, White A, Westwood M. Regulation of IGF bioavailability in pregnancy. Mol Hum Reprod 2001;7:79–87.
32. Gilbert-Barness E, Opitz J. Chromosomal abnormalities. In: Wigglesworth JS, Singer DB, eds. Textbook of fetal and perinatal pathology. Boston: Blackwell Scientific Publications; 199:339–79.
33. Giles WB, Trudiner BJ, Baird PJ. Fetal umbilical artery flow velocity waveforms and placental resistance: pathological correlation. Br J Obstet Gynaecol 1985;92:31–8.
34. Greenberg JA, Sorem KA, Shifren JL, Riley LE. Placenta membranacea with placenta increta: a case report and literature review. Obstet Gynecol 1991;78(Pt 2):512–4.
35. Haddow JE, Palomaki GE, Knight GJ, et al. Prenatal screening for Down's syndrome with use of maternal serum markers. N Engl J Med 1992;327:588–93.
36. Jacques SM, Qureshi F. The significance of placental basal plate myometrial fibers: a clinicopathologic study of 147 cases. Mod Pathol 1999;12:118A.
37. Jauniaux E, Hempstock J, Greenwold N, Burton GJ. Trophoblastic oxidative stress in relation to temporal and regional differences in maternal placental blood flow in normal and abnormal early pregnancies. Am J Pathol 2003;162:115–25.
38. Jauniaux E, Nicolaides KH, Hustin J. Perinatal features associated with placental mesenchymal dysplasia. Placenta 1997;18:701–6.
39. Jauniaux E, Watson AL, Hempstock J, Bao YP, Skepper JN, Burton GJ. Onset of maternal arterial blood flow and placental oxidative stress. A possible factor in human early pregnancy failure. Am J Pathol 2000;157:2111–22.
40. Jauniaux E, Zucker M, Meuris S, Verhest A, Wilkin P, Hustin J. Chorangiocarcinoma: an unusual tumour of the placenta. The missing link? Placenta 1988;9:607–13.
41. Johnson A, Wapner RJ, Davis GH, Jackson LG. Mosaicism in chorionic villus sampling: an association with poor perinatal outcome. Obstet Gynecol 1990;75:573–7.
42. Johnstone FD, Nasrat AA, Prescott RJ. The effect of established and gestational diabetes on pregnancy outcome. Br J Obstet Gynaecol 1990;97:1009–15.
43. Jones CE, Rivers RP, Taghizadeh A. Disseminated intravascular coagulation and fetal hydrops in a newborn infant in association with a chorangioma of placenta. Pediatrics 1972;50:901–5.
44. Kadyrov M, Kosanke G, Kingdom J, Kaufmann P. Increased fetoplacental angiogenesis during first trimester in anaemic women. Lancet 1998;352:1747–9.
45. Kadyrov M, Schmitz C, Black S, Kaufmann P, Huppertz B. Pre-eclampsia and maternal anaemia display reduced apoptosis and opposite invasive phenotypes of extravillous trophoblast. Placenta 2003;24:540–8.
46. Kalousek DK, Barrett IJ, McGillivray BC. Placental mosaicism and intrauterine survival of trisomies 13 and 18. Am J Hum Genet 1989;44:338–43.
47. Kalousek DK, Dill FJ. Chromosomal mosaicism confined to the placenta in human conceptions. Science 1983;221:665–7.
48. Kalousek DK, Howard-Peebles P, Barrett I, Schulman J, Wilson D. Chromosomal mosaicism in term placentas and its association with high incidence of abnormal intrauterine development [Abstract]. Lab Invest 1991;64:6P.
49. Khong TY. Acute atherosis in pregnancies complicated by hypertension, growth retardation, and diabetes mellitus. Arch Pathol Lab Med 1991;115:722–5.
50. Khong TY. Chorangioma with trophoblastic proliferation. Virchows Arch 2000;436:167–71.
51. Kingdom JC, Rodeck CH, Kaufmann P. Umbilical artery Doppler—more harm than good? Br J Obstet Gynaecol 1997;104:393–6.
52. Kjos SL, Buchanan TA. Gestational diabetes mellitus. N Engl J Med 1999;341:1749–56.
53. Kouyoumdijian A. Velamentous insertion of the umbilical cord. Obstet Gynecol 1980;56:737–42.
54. Lake BD, Young EP, Winchester BG. Prenatal diagnosis of lysosomal storage diseases. Brain Pathol 1998;8:133–49.
55. Lim KH, Zhou Y, Janatpour M, et al. Human cytotrophoblast differentiation/invasion is abnormal in pre-eclampsia. Am J Pathol 1997;151:1809–18.
56. Madazli R, Somunkiran A, Calay Z, Ilvan S, Aksu MF. Histomorphology of the placenta and the placental bed of growth restricted foetuses and correlation with the Doppler velocimetries of the uterine and umbilical arteries. Placenta 2003;24:510–6.

57. Maher ER, Reik W. Beckwith-Wiedemann syndrome: imprinting in clusters revisited. J Clin Invest 2000;105:247–52.
58. Maynard SE, Min JY, Merchan J, et al. Excess placental soluble fms-like tyrosine kinase 1 (sFlt1) may contribute to endothelial dysfunction, hypertension, and proteinuria in preeclampsia. J Clin Invest 2003;111:649–58.
59. McKusick V. Mendelian inheritance in man, 12th ed. Baltimore, MD: Johns Hopkins University Press, 1998.
60. Mengert W, Goodson J, Campbell R, Haynes D. Observations of the pathogenesis of premature separation of the normally implanted placenta. Am J Obstet Gynecol 1953;66:1104–12.
61. Morgan T, Craven C, Lalouel JM, Ward K. Angiotensinogen Thr235 variant is associated with abnormal physiologic change of the uterine spiral arteries in first-trimester decidua. Am J Obstet Gynecol 1999;180(Pt 1):95–102.
62. Mucitelli DR, Charles EZ, Kraus FT. Chorio-angiomas of intermediate size and intrauterine growth retardation. Pathol Res Pract 1990;186:455–8.
63. Mutema G, Stanek J. Increased prevalence of chorangiosis in placentas from multiple gestation [Abstract]. Am J Clin Pathol 1998;108:341.
64. Naftolin F, Khudr G, Benirschke K, Hutchinson DL. The syndrome of chronic abruptio placentae, hydrorrhea, and circumvallate placenta. Am J Obstet Gynecol 1973;116:347–50.
65. Novak R, Agamanolis D, Dasu S, et al. Histologic analysis of placental tissue in first trimester abortions. Pediatr Pathol 1988;8:477–82.
66. Ogino S, Redline RW. Villous capillary lesions of the placenta: distinctions between chorangioma, chorangiomatosis, and chorangiosis. Hum Pathol 2000;31:945–54.
67. Ong K, Kratzsch J, Kiess W, Costello M, Scott C, Dunger D. Size at birth and cord blood levels of insulin, insulin-like growth factor I (IGF-I), IGF-II, IGF-binding protein-1 (IGFBP-1), IGFBP-3, and the soluble IGF-II/mannose-6-phosphate receptor in term human infants. The ALSPAC Study Team. Avon Longitudinal Study of Pregnancy and Childhood. J Clin Endocrinol Metab 2000;85:4266–9.
68. Oppenheimer EH, Esterly JR. Thrombosis in the newborn: comparison between infants of diabetic and nondiabetic mothers. J Pediatr 1965;67:549–56.
69. Paria BC, Ma W, Tan J, et al. Cellular and molecular responses of the uterus to embryo implantation can be elicited by locally applied growth factors. Proc Natl Acad Sci U S A 2001;98:1047–52.
70. Pfarrer C, Macara L, Leiser R, Kingdom J. Adaptive angiogenesis in placentas of heavy smokers. Lancet 1999;354:303.
71. Ramsey EM. The placenta of laboratory animals and man. New York: Holt, Rinehart & Winston; 1975. Holt, Rinehart & Winston Developmental Biology Series.
72. Read JA, Cotlon DB, Miller FC. Placenta accreta: changing clinical aspects and outcome. Obstet Gynecol 1980;56:31–4.
73. Redline RW. Role of uterine natural killer cells and interferon gamma in placental development. J Exp Med 2000;192:F1–4.
74. Redline RW, Hassold T, Zaragoza MV. Determinants of trophoblast hyperplasia in spontaneous abortions. Mod Pathol 1998;11:762–8.
75. Redline RW, Hassold T, Zaragoza MV. Prevalence of the partial molar phenotype in triploidy of maternal and paternal origin. Hum Pathol 1998;28:505–11.
76. Redline RW, O'Riordan MA. Placental lesions associated with cerebral palsy and neurologic impairment following term birth. Arch Pathol Lab Med 2000;124:1785–91.
77. Redline RW, Patterson P. Preeclampsia is associated with an excess of proliferative immature intermediate trophoblast. Hum Pathol 1995;26:594–600.
78. Redline RW, Shah D, Sakar H, Schluchter M, Salvator A. Placental lesions associated with abnormal growth in twins. Pediatr Dev Pathol 2001;4:473–81.
79. Redline RW, Wilson-Costello D. Chronic peripheral separation of placenta. The significance of diffuse chorioamnionic hemosiderosis. Am J Clin Pathol 1999;111:804–10.
80. Redline RW, Zaragoza MV, Hassold T. Prevalence of developmental and inflammatory lesions in non-molar first trimester spontaneous abortions. Hum Pathol 1999;30:93–100.
81. Redman CW, Sargent IL. Placental debris, oxidative stress and pre-eclampsia. Placenta 2000;21:597–602.
82. Reshetnikova OS, Burton GJ, Milovanoc AP, Fokin EI. Increased incidence of placental chorioangioma in high-altitude pregnancies: hypobaric hypoxia as a possible etiologic factor. Am J Obstet Gynecol 1996;174:557–61.
83. Roberts DJ, Ampola MG, Lage JM. Diagnosis of unsuspected fetal metabolic storage disease by routine placental examination. Pediatr Pathol 1991;11:647–56.

84. Robertson WB, Khong TY, Brosens I, De Wolf F, Sheppard BL, Bonnar J. The placental bed biopsy: review from three European centers. Am J Obstet Gynecol 1986;155:401–12.
85. Robinson WP, Barrett IJ, Bernard L, et al. Meiotic origin of trisomy in confined placental mosaicism is correlated with presence of fetal uniparental disomy, high levels of trisomy in trophoblast, and increased risk of fetal intrauterine growth restriction. Am J Hum Genet 1997;60:917–27.
86. Rochelson B, Kaplan C, Guzman E, Arato M, Hansen K, Trunca C. A quantitative analysis of placental vasculature in the third-trimester fetus with autosomal trisomy. Obstet Gynecol 1990;75:59–63.
87. Saftlas AF, Olson DR, Franks AL, Atrash HK, Pokras R. Epidemiology of preeclampsia and eclampsia in the United States, 1979-1986. Am J Obstet Gynecol 1990;163:460–5.
88. Singer DB. The placenta in pregnancies complicated by diabetes mellitus. Perspect Pediatr Pathol 1984;8:199–212.
89. Soma H, Watanabe Y, Hata T. Chorangiosis and chorangioma in three cohorts of placentas from Nepal, Tibet and Japan. Reprod Fertil Devel 1996;7:1533–8.
90. Stallmach T, Hebisch G, Meier K, Dudenhausen JW, Vogel M. Rescue by birth: defective placental maturation and late fetal mortality. Obstet Gynecol 2001;97:505–9.
91. Takayama M, Soma H, Yaguchi S, et al. Abnormally large placenta associated with Beckwith-Wiedemann syndrome. Gynecol Obstet Invest 1986;22:165–8.
92. Todros T, Sciarrone A, Piccoli E, Guiot C, Kaufmann P, Kingdom J. Umbilical Doppler waveforms and placental villous angiogenesis in pregnancies complicated by fetal growth restriction. Obstet Gynecol 1999;93:499–503.
93. Tonkin IL, Setzer ES, Ermocilla R. Placental chorangioma: a rare cause of congestive heart failure and hydrops fetalis in the newborn. Am J Roentgenol 1980;134:181–3.
94. Torpin R. Evolution of a placenta circumvallata. Obstet Gynecol 1966;27:98–101.
95. Trask C, Lage JM, Roberts DJ. A second case of "chorangiocarcinoma" presenting in a term asymptomatic twin pregnancy: choriocarcinoma in situ with associated villous proliferation. Int J Gynecol Pathol 1994;3:87–91.
96. van der Molen EF, Verbruggen B, Novakova I, Eskes TK, Monnens LA, Blom HJ. Hyperhomocysteinemia and other thrombotic risk factors in women with placental vasculopathy. BJOG 2000;107:785–91.
97. Van Lijschoten G, Arends JW, De La Fuente AA, Schouter HJ, Geraedts JP. Intra- and inter-observer variation in the interpretation of histological features suggesting chromosomal abnormality in early abortion specimens. Histopathology 1993;22:25–9.
98. Williams MA, Hickok DE, Zingheim RW, Mittendorf R, Kimelman J, Mahony BS. Low birth weight and preterm delivery in relation to early-gestation vaginal bleeding and elevated maternal serum alpha-fetoprotein. Obstet Gynecol 1992;80:745–9.
99. Wolstenholme J, White I, Sturgiss S, Carter J, Plant N, Goodship JA. Maternal uniparental heterodisomy for chromosome 2: detection through 'atypical' maternal AFP/hCG levels, with an update on a previous case. Prenat Diagn 2001;21:813–7.
100. Yeruchimovich M, Mimouni FB, Green DW, Dollberg S. Nucleated red blood cells in healthy infants of women with gestational diabetes. Obstet Gynecol 2000;95:84–6.
101. Zhang J, Zeisler J, Hatch MC, Berkowitz G. Epidemiology of pregnancy-induced hypertension. Epidemiol Rev 1997;19:218–32.
102. Zhou Y, Chiu K, Brescia RJ, et al. Increased depth of trophoblast invasion after chronic constriction of the lower aorta in rhesus monkeys. Am J Obstet Gynecol 1993;169:224–9.
103. Zhou Y, Damsky CH, Chiu K, Roberts JM, Fisher SJ. Preeclampsia is associated with abnormal expression of adhesion molecules by invasive cytotrophoblasts. J Clinical Invest 1993;91:950–60.

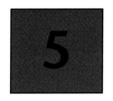

5 INFLAMMATION AND INFECTION

INTRODUCTION

Inflammatory responses in the uterus of a pregnant woman must be strictly regulated to strike a balance between two opposing threats to the fetus. The first threat, infection, usually gains entry to the sterile uterine environment from adjacent sites that are colonized by microorganisms, such as the vagina, cervix, and gastrointestinal tract. Other sources include the contiguous spread from local processes such as chronic salpingitis or acute cystitis, and hematogenous seeding by organisms circulating in the maternal bloodstream (11). There are only two effective defenses against infection: 1) anatomic barriers that limit access (cervical os, decidualized endometrium, uterine wall, and the continuous layer of trophoblast separating maternal from fetal tissues) and 2) preexisting maternal immunity, generally in the form of protective antibodies.

The second threat to the fetus comes from the maternal immune system, which may react against foreign fetal antigens in the placenta or against novel antigenic determinants generated during the processes of implantation and vascular remodeling (8). Control of maternal immune reactivity during pregnancy occurs via a number of overlapping mechanisms, including active regulation of lymphocyte homing, cytokine release, antigen presentation, and complement activation (32,60,71,75,97,118). The effectiveness of these mechanisms, together with the immaturity of the fetal immune system, compromise effective local responses to infection (96). Conversely, failure of these mechanisms can lead to inappropriate local immune responses, with placental inflammation and, in some cases, recurrent pregnancy failure.

Several generalizations apply to inflammation in the pregnant uterus. First, the response to microorganisms is usually restricted to antigen nonspecific cells such as neutrophils and macrophages. Second, inflammation tends to be confined to peripheral areas of the placenta, such as the membranes and terminal villi, reducing the chances that infectious organisms will gain access to the fetus. Third, the fetal inflammatory response elicited by microbial antigens and other bacterial products can damage fetal placental vessels and developing fetal organs. These responses include cellular activation via toll-like receptors, which bind bacterial structural proteins (lipopolysaccharide, other bacterial cell wall components, and exotoxins) (35); cytokine release (interleukin [IL]-6, IL-8, tumor necrotic factor [TNF]-alpha, and others) (30); activation of the coagulation cascade (78); and secretion of acute phase reactant proteins by the fetal liver (69). Finally, because of the closed environment of the pregnant uterus and the tightly regulated host response in this region, the only effective way for the mother (or the obstetrician) to deal with fetoplacental infection is to empty the uterus. This most commonly occurs spontaneously by rupture of the membranes or the onset of labor, irrespective of gestational age and fetal maturity. A summary of the terminology, etiology, location, and clinical implications of the different patterns of placental inflammation is given in Table 5-1.

INFECTIONS

Acute Chorioamnionitis (Histologic)

Definition. Acute chorioamnionitis is the stereotypical pattern of inflammatory changes in the placenta, umbilical cord, and membranes seen in response to microorganisms in the amniotic fluid.

Maternal Inflammatory Response. There is diffuse infiltration of the chorionic plate and membranous chorioamnion by maternal neutrophils derived from the intervillous space and the venules of the decidua capsularis, respectively. An absence of neutrophils in the subchorionic fibrin layer essentially excludes the diagnosis of chorioamnionitis.

Table 5-1
PATTERNS OF PLACENTAL INFLAMMATION[a]

Anatomic Location/Lesions	Etiology/Significance
Chorioamnion	
Acute subchorionitis/chorionitis	?Early ascending amnionic fluid infection
Acute chorioamnionitis	Stereotypical response, amnionic fluid infection
Necrotizing chorioamnionitis	?Prolonged amnionic fluid infection (days)
Subacute chorioamnionitis	?Prolonged amnionic fluid infection (weeks)
Chorionic microabsesses	Severe maternal response, increased risk fetal sepsis
Chronic chorioamnionitis	Idiopathic
Umbilical Cord/Chorionic Plate	
Umbilical phlebitis/chorionic vasculitis	Fetal inflammatory response
Umbilical arteritis	?Increased risk neurologic impairment, increased fetal sepsis
Intense chorionic vasculitis	Increased risk neurologic impairment
Necrotizing funisitis	Any prolonged fetal immune response, also herpes simplex virus
Necrotizing periphlebitis	Congenital syphilis
Eosinophilic/T-cell chorionic vasculitis	Idiopathic
Stem Villi	
VUE-associated stem villous vasculitis[b]	Vascular obliteration and avascular villi; increased risk of neurologic impairment
Proliferative endovasculitis	Congenital syphilis
Terminal Villi	
VUE	?Host versus graft reaction, IUGR[b], IUFD[b], recurrent fetal loss
Fibrosclerosing villitis	TORCH[b] infection: HSV[b] and varicella-zoster
Plasma cell villitis	TORCH infection: CMV[b], EBV[b]
Histiocyte-predominant villitis	TORCH infection: toxoplasmosis, syphilis, Chagas' disease
Active chronic villitis/intervillositis	Some VUE, infections: HSV, intestinal spirochetes, others
Actute villitis	Fetal bacterial sepsis: usually coliforms or streptococci
Intervillous Space	
Acute intervillositis/intervillous absesses	*Listeria monocytogenes, Campylobacter fetus,* others (maternal sepsis)
Chronic (histiocytic) intervillositis	Malaria (with malarial pigment), idiopathic with recurrent loss, IUGR, IUFD
Decidua	
Diffuse chronic deciduitis	Some VUE, idiopathic
Decidual plasma cells	Some VUE, subclinical (infectious) chronic endometritis
Chronic decidual perivasculitis	Preeclampsia, related disorders
Granulomatous deciduitis	*Mycobacterium tuberculosis,* sarcoidosis, postoperative change, idiopathic giant cell endometritis

[a]See text for detailed description and references.
[b]VUE = villitis of unknown etiology; IUGR = intrauterine growth restriction; IUFD = intrauterine fetal distress; TORCH = *Toxoplasma*, rubellavirus, cytomegalovirus, herpes simplex virus, others; HSV = herpes simplex virus; CMV = cytomegalovirus; EBV = Epstein-Barr virus.

Fetal Inflammatory Response. Neutrophils (and occasionally eosinophils) transmigrate from the fetal circulation through the wall of the large fetal vessels in the chorionic plate and umbilical cord. Neutrophils are most dense on the side facing the amnionic cavity. Involvement is more common for umbilical vessels near the insertion of the umbilical cord into the chorionic plate. Upon leaving the vessel wall, neutrophils spread to the connective tissues of the chorionic plate and umbilical cord (Wharton's jelly).

Clinical Chorioamnionitis. Pregnant women with premature rupture of membranes, fever, and leukocytosis during labor often receive a clinical diagnosis of chorioamnionitis (see chapter 3, Clinical (versus Pathologic) Chorioamnionitis). However, this "clinical chorioamnionitis" correlates poorly with histologic chorioamnionitis, which remains the "gold standard" for the diagnosis of amnionic fluid infection (Table 5-2 and discussion below).

Incidence. The incidence of chorioamnionitis is inversely proportional to gestational age, varying from 67 percent at less than 24 weeks to about 20 percent at term (74). The prevalence of chorioamnionitis and other common

Table 5-2
CORRELATION OF HISTOLOGIC CHORIOAMNIONITIS WITH CLINICAL CHORIOAMNIONITIS AND EARLY ONSET NEONATAL SEPSIS IN 119 VERY LOW BIRTH WEIGHT INFANTS[a]

Histologic Chorioamnionitis Maternal IR[b]	Fetal IR	Number	Clinical Chorioamnionitis[c]	Neonatal Sepsis at <7 days
none	none	47	4 (9)[d]	0 (0)
+	none	14	1 (7)	0 (0)
+	mild-moderate	41	6 (15)	5 (12)
+	severe (intense)	17	13 (77)	2 (12)
	Total:	119	24 (20)	7 (6)

[a]Modified from reference 102.
[b]IR = inflammatory response.
[c]See text, Clinical Features, page 78.
[d]Number (percent positive).

Table 5-3
PREVALENCE OF COMMON PLACENTAL INFLAMMATORY LESIONS BY GESTATIONAL AGE[a]

Gest. Age[b]	N	Acute Chorioamnionitis				Chronic Deciduitis		Villitis of Unknown Etiology			
		Any	St. 1[c]	St. 2	St. 3	Any	Plasma Cell	Any	Focal	Diffuse	Basal
20-31 6/7	229	115 (50)[d]	33 (14)	47 (21)	35 (15)	30 (13)	25 (11)	2 (1)	0 (0)	2 (1)	0 (0)
32-36 6/7	303	67 (22)	16 (5)	40 (13)	11 (4)	26 (9)	18 (6)	13 (4)	3 (1)	8 (3)	2 (1)
37-42	759	133 (18)	44 (6)	76 (10)	13 (2)	21 (3)	18 (2)	62 (8)	28 (4)	30 (4)	4 (1)
Total	1291	315 (24)	93 (7)	163 (13)	59 (5)	77 (6)	61 (5)	77 (6)	31 (2)	40 (3)	6 (1)

[a]Submitted to pathology at the MacDonald Women's Hospital, 1992-1996.
[b]Gestational age range in weeks from LMP.
[c]Maternal stage 1 = acute subchorionitis and acute chorionitis; maternal stage 2 = acute chorioamnionitis; maternal stage 3 = necrotizing chorioamnionitis.
[d]Number (percent positive).

inflammatory lesions among placentas submitted to pathology at the MacDonald Women's Hospital, Cleveland, Ohio, is given in Table 5-3. The high rate of chorioamnionitis observed in preterm births is one of many arguments suggesting that these infections are a leading cause of preterm delivery.

Etiology. Most cases are due to bacteria or mycoplasma originating in the cervicovaginal tract that breach the normal barrier at the cervical os, and gain access to the amnionic cavity (11,38,126). Causative organisms include normal endogenous flora, the abnormal flora associated with bacterial vaginosis, and organisms colonizing the vagina from gastrointestinal sites (group B streptococci, *Listeria monocytogenes*). Factors facilitating spread to the amnionic cavity include premature rupture of membranes, uterine contractions, cervical dilatation, and presence of a foreign body (intrauterine device [IUD] or cerclage). The role of coitus or selective maternal antibody deficiency is controversial (7,76). A few cases are due to contiguous spread of bacteria from adjacent pelvic organs (bladder, fallopian tube, intraabdominal abscess) or hematogenous spread to the membranes. A subgroup of women with recurrent preterm labor and chorioamnionitis in multiple pregnancies may have subclinical endometritis, with spread to the membranes at the time of fusion with the endometrial wall at 20 to 24 weeks (29). There is some current interest in the potential role of oral flora in women with periodontal disease (36). These organisms could either colonize the cervicovaginal tract or seed the placenta hematogenously.

Clinical Features. No single definition of clinical chorioamnionitis exists. One definition that the authors have used in correlation studies is as follows: premature rupture of membranes with a maternal temperature of either greater than 37.8°C on two occasions at least 1 hour apart, or greater than 38.3°C on one occasion with no other known sources for the fever plus one or more of the following—maternal tachycardia (100 beats per minute or more), fetal tachycardia (160 beats per minute or more), maternal leukocytosis (more than 11,000/mm white blood cells), or foul smelling amnionic fluid (102).

Unfortunately, the sensitivity and specificity of these criteria for predicting true histologic chorioamnionitis are poor (112). Table 5-1 shows that the majority of cases with histologic chorioamnionitis (72 percent) fail to reach the diagnostic threshold. Conversely, a substantial number of patients with clinical chorioamnionitis (9 percent) have no histologic inflammation in the placenta. Laboratory tests, such as amnionic fluid culture or Gram stain, and cytokine assays of amnionic fluid or fetal blood, provide better agreement with histologic chorioamnionitis (106,125,127).

Only a small proportion of infants whose placentas show histologic chorioamnionitis have early onset neonatal sepsis (Table 5-2). The risk of neonatal sepsis is increased with highly pathogenic organisms, such as group B streptococci, and specific clinical algorhythms have been developed for the management of women known to harbor this organism in their cervicovaginal tract (62).

Most placentas with histologic chorioamnionitis have a fetal inflammatory component (Table 5-2). Recent data suggest that enhanced fetal cytokine release, as part of a fetal inflammatory response syndrome (FIRS), may directly injure the developing brain and lung (18, 30,123). One particularly sensitive target tissue is the developing white matter of the cerebral cortex (17). Several studies have related acute chorioamnionitis to white matter lesions, including sonographically defined echolucencies and other forms of periventricular leukomalacia (see case presented in figure 5-1). Studies correlating specific features of histologic chorioamnionitis with adverse outcome have shown that fetal inflammatory responses in umbilical or chorionic plate vessels are particularly important risk factors (20,59,78,98,120). Increased severity of fetal inflammation in these locations has been associated with vessel wall damage, mural thrombosis, and increased circulating fetal IL-6 levels (101,106). Involvement of umbilical arteries has been shown to be more significant than involvement of the vein alone (45,48,106).

It has long been known that chorioamnionitis is associated with premature rupture of the membranes and that rupture can either be the cause or the result of chorioamnionitis. An interesting dichotomy has emerged suggesting that damage to the white matter of the central nervous system (CNS) is increased in infants with rupture of membranes within 1 hour of delivery, but not in those with longstanding rupture of membranes (59,67). This suggests that chorioamnionitis associated with intact membranes may be a different entity than chorioamnionitis developing after prolonged rupture of membranes.

The growth of bacteria in the amnionic cavity is facilitated by meconium, and the combination of longstanding meconium and severe fetal chorioamnionitis appears to be especially deleterious to the fetus (85). It is controversial whether meconium alone without infection can cause histologic chorioamnionitis, but the finding of isolated umbilical phlebitis (see below) in meconium-stained placentas is not infrequent (13).

Gross Findings. The neutrophilic exudate in maternal chorioamnionitis imparts a diffuse dullness and opacity to the membranes covering the chorionic plate. This opacity is prominent and may obscure chorionic vessels in cases with a fetal inflammatory response (fig. 5-2, top; fig. 5-3). Marked neutrophilic exudation can result in a green-yellow discoloration of the membranes (fig. 5-2, bottom), that can mimic meconium (see fig. 7-3) or biliverdin staining (seen in cases of chronic abruption, chapter 4, fig. 4-3).

Microscopic Findings. The most widely used pathologic staging system for chorioamnionitis relies on the maternal inflammatory response alone (11). Recent clinical data (summarized above) regarding the importance of the fetal inflammatory response has made this an important aspect of pathologic diagnosis. The following

Placental Pathology

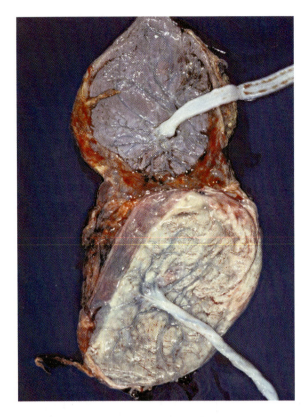

Figure 5-2

ACUTE CHORIOAMNIONITIS

There is a diffuse, green-stained purulent exudate on the fetal surface of twin A (bottom) and more typical acute chorioamnionitis with opacity near the chorionic plate vessels of twin B (top). The opacity in twin B is due to extravasated fetal neutrophils.

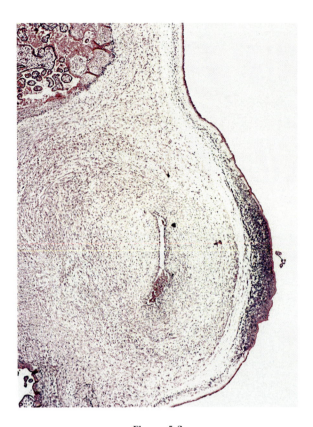

Figure 5-3

ACUTE CHORIOAMNIONITIS

The chorionic plate shows acute chorioamnionitis with a maternal inflammatory response (maternal stage 2) plus a fetal inflammatory response (chorionic vasculitis, fetal stage 1). Note the increased intensity of inflammation near the fetal vessels which corresponds to the opacity seen by gross examination.

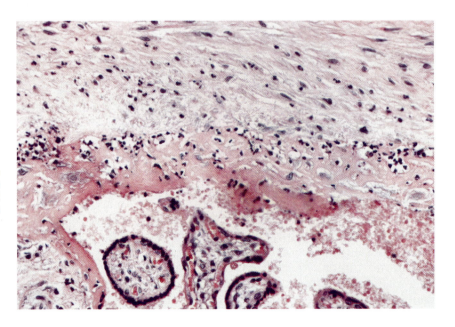

Figure 5-4

ACUTE CHORIOAMNIONITIS, MATERNAL FETAL INFLAMMATORY RESPONSE, STAGE 1 (ACUTE SUBCHORIONITIS)

Maternal neutrophils from the intervillous space marginate in the subchorionic fibrin and enter the lower portions of the chorionic plate.

Inflammation and Infection

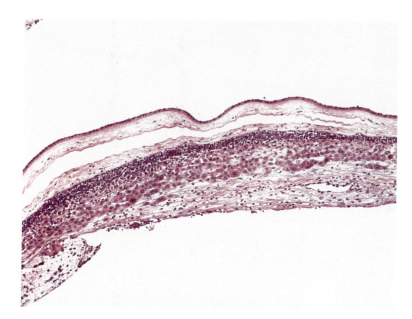

Figure 5-5
ACUTE CHORIOAMNIONITIS, MATERNAL INFLAMMATORY RESPONSE, STAGE 1 (ACUTE CHORIONITIS)
Maternal neutrophils extravasating from postcapillary venules in the membranous decidua first accumulate at the choriodecidual margin and among chorion laevae trophoblast cells.

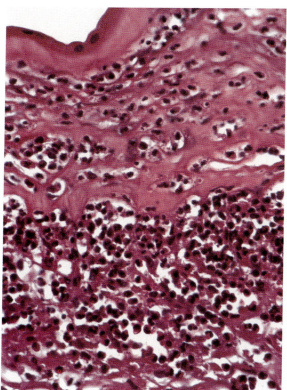

Figure 5-6
ACUTE CHORIOAMNIONITIS, MATERNAL INFLAMMATORY RESPONSE, STAGE 2 (ACUTE CHORIOAMNIONITIS)
Maternal neutrophils cross the chorion laevae and enter the chorionic and amnionic connective tissues.

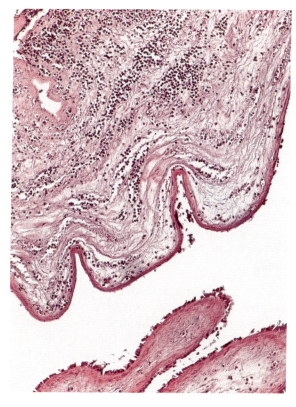

Figure 5-7
ACUTE CHORIOAMNIONITIS, MATERNAL INFLAMMATORY RESPONSE, STAGE 3 (NECROTIZING CHORIOAMNIONITIS)
Maternal neutrophils undergo karyorrhexis, fibrin accumulates in a thick homogeneous layer in the amnionic epithelial basement membrane, and amnionic epithelial cells become necrotic and slough into the amnionic fluid.

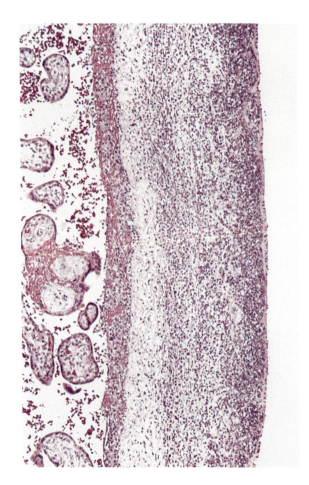

Figure 5-8

ACUTE CHORIOAMNIONITIS, SEVERE MATERNAL INFLAMMATORY RESPONSE

The chorionic plate shows a diffuse, maternally-derived, inflammatory infiltrate containing more than 30 neutrophils per high-power field.

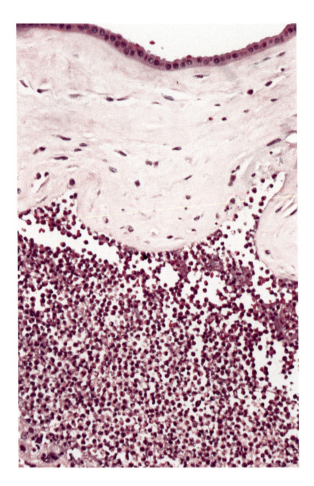

Figure 5-9

ACUTE CHORIOAMNIONITIS, WITH (MATERNAL) MICROABSCESS FORMATION (SEVERE, GRADE 2)

Aggregates of confluent neutrophils at least 20 cells in minimum diameter are seen beneath the chorion.

formation, was associated with an increased risk of clinical neonatal infection (possible, probable, and proven sepsis) in one study (45). Although the lesion was not defined in the study, illustrations demonstrate confluent clusters of neutrophils, approximately 10 to 20 cells in extent, aggregating between chorion and amnion in the membranes (fig. 5-9).

Fetal Inflammatory Response. The stage (duration) of the fetal inflammatory response is also subclassified into stages and grades as follows. In stage 1 (early), *chorionic vasculitis and/or umbilical phlebitis* (figs. 5-3, 5-10), fetal neutrophils are seen in the wall of a chorionic vessel or the umbilical vein. In stage 2 (intermediate), *umbilical arteritis* (fig. 5-11), fetal neutrophils are in the wall of one or both umbilical arteries (48). At this stage, a few neutrophils may also be present in Wharton's jelly (fig. 5-12). Stage 3 (late), *necrotizing funisitis or concentric umbilical perivasculitis* (fig. 5-13), bands of degenerating neutrophils and eosinophilic debris are arranged in concentric arcs surrounding one or more umbilical vessels. In some cases, capillary neovascularization is also present. This lesion is seen with longstanding bacterial, fungal, protozoal, and viral infections (34,65). On occasion, the band-like infiltrates undergo pronounced calcification (fig. 5-14). Calcification imparts a chalky white appearance to the arcs on gross

Inflammation and Infection

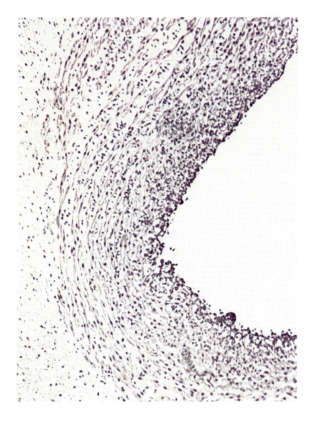

Figure 5-10

ACUTE CHORIOAMNIONITIS, FETAL INFLAMMATORY RESPONSE, STAGE 1 (UMBILICAL PHLEBITIS)

Fetal neutrophils migrate through the widely separated fascicles of vascular smooth muscle cells that characterize the umbilical vein.

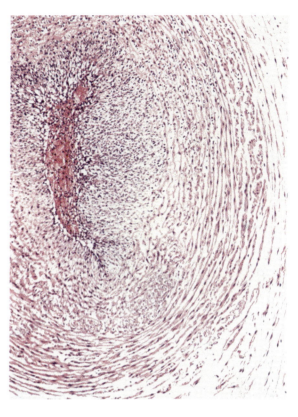

Figure 5-11

ACUTE CHORIOAMNIONITIS, FETAL INFLAMMATORY RESPONSE, STAGE 2 (UMBILICAL ARTERITIS)

Fetal neutrophils migrate through two layers of closely packed vascular smooth muscle cells: an inner haphazardly arranged subintimal layer and an outer circular layer. These two layers typify the umbilical arteries.

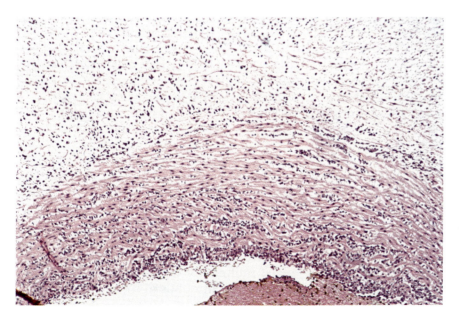

Figure 5-12

ACUTE CHORIOAMNIONITIS, FETAL INFLAMMATORY RESPONSE, STAGE 2 (UMBILICAL PERIVASCULITIS)

Fetal neutrophils migrate in substantial numbers into the umbilical cord stroma (Wharton's jelly) adjacent to inflamed vessels.

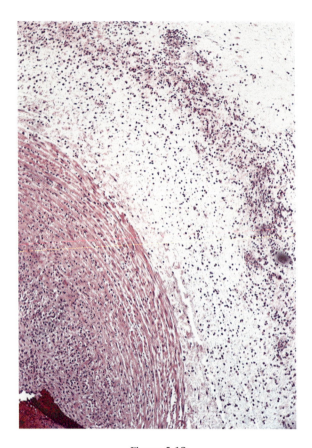

Figure 5-13

NECROTIZING FUNISITIS, STAGE 3 (CONCENTRIC PERIVASCULITIS)

Clusters of degenerating fetal neutrophils in the umbilical cord stroma are arranged in a semicircular arc around the vessel.

examination. In such cases, the cord may have the spiraled appearance of a "barber's pole" on radiographs of the maternal abdomen. The pathogenesis of necrotizing funisitis is tissue precipitation of immune complexes, formed when microbial antigens from the amniotic fluid are bound by maternal antibodies (acquired by transplacental passage) from the fetal umbilical vessels. These aggregates are analogous to the precipitin arcs seen in an Ouchterlony immunodiffusion assay (11,39).

Although entrenched in the literature, the use of the generic term "funisitis" without qualifiers to describe any fetal inflammatory response in umbilical vessels is discouraged. As discussed below, inflammation of the umbilical cord includes many specific patterns, each of which has significant and different implications for the etiology and timing of infection.

The grade (intensity) of fetal inflammation has important associations with adverse clinical outcome. Severe (grade 2) fetal inflammation, particularly in chorionic plate vessels *(intense chorionic vasculitis)*, can lead to vascular damage (fig. 5-15) or chorionic vessel thrombi (fig. 5-16), which may be harbingers of a fetal thrombotic diathesis that can affect other fetal organs (98,101). Severe fetal inflammation is an independent predictor of neurologic impairment at term and has been correlated with cerebral palsy, early onset fetal sepsis, and the clinical signs and symptoms of maternal chorioamnionitis in very low birth weight infants (98, 102). It can either be transmural or localized just below the endothelial layer. In our experience, the latter pattern is often seen with group B streptococcal sepsis (fig. 5-17).

Identification of Causative Organisms. Placental cultures and special stains in cases of routine acute chorioamnionitis do not generally guide clinical management. They can also be misleading if not performed correctly (see chapter 13) because of contamination from the cervicovaginal canal. Many placental infections are polymicrobial, involving mycoplasma and anaerobic bacteria that are difficult to stain and culture (5, 51,84). Organisms infrequently cross into the fetal circulation, and blood cultures are routinely obtained in infants with suspected sepsis prior to treatment with broad spectrum antibiotics. One scenario in which special stains or placental cultures may be helpful is in the depressed newborn with occult sepsis whose neonatal cultures are negative due to maternal antibiotic therapy prior to delivery. Silver impregnation stains (Steiner, Dieterle, Warthin-Starry) generally have the highest sensitivity for demonstrating bacteria in tissue sections, often showing a mixture of cocciform and bacilliform organisms. One distinctive pattern of staining is a confluent meshwork of filamentous bacilli, indicative of *Fusobacterium* sp (fig. 5-18) (3), one of the organisms associated with periodontal disease (see above).

Subacute Chorioamnionitis

Definition. Subacute chorioamnionitis is a mixed infiltrate of mononuclear cells and degenerating neutrophils in the chorionic plate.

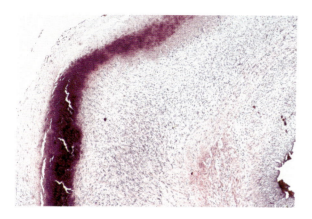
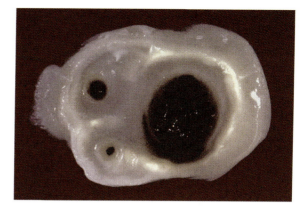

Figure 5-14

NECROTIZING FUNISITIS (CALCIFYING CONCENTRIC PERIVASCULITIS)

Left: Microscopic view of calcified arc of cellular debris and immune complexes surrounding an umbilical vessel.
Right: Gross specimen shows chalky white calcifications spiraling around the umbilical vessels ("barber pole lesion").

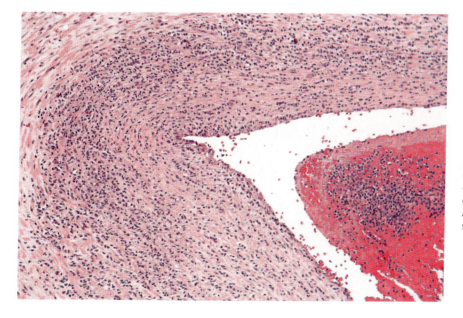

Figure 5-15

ACUTE CHRIOAMNIONITIS WITH SEVERE FETAL INFLAMMATORY RESPONSE (FETAL GRADE 2)

Near confluent fetal neutrophils are seen on the upper lateral (amnionic) aspect of the chorionic vessel wall, with endothelial fibrin deposition and disarray of vascular smooth muscle.

Incidence. Subacute chorioamnionitis was found in 6 percent of placentas from very low birth weight infants in the one published study of this recently defined entity (81).

Etiology. It has been proposed that subacute chorioamnionitis is the result of either infection by organisms of low pathogenicity that fail to elicit immediate delivery or repetitive bouts of mild infection in women with recurrent second and third trimester bleeding.

Clinical Features. The maternal history is remarkable only for repetitive vaginal bleeding. Very low birth weight infants with placentas showing subacute chorioamnionitis have higher white blood cell counts, higher immunoglobulin (Ig) M titers, and elevated C-reactive protein (CRP) levels. Chronic lung disease was increased in a subgroup of very low birth weight infants with both subacute chorioamnionitis and amnion necrosis (maternal stage 3 chorioamnionitis, above) (81). Firm conclusions regarding the relative significance of this lesion await further studies.

Gross and Microscopic Findings. Subacute chorioamnionitis has no specific gross features. The histologic features are as listed above (fig. 5-

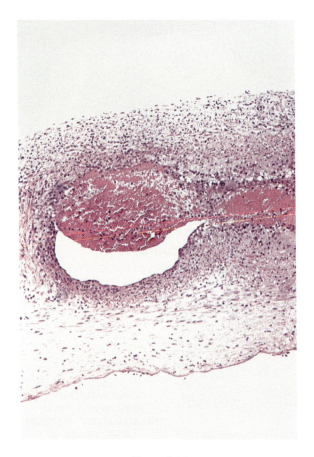

Figure 5-16

ACUTE CHORIOAMNIONITIS WITH SEVERE FETAL INFLAMMATORY RESPONSE AND RECENT NONOCCLUSIVE MURAL THROMBOSIS

Laminated fibrin is seen on the amnionic aspect of the lumen of the chorionic vessel. This 950-g infant had variable decelerations and clinically diagnosed amnionitis. The infant developed severe periventricular leukomalacia and subsequent spastic quadriplegia. Blood cultures at birth were negative.

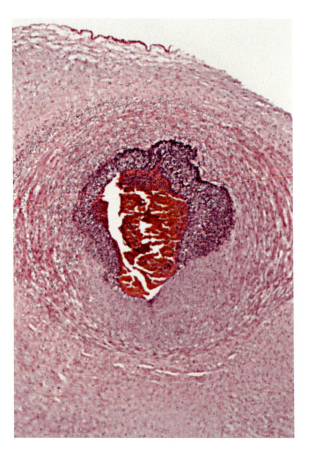

Figure 5-17

ACUTE CHORIOAMNIONITIS: GROUP B STREPTOCOCCI

The intense, subendothelial, fetal neutrophilic infilrate, has been seen in other cases of group B streptococcal chorioamnionitis. The patient was a 28-year-old G3 P2002 who presented at 21 weeks with fever and leukocytosis, premature labor, and ruptured membranes. The 398-g infant, with blood cultures positive for group B streptococci, died at 1 1/2 hours of life.

19). In contrast to acute chorioamnionitis, inflammatory cells are most numerous in the amnion and upper chorion rather than subchorionic fibrin and lower chorion. This entity should be distinguished from chronic chorioamnionitis, which contains predominantly small lymphocytes (discussed later in this chapter).

Acute Chorioamnionitis with Peripheral Funisitis

Definition. This entity is characterized by diffusely scattered, punctate microabscesses on the surface of the umbilical cord in a placenta with acute chorioamnionitis (39,89).

Incidence. The incidence of peripheral funisitis at the Hutzel Hospital was reported as 1.4 in 1,000 placentas examined over a 10-year period (89).

Etiology. Most reported cases have been associated with fungi of the *Candida* genus, including *C. albicans, C. parapsilosis,* and *C. glabrata.* Individual cases due to *Corynebacterium kutscheri, Haemophilus influenza,* and *Listeria monocytogenes* have also been reported.

Clinical Features. In one study, approximately 75 percent of the cases were from preterm deliveries and most of these were delivered prior to 25 weeks (89). An association with intrauterine contraceptive devices or cervical cerclages was

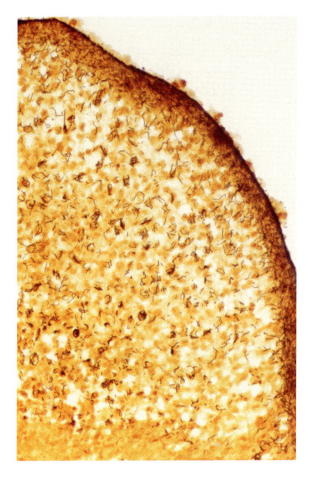

Figure 5-18

FUSOBACTERIUM NUCLEATUM CHORIOAMNIONITIS

Filamentous bacteria coat the denuded surface of the amnion (Steiner stain).

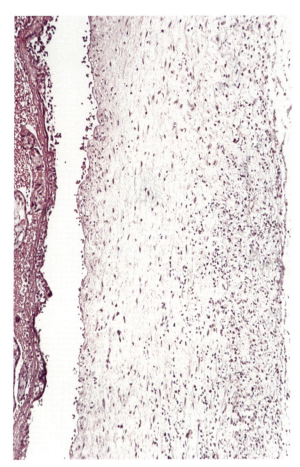

Figure 5-19

SUBACUTE CHORIOAMNIONITIS

There is a mixed mononuclear cell-neutrophilic exudate, indicative of prolonged duration of infection.

found in 16 percent of cases. Candidal vaginitis was a risk factor. Fetal infection by *Candida* was documented in 16 percent of cases. The specificity of peripheral funisitis as an indicator of congenital candidiasis is high. Reports in the literature also suggest a high sensitivity, but in our experience some clinical cases of candidiasis lack the placental lesion. Special stains for fungi are not generally helpful in placentas that lack peripheral funisitis.

Gross Findings. Slightly raised and well-circumscribed, 1- to 2-mm yellow-white plaques are observed diffusely studding the surface of the umbilical cord (fig. 5-20). Membrane opacity and discoloration suggestive of severe acute chorioamnionitis are common.

Microscopic Findings. Triangular-shaped microabscesses containing neutrophils and budding yeasts, with or without pseudohyphae, are seen subjacent to the amnionic covering of the cord (fig. 5-21). The lesions are present in virtually every section. Chorioamnionitis with a maternal inflammatory response is always present. A fetal inflammatory response is common and necrotizing funisitis is frequent.

Acute Intervillositis with Intervillous Abscesses

Definition. Neutrophils infiltrate the intervillous space, usually accompanied by chorioamnionitis. Severe acute intervillositis merges with intervillous abscess formation. Contiguous

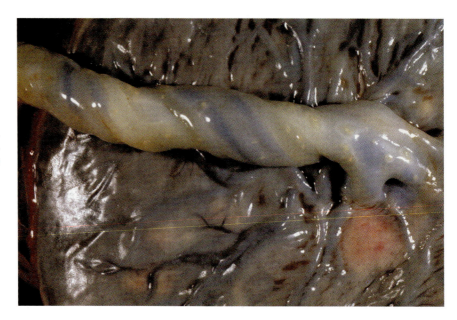

Figure 5-20

CANDIDA ALBICANS PERIPHERAL FUNISITIS

Small, punctate, yellow-white plaques are seen studding the outer surface of the umbilical cord.

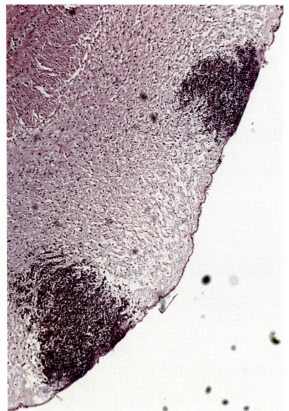 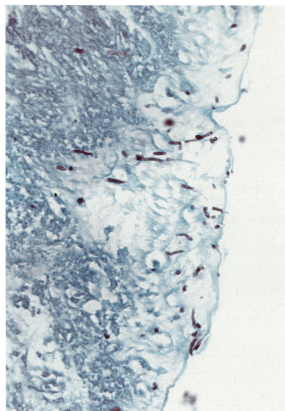

Figure 5-21

CANDIDA ALBICANS PERIPHERAL FUNISITIS

Left: Triangular microabscesses are composed of neutrophils and debris, with their bases adjacent to the perimeter of the umbilical cord (hematoxylin and eosin stain).

Right: Candidal pseudohyphae and budding yeast are within a peripheral umbilical cord microabscess (Gomori's methenamine silver stain).

spread to the villous stroma may be seen in severely affected areas.

Incidence. This histologic pattern is most commonly seen with infections caused by *Listeria monocytogenes* (23,121). The incidence of human listeriosis in pregnancy is 12 in 100,000. However, infections occur in clusters and the detection of one case may be a harbinger for others in the same community, generally related to the same contaminated food source (117).

Etiology. In addition to *L. monocytogenes*, other less common causative agents include *Campylobacter fetus*, *Chlamydia psittaci*, *Francisella tularensis*, and *Coccidioides immitis* (4,15, 40,41). A lesion with overlapping features may be seen in cases of maternal septicemia (9).

Clinical Features. Infection with *Listeria* has been associated with abortion and pregnancy loss in a wide variety of animal species. Host defenses against *Listeria* require local cell-mediated immunity, which is conspicuously deficient in the placental environment. *L. monocytogenes* can be found in soil, sewage, and animal silage. Perinatal infections are generally traced to contaminated food, principally dairy products and fresh produce, from farms with heavy environmental colonization (115). Human epidemics are food borne and person-person spread is rare.

Following ingestion, *Listeria* are phagocytosed by intestinal epithelial cells (117). After a brief hematogenous phase, organisms persist in the intestine, shedding into the feces, until systemic immunity is elicited. Early in the course of *Listeria* infection, mothers often have a transient flu-like illness with features similar to those of mononucleosis. Placental infection can occur either hematogenously during the hematogenous phase of maternal infection or by the ascending route in patients with intestinal carriage. Twin and triplet pregnancies are more commonly affected than singletons during *Listeria* epidemics (64). Unlike most bacterial infections, spread to the fetus is rapid and common, and leads to disseminated granulomas and microabscesses in liver, adrenal gland, lung, kidney, bone marrow, ileum, and thymus (granulomatosis infantiseptica) (121).

Gross Findings. Placentas often show opacity and green staining of the membranes. The basal plate may be abnormally pale due to an associated acute deciduitis. Occasionally, inter-

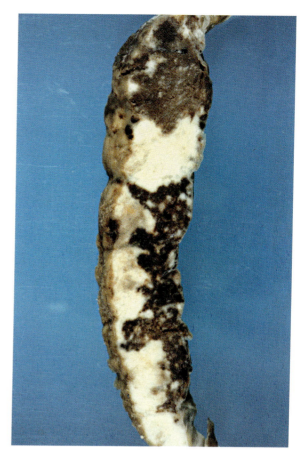

Figure 5-22

LISTERIA MONOCYTOGENES INTERVILLOUS ABSCESSES ("SEPTIC INFARCTS")

Irregularly distributed foci of consolidation with yellow-white discoloration, central degeneration, and a geographic border are distributed throughout the intervillous space.

villous abscesses and so-called septic infarcts are apparent as irregularly outlined, firm, yellow foci on the cut surface of the villous parenchyma (fig. 5-22).

Microscopic Findings. The maternal intervillous space contains a patchy neutrophilic exudate accompanied by necrosis and fibrin deposition, centered about small groups of tertiary stem and terminal villi (fig. 5-23). A second, smaller population of histiocytes is present in some areas, but lymphocytes, eosinophils, plasma cells, and histiocytic giant cells are generally absent. Accompanying areas of acute villitis are less common and are characterized by accumulation of neutrophils in the space between the trophoblastic basement membrane

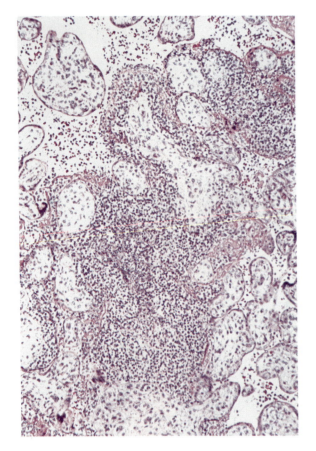

Figure 5-23

LISTERIA MONOCYTOGENES ACUTE INTERVILLOSITIS AND INTERVILLOUS ABSCESSES

Sheets of neutrophils with occasional foci of immature monocytes fill the intervillous space; villi are focally involved (acute villitis).

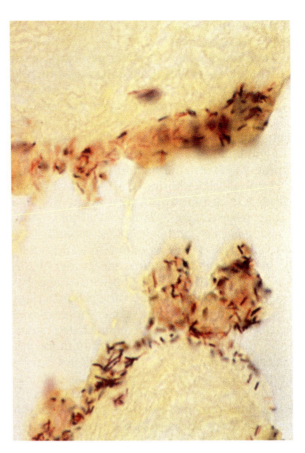

Figure 5-24

LISTERIA MONOCYTOGENES ACUTE PERIVILLITIS

Short Gram-positive cocci with diphtheroidal morphology are arranged at oblique angles to one another ("Chinese character" arrangement) (Brown and Brenn stain).

and villous stroma. Stem villous vasculitis may be present in some cases. Organisms are easily demonstrated by tissue Gram stain (fig. 5-24).

A overlapping histologic picture is seen in placentas with maternal-fetal septicemia (fig. 5-25). In this variant, the acute intervillositis is less prominent and there is a predominance of fibrin deposition and villous agglutination (9). Organisms are often easily seen in routine hematoxylin and eosin (H&E)-stained sections.

Acute Villitis

Definition. Neutrophils occur in fetal capillaries and stroma of distal villi, often accompanied by stainable microorganisms (57).

Etiology. This lesion is seen with in utero fetal sepsis. It is most commonly associated with *Escherichia coli* or group B and other streptococci. It is believed to represent hematogenous infection of the fetus followed by secondary bacteremic spread to villi.

Gross and Microscopic Findings. There are no typical gross findings. Most cases are accompanied by chorioamnionitis. Microscopically, neutrophils and bacteria are seen within villous capillaries (acute capillaritis) and there is often a prominent accumulation of neutrophils beneath the trophoblast basement membrane (fig. 5-26).

Active Chronic Villitis and Intervillositis with Villous Necrosis

Definition. The villous stroma and adjacent intervillous space are infiltrated by a polymorphous inflammatory composition of neutrophils,

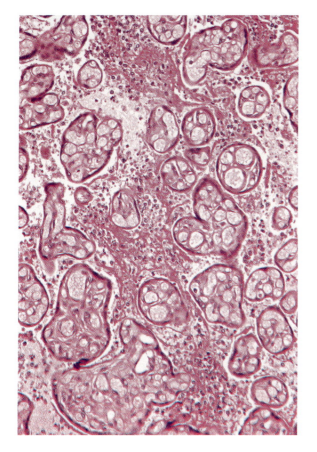

Figure 5-25

MATERNAL SEPSIS, GROUP A STREPTOCOCCI

A loose perivillous fibrin deposition contains neutrophils and scattered Gram-positive cocci. The mother died shortly after delivery from shock and disseminated intravascular coagulation.

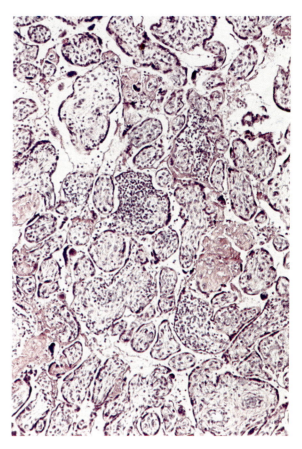

Figure 5-26

ACUTE VILLITIS, FETAL *ESCHERICHIA COLI* SEPSIS

Neutrophils accumulate between the villous stroma and the trophoblastic basement membrane.

lymphocytes, monocyte-macrophages, and occasional eosinophils. Common accompanying features include fetal stem villous vasculitis, villous necrosis, diffuse perivillous fibrin deposition, and villous infarcts. Acute chorioamnionitis is not generally present.

Incidence. A specific incidence figure is not available, but the pattern is uncommon.

Etiology. The differential diagnosis is infection versus a fulminant presentation of idiopathic chronic villitis (discussed below). Microorganisms to be considered include nonsyphilitic spirochetes, some Gram-negative bacteria, Rickettsia (*Coxiella burnetii*, Q fever) (27), and both herpes simplex and varicella-zoster viruses (1,4,92).

Clinical Features. These depend on the etiologic agent. Patients often give a history of recent infectious symptoms. The pattern may occasionally be seen in multiple specimens from patients with recurrent fetal loss (92). It is particularly important in these latter cases to distinguish treatable infections from the much more common cases of recurrent idiopathic chronic villitis.

Gross and Microscopic Findings. Placentas may be small for gestational age, but otherwise have no distinctive gross features. The microscopic pattern is as described above. Unlike acute villitis and intervillositis (discussed above), acute chorioamnionitis is absent and mononuclear cells predominate. Features favoring infection as opposed to idiopathic inflammation (discussed below) include the presence of neutrophils, eosinophils, immature monocyte-macrophages,

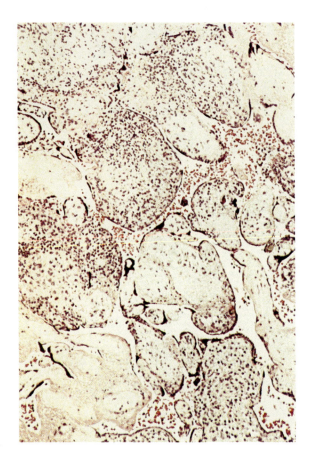
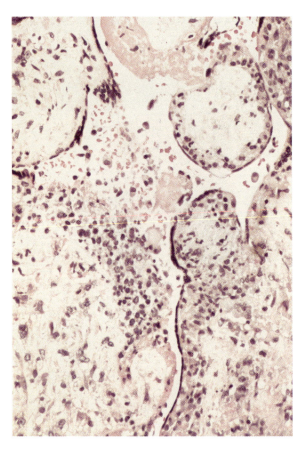

Figure 5-27

ACTIVE CHRONIC BACTERIAL VILLITIS AND INTERVILLOSITIS

A polymorphous inflammatory infiltrate composed of lymphocytes, macrophages, plasma cells, eosinophils, and neutrophils is seen in the villous stroma and intervillous space (left = low-power; right = high-power view). Steiner stain revealed bacterial rods.

tissue necrosis, and prominent intervillous inflammation and fibrin deposition (fig. 5-27). Silver stains (Steiner, Dieterle, Warthin-Starry) are often required to demonstrate organisms (fig. 5-28).

Chronic Placentitis, TORCH Type

Definition. This placental infection is characterized by chronic villous inflammation with fibrosis or edema, commonly accompanied by inflammation of the chorion, decidua, or umbilical cord stroma (4).

Incidence. Incidence figures vary, but over 90 percent of cases in the United States are attributable to cytomegalovirus and *Treponema pallidum*.

Etiology. The acronym TORCH stands for *Toxoplasma gondii*, rubella virus, cytomegalovirus, and herpes simplex virus plus certain other organisms associated with fetal infection. The other organisms encountered most frequently in the United States are *Treponema pallidum* (syphilis), varicella-zoster virus, and Epstein-Barr virus (83, 88,105). These organisms all cause histologic chronic placentitis (31). Rubella virus, once a leading cause of pregnancy loss and congenital heart disease, is so rare today that many perinatal pathologists have not seen a case. This dramatic success story is a testament to routine childhood immunization and antenatal screening. The poxviruses, variola (small pox) and vaccinia (small pox vaccine), are other historically interesting causes of congenital placentitis that are no longer seen in the United States. A rare cause of chronic placentitis in the United States is Chagas' disease (caused by *Trypanosoma cruzi*) which may be encountered among immigrants from Latin America (fig. 5-29), mothers with appropriate travel histories, and patients from southern Texas where the disease is endemic (4).

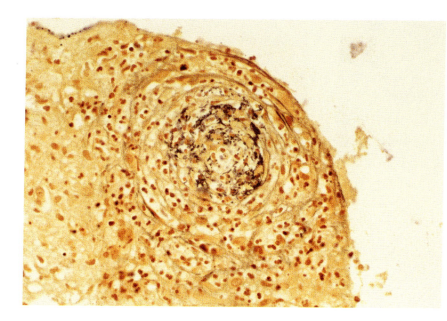

Figure 5-28

ACTIVE CHRONIC VILLITIS WITH VILLOUS VASCULITIS

Unclassified curved bacilli are seen in the villous vessel wall and adjacent stroma (Steiner stain).

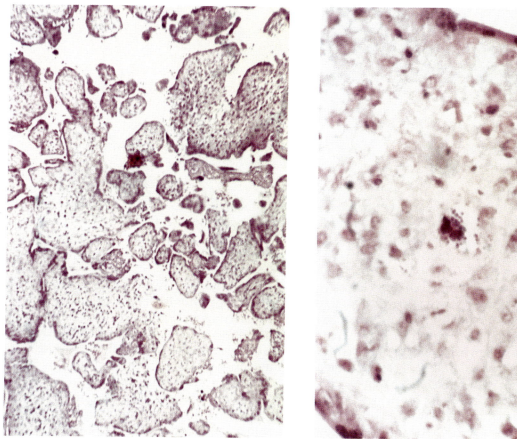

Figure 5-29

CHAGAS' DISEASE (*TRYPANOSOMA CRUZI*) PLACENTITIS

Left: Chronic necrotizing villitis.
Right: *T. cruzi* amastigotes in a fetal villous capillary.

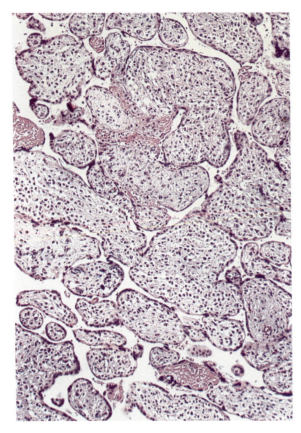

Figure 5-30

SYPHILIS PLACENTITIS

Edematous villi with diffuse histiocyte-predominant villitis.

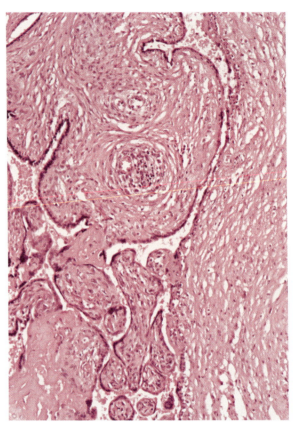

Figure 5-31

SYPHILIS PLACENTITIS

Proliferative periarteritis involving stem villi.

Clinical Features. The characteristics of the individual TORCH infections are beyond the scope of this discussion and are summarized elsewhere (16,108). Shared maternal features include lack of protective antibodies (primary infection), history of a flu-like illness, and the gradual onset of fetal growth restriction (or less commonly, hydrops fetalis). In some instances, antenatal ultrasound demonstrates typical patterns of fetal organ involvement such as the hyperechogenic bowel wall, liver calcifications, and ascites seen with congenital cytomegalovirus or the CNS calcifications seen with toxoplasmosis. Shared neonatal features of TORCH infections include low birth weight, hepatosplenomegaly, interstitial pneumonitis, pancytopenia, increased nucleated red blood cells, and petechial rash. The definitive diagnosis relies on serologic testing and assays for either organism-specific antigens (enzyme-linked immunosorbent assay [ELISA]) or nucleic acids (polymerase chain reaction [PCR]). Placental inflammation is ubiquitous and subclassification by histologic pattern can be an important adjunct to diagnosis.

Gross Findings. Two distinct gross patterns are seen with chronic placentitis: relatively large pale placentas with evidence of villous hydrops (*histiocyte-predominant villitis*) and relatively small firm placentas with villous fibrosis and mineralization (*fibrosclerosing villitis*).

Microscopic Findings. *Congenital Syphilis (Treponema pallidum).* Placentas are large and pale (49,90,110). Three important microscopic features may be seen: histiocytic-predominant villitis, which can be difficult to appreciate and is essentially just an increase in villous Hofbauer cells (fig. 5-30); proliferative endovasculitis, a stem villous perivasculitis with concentric mural vascular sclerosis (fig. 5-31); and necrotizing

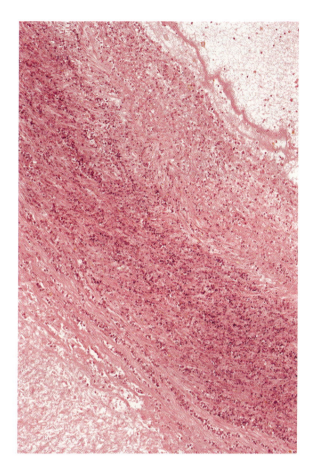

Figure 5-32

SYPHILIS PLACENTITIS

Necrotizing umbilical periphlebitis, with a broad ill-defined band of eosinophilic precipitate and cellular debris, extends from the margin away from the umbilical vein into the cord stroma.

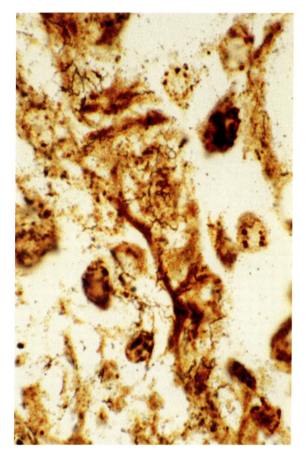

Figure 5-33

SYPHILIS PLACENTITIS (TREPONEMA PALLIDUM)

Spirochetes with corkscrew morphology are demonstrated in a focus of necrotizing umbilical periphlebitis (Warthin-Starry stain).

umbilical periphlebitis (fig. 5-32). The latter lesion consists of necrotic cell debris and nonspecific eosinophilic precipitation surrounding the umbilical vein, and is virtually pathognomonic for syphilis. The umbilical cord is the best location in the placenta to demonsrate spirochetes by special stains (Warthin-Starry, Dieterle, or Steiner) (fig 5-33).

Congenital Cytomegalovirus Infection. The placenta is either large and pale or small and fibrotic (73). In either case, three important features should be sought: prominent villous fibrosis and mineralization, plasma cell infiltrates in the villous stroma (fig. 5-34), and diagnostic large intranuclear inclusions with or without smaller basophilic cytoplasmic inclusions (fig. 5-35).

Villous stromal plasma cell infiltrates are virtually diagnostic for cytomegalovirus (or the much rarer Epstein-Barr virus placentitis). Placentas with plasma cells but no inclusions should be further evaluated by immunoperoxidase staining for cytomegalovirus early and late antigen or other virus-specific methods.

Congenital Toxoplasmosis. Placentas are generally large and pale with a subtle villous infiltrate, similar to that seen in syphilis, plus rare foci of necrotizing chronic villitis (fig. 5-36) (24). Intense chronic deciduitis in the placental membranes is a common, but nonspecific, feature (fig. 5-37). The diagnostic finding, readily apparent by light microscopy, is the presence of pseudocysts in the umbilical cord stroma (fig. 5-38).

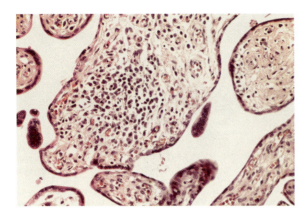
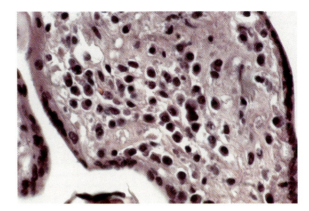

Figure 5-34

CYTOMEGALOVIRUS PLACENTITIS

Focal aggregates of lymphocytes and plasma cells are in the villous stroma.

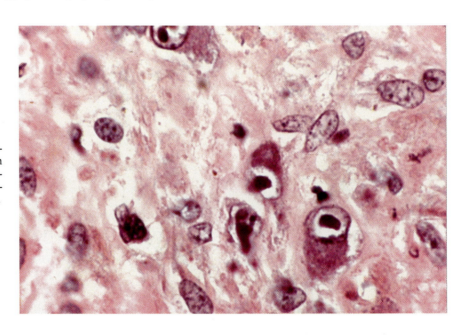

Figure 5-35

CYTOMEGALOVIRUS INCLUSION IN VILLOUS STROMA

Large, 7- to 9-μm, eosinophilic nuclear inclusions with a perinuclear halo, plus clusters of small 1- to 2-μm basophilic cytoplasmic inclusions.

Congenital Herpes Simplex and Varicella-Zoster Infections. These are morphologically similar (34,88). Placentas with longstanding infection are generally small and fibrotic. Placentas from more recent infections are described above in the section, Active Villitis and Intervillositis. Villous fibrosis and calcification are prominent (figs. 5-39, 5-40). Villous vasculitis, with subsequent hemorrhage, can lead to hemosiderin deposition. The umbilical cord may show necrotizing funisitis, as described above. An accompanying chorioamnionitis is more common with herpes simplex and varicella-zoster virus infections than with other TORCH-type infections. Small eosinophilic intranuclear inclusions of either Cowdry type A (with halos) or B (smudgy eosinophilic chromatin) are usually equivocal and ancillary immunocytochemical stains should be performed when the clinical index of suspicion is high.

Chronic Intervillositis with Malarial Pigment

Definition. Chronic intervillositis with malarial pigment occurs when there is a massive infiltration of the intervillous space by a monomorphous population of monocyte-macrophages, accompanied by fibrin, red blood cells with malarial organisms, black extracellular malarial

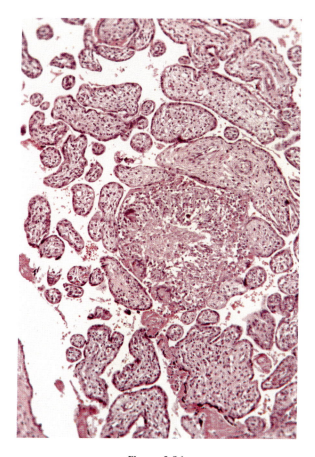 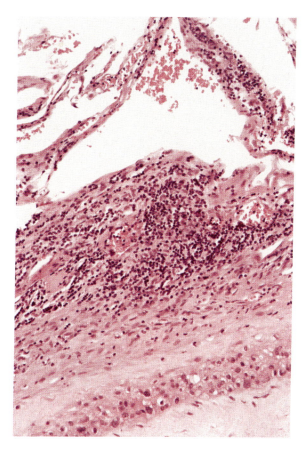

Figure 5-36

TOXOPLASMA PLACENTITIS

A central area of necrotizing villitis with focal giant cells surrounds cellular villi with increased villous Hofbauer cells and occasional small lymphocytes.

Figure 5-37

TOXOPLASMA PLACENTITIS

An intense lymphoplasmocytic infiltrate is in the membranous decidua.

pigment, variable amounts of necrotic cellular debris, and occasional neutrophils (42,122).

Incidence. It has been estimated that 25 percent of pregnant women in sub-Saharan Africa harbor placental malarial infection and that 5.7 percent of all infant deaths in endemic areas are attributable to the perinatal sequelae of maternal infection (33).

Etiology. Chronic intervillositis associated with malaria is a specific immune response to red blood cells parasitized by immature stages of *Plasmodium falciparum*, which are sequestered in the intervillous space. Sequestration is the consequence of specific molecular interactions between syncytiotrophoblast ligands, the most prominent of which are the low sulfated chondroitin sulfate proteoglycans, and antigens expressed by infected red blood cells (66,86).

Women from low endemic areas who have no preexisting immunity mount a fulminant immune response to parasite antigens, resulting in impaired uteroplacental perfusion and gas exchange (63). Women from high endemic areas have a three-fold increase in the frequency of parasitemia beginning in the late first and early second trimesters when arterial perfusion of the intervillous space begins (see chapter 1); this persists until about 2 months after delivery (21). This three-fold frequency increase may underestimate the true increase in infection since sequestration in the intervillous space is so extensive that many women have few parasites in the systemic circulation. Intervillositis and parasite load are greatest in the late second and early third trimesters; thus, postpartum flares of infection may represent release of parasites into the systemic circulation at the time of delivery.

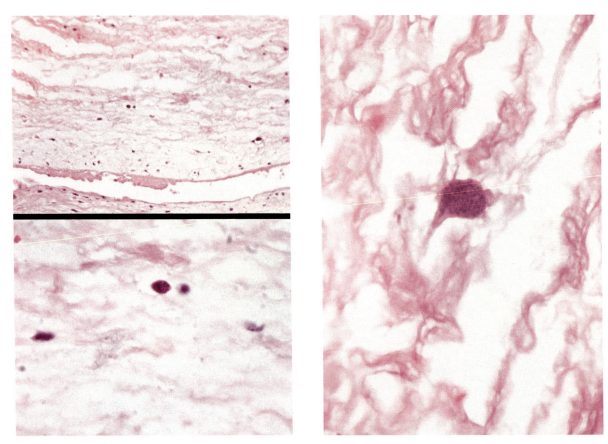

Figure 5-38

***TOXOPLASMA* PLACENTITIS (FUNISITIS)**

Scattered *Toxoplasma* pseudocysts containing numerous intracellular tachyzoites are seen in the umbilical cord stroma (Wharton's jelly).

Clinical Features. Women from low endemic areas with placental malaria have an increased risk of abortion, preterm delivery, fetal growth restriction, stillbirth, acute maternal illness, and maternal mortality. Serious morbidity is attributable to a lack of protective antibodies, including those that block the binding of parasitized red blood cells to syncytiotrophoblast. Women from high endemic areas mount secondary immune responses of lesser magnitude and hence have milder symptoms, such as fetal growth restriction and maternal anemia. The prevalence of all adverse outcomes with malaria is highest in the first pregnancy and decreases with each successive pregnancy. Fetal infection with malaria is relatively uncommon: cord blood parasitemia is seen in 3 to 6 percent of affected pregnancies.

Gross and Microscopic Findings. There are no typical gross features of chronic intervillositis in malaria, but placentas may be pale and firm when intervillous fibrin is extensive. Parasitized red blood cells in the intervillous space contain ring-shaped trophozoites. Hemozoin pigment from the breakdown of hemoglobin is deposited in the intervillous space, where it appears dark brown-black by light microscopy and fluoresces upon polarization (fig. 5-41, left).

Placental malaria is separated into three categories: acute infection, characterized by parasitized red blood cells with minimal malarial pigment; chronic infection, with both parasitized red blood cells and malarial pigment; and (inactive) past infection, with malarial pigment and no parasites. One large study of over 1,000 placentas in a high endemic area found acute

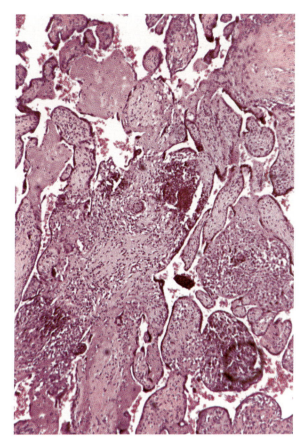

Figure 5-39

HERPES SIMPLEX VIRUS PLACENTITIS

Immature placenta with severe chronic villitis and numerous large villous stromal calcifications.

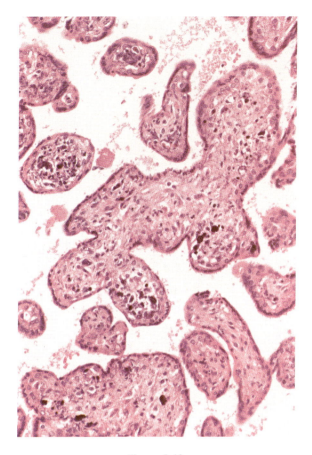

Figure 5-40

VARICELLA-ZOSTER PLACENTITIS

Sclerotic contracted villi with punctate calcifications and a subtle chronic inflammatory infiltrate.

infection in 10 percent, chronic infection in 25 percent, past infection in 40 percent, and no evidence of malaria in 24 percent (42). Massive chronic intervillositis is most frequent in primigravidas and is limited to the chronic stage, where it is seen in 59 percent of cases (fig. 5-41, right). The inflammatory infiltrate is composed of CD68-positive immature monocyte-macrophages, similar to those seen with idiopathic chronic histiocytic intervillositis (see below). The histologic findings in malaria which distinguish it from chronic histiocytic intervillositis (see below) include abundant perivillous fibrin, occasional neutrophils, focal syncytiotrophoblast necrosis, trophoblast basement membrane thickening, and malarial pigment.

Perinatal Infections with Minimal or No Placental Inflammation

Placental Infection without Inflammation. In several perinatal infections, organisms found in the intervillous space or syncytiotrophoblast are associated with fibrin deposition or necrosis, but little or no accompanying inflammation. Examples include infection from rubeola virus (measles) (80), *Schistosoma* sp (104), *Cryptococcus neoformans* (47), and *Borrelia burgdorferi* (Lyme disease) (25). Fetoplacental transmission in these circumstances is rare.

Transplacental infection refers to situations in which organisms cross the placenta and infect the fetus without eliciting an inflammatory response in the placenta. The most important

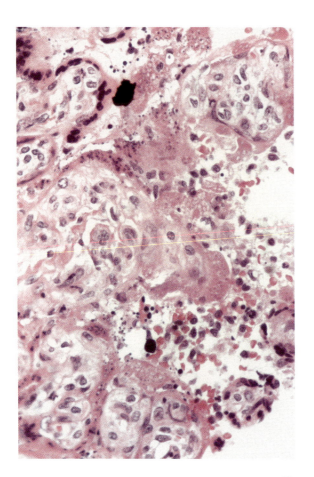
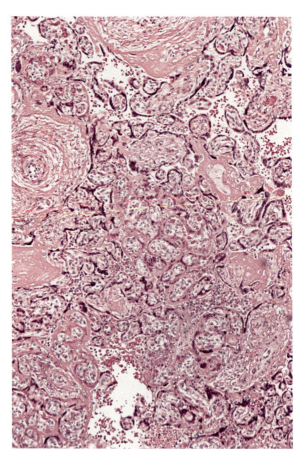

Figure 5-41

PLACENTAL MALARIA

There is a blue-black granular pigment in the intervillous space (left) with a background (right) of trophoblast necrosis, perivillous fibrin, and clusters of typical intervillous histiocytes. This 32-year-old Nigerian female at 33 weeks' pregnancy was admitted with anemia, chest pain, hypotension, and diaphoresis. Stillborn, growth restricted twins were delivered.

organisms spread by this route are parvovirus B19, human immunodeficiency virus, hepatitis viruses, and enteroviruses (14,58,61,72). The exact mode of transmission in transplacental infection is not known and may differ between organisms. Possible mechanisms include phagocytosis by villous macrophages, direct maternal-fetal blood transfusion following villous epithelial denudation, and receptor-mediated uptake by the syncytiotrophoblast. Although parvovirus B19 does not elicit inflammation within the placenta, placental pathology is an important adjunct to its diagnosis (see chapter 10, Fetal Anemias) (70).

Microscopic examination shows diffusely edematous and histologically immature villi, with a thick cellular layer of surrounding trophoblast. These features are shared by other causes of hydrops fetalis. Most useful is the finding of increased nucleated red blood cell precursors with pathognomonic intranuclear inclusions (see chapter 10, figs. 10-4, 10-5). PCR or immunocytochemistry can be performed on paraffin-embedded placental tissue for a definitive diagnosis (see fig. 10-6) (107).

Infections Acquired at Delivery. Another distinct group of perinatal infections are caused by organisms that do not involve the placenta, but are acquired by the infant during passage through an infected birth canal. This category includes many proportion of the neonatal infections caused by herpes simplex virus, group

B streptococci, and other highly virulent bacteria and fungi. Organisms whose perinatal transmission occurs exclusively by this route include *Neisseria gonorrhea* (conjunctivitis), *Chlamydia trachomatis* (pneumonia and conjunctivitis), *Mycoplasma hominis* (pneumonia), and human papilloma virus (tracheobronchial papillomatosis) (16). The prevention of many of these infections is facilitated by clinical testing algorhythms that may lead to antimicrobial treatment of the mother, avoidance of vaginal delivery, and screening of the newborn.

IDIOPATHIC INFLAMMATORY LESIONS

Chronic Villitis (Villitis of Unknown Etiology)

Definition. Lymphohistiocytic inflammation predominantly localized to the stroma of terminal villi, but often extending to the adjacent intervillous space and the small vessels of upstream stem villi.

Incidence. Villitis of unknown etiology (VUE) is a common lesion occurring in approximately 3 to 5 percent of all term placentas (50, 109). Involvement of placentas at less than 35 weeks is uncommon (Table 5-3).

Etiology. Hematogenous infection by some organism similar to those causing chronic placentitis of the TORCH type (see above) has been touted as the cause of VUE for many years. Despite the high prevalence of VUE and the many years of study, no causative organisms have been identified, no maternal infectious symptoms have been described, no seasonal or geographic pattern of occurrence has been shown, no neonatal inflammatory response has been found, and no infants have had documented congenital infection. Furthermore, VUE lacks many features of chronic infectious placentitis such as uniform involvement of villi, predominance of histiocytes, villous edema, villous plasma cells, fibrosis, mineralization, and prominent inflammation of the membranes and umbilical cord.

Immunohistochemical and in situ hybridization studies have shown that VUE represents a maternal immune response occurring within fetal tissue (54,55,100). The infiltrating maternal cells are primarily T lymphocytes. These observations suggest that VUE may be initiated by the chance entry of a small number of maternal lymphocytes into the antigenically foreign fetal villous stroma. Depending on the degree of intrinsic maternal alloreactivity and the local availability of costimulatory factors, a host versus graft–type response is initiated. In some cases, the magnitude of this response is sufficient to facilitate entry of lymphocytes into adjacent villi, eventually leading to recognizable disease (54). One possible adaptive advantage of the vigorous local response in VUE is to prevent maternal lymphocytes from entering the fetal circulation, a situation associated with severe failure to thrive in experimental animals and autoimmune diseases in humans (6).

Clinical Features. VUE is the most common placental lesion identified in nonhypertensive term pregnancies with significant fetal growth restriction (FGR) (53,99). The recurrence risk for diffuse villitis is 10 to 25 percent and women with recurrences are especially prone to severe FGR, premature delivery, and intrauterine fetal death. Cases of recurrent VUE are more commonly associated with maternal autoimmune disease, recurrent spontaneous abortion, and infertility (94,111). Empiric treatment for persistent fetal loss in association with recurrent VUE has included immunosuppressive agents such as progesterone, intravenous immunoglobulin, or corticosteroids. An association of VUE with elevated midtrimester maternal serum alpha-fetoprotein has been reported (113). Antenatal fetal monitoring abnormalities are more common in pregnancies with diffuse VUE (99). High-grade VUE is significantly more frequent in the placentas of term infants with cerebral palsy and other forms of neurologic impairment (see case presented in figure 5-42) (98).

Gross Findings. Placentas are often small for gestational age. There may be pale discoloration and irregular consolidation of the villous parenchyma in cases with severe involvement (fig. 5-43).

Microscopic Findings. The histologic extent of involvement and severity of VUE vary widely. Approximately two thirds of cases involve small clusters of 5 to 10 villi in either a single (focal) or multiple (multifocal) slides (figs. 5-44, 5-45). These low-grade patterns are usually clinically silent. The remaining cases are those with larger (more than 10 villi) foci (patchy) and those with diffuse involvement of all sections by groups of more than 10 inflamed villi (diffuse) (figs. 5-46, 5-47). These high-grade

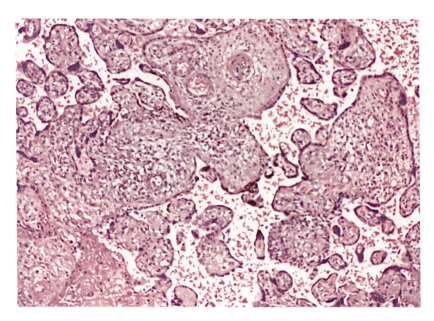

Figure 5-42

VILLITIS OF UNKNOWN ETIOLOGY

Clusters of chronically inflamed villi. This 27-year-old had a normal pregnancy. Decreased fetal movements were appreciated just prior to labor. Late decelerations resulted in an emergency cesarean section. Cord pH was 6.9. Neonatal seizures and poor growth and development occurred in the first 6 months of life.

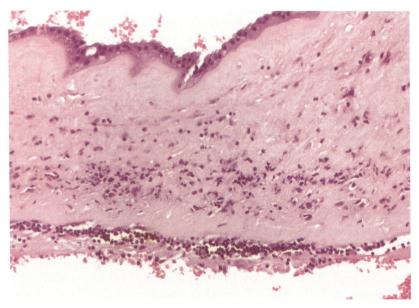

Figure 5-43

VILLITIS OF UNKNOWN ETIOLOGY

Chronic chorioamnionitis associated with the clusters in figure 5-42.

patterns have a strong relationship to FGR and other clinical complications. Other histologic features that may accompany VUE include decidual plasma cells, chronic chorioamnionitis, perivillous fibrin deposition, and avascular villi related to upstream villous vasculitis (figs. 5-48–5-50) (2). The latter pattern is particularly common in cases of later neurologic impairment (RWR, unpublished data, 2004).

CD3-positive T lymphocytes (fig. 5-51) and macrophages are the predominant cells. Occasional granulomatous foci with giant cells are common and are not indicative of infection (fig. 5-52). Acute (active) perivillitis may be a component of diffuse VUE (fig. 5-53). Its presence may in some cases be associated with infection (see above) and special stains for bacteria (Gram, Steiner, Dieterle, Warthin-Starry) should be considered.

Placentas in which involvement of anchoring villi (basal villitis) predominates represent a distinct subgroup of VUE (fig. 5-54). Basal villitis is more commonly associated with plasma cell deciduitis (47 percent compared to 19 percent

Inflammation and Infection

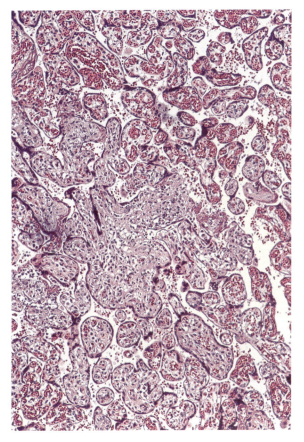

Figure 5-44

VILLITIS OF UNKNOWN ETIOLOGY, FOCAL

A single cluster of 5 to 10 villi with lymphocytic inflammation.

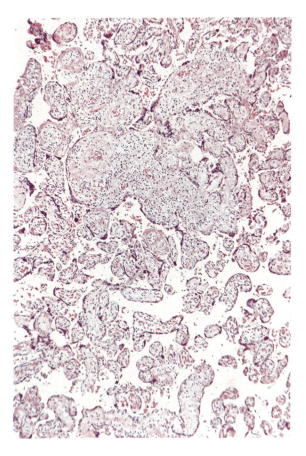

Figure 5-45

VILLITIS OF UNKNOWN ETIOLOGY, MULTIFOCAL

Widely scattered small clusters of partially agglutinated villi with lymphocytic infiltrate.

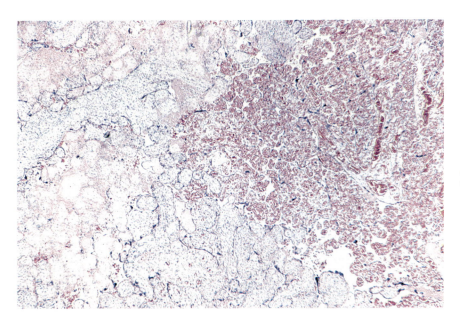

Figure 5-46

VILLITIS OF UNKNOWN ETIOLOGY, PATCHY

Large confluent zones of chronic inflammation and villous fibrosis.

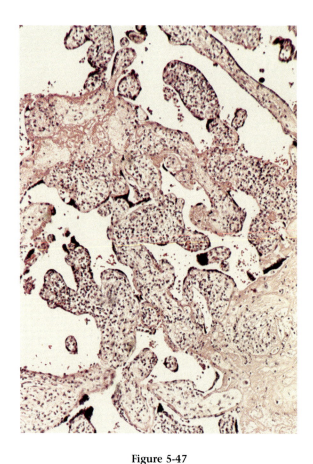

Figure 5-47

VILLITIS OF UNKNOWN ETIOLOGY, DIFFUSE
Chronically inflamed villi affected all placental regions sampled.

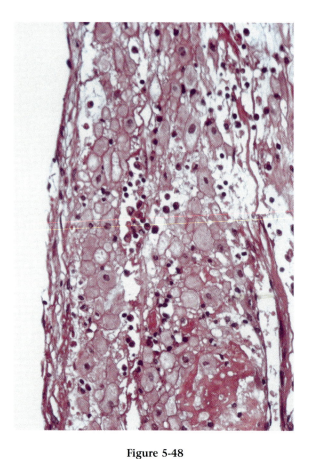

Figure 5-48

VILLITIS OF UNKNOWN ETIOLOGY WITH DECIDUAL PLASMA CELLS
A chronic decidual infiltrate shows definitive plasma cells with cartwheel nuclei, perinuclear halos, and eccentric purple cytoplasm.

Figure 5-49

VILLITIS OF UNKNOWN ETIOLOGY WITH EXTENSIVE PERIVILLOUS FIBRIN DEPOSITION

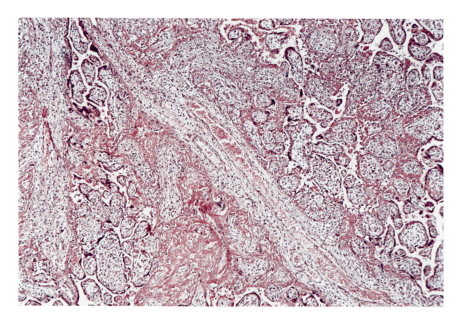

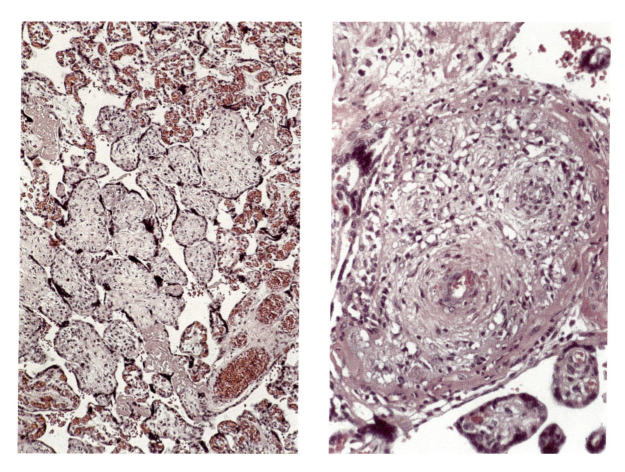

Figure 5-50

VILLITIS OF UNKNOWN ETIOLOGY WITH AVASCULAR VILLI

Villi may become avascular due to direct inflammatory damage (left) or upstream vascular occlusion secondary to chronic stem villous vasculitis (right).

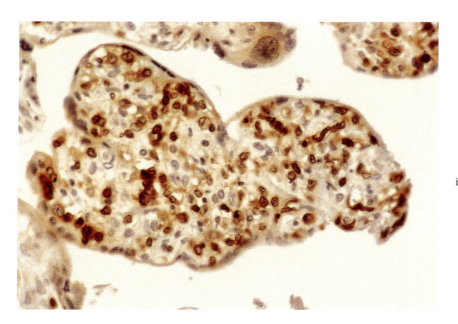

Figure 5-51

VILLITIS OF UNKNOWN ETIOLOGY, CD3 IMMUNOSTAIN

CD3-positive T lymphocytes in a terminal villus.

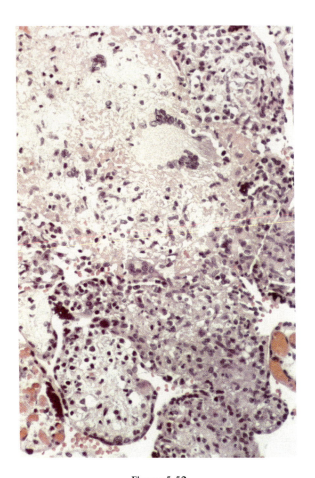

Figure 5-52

VILLITIS OF UNKNOWN ETIOLOGY WITH MULTINUCLEATE HISTIOCYTES

Foci of granulomatous inflammation with giant cells.

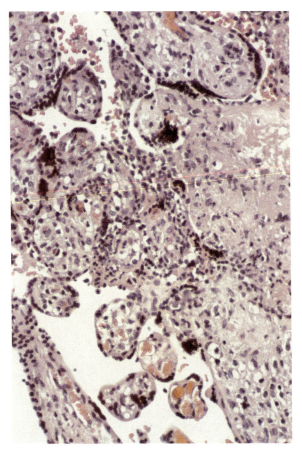

Figure 5-53

VILLITIS OF UNKNOWN ETIOLOGY, ACTIVE, WITH ASSOCIATED INTERVILLOSITIS

Otherwise typical villitis of unknown etiology with occasional neutrophils and involvement of the intervillous space.

Figure 5-54

CHRONIC BASAL VILLITIS

Chronic inflammation of basal anchoring villi in contiguity with decidua basalis. This pattern is usually associated with decidual plasma cells.

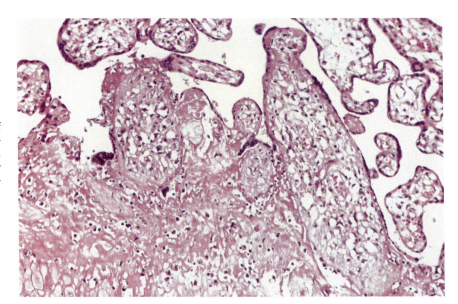

for all VUE) and has been associated with a past history of upper and lower genital tract infections (94). The prevalence of different histologic subtypes of villitis at the MacDonald Women's Hospital is shown in Table 5-3.

Chronic (Histiocytic) Intervillositis (Massive Chronic Intervillositis)

Definition. Chronic (histiocytic) intervillositis is the diffuse infiltration of the intervillous space by a monomorphic population of CD68-positive monocyte-macrophages, accompanied by a variable component of perivillous matrix-type fibrinoid containing intermediate trophoblast (12,22,44,52,79,82,119).

Incidence. This idiopathic lesion is most common in spontaneous abortions. In one study the overall prevalence in the first trimester was 9.6 in 1,000 pregnancies. The prevalence was higher in abortions with a normal karyotype (22 in 1,000) and in women with recurrent spontaneous abortions (80 in 1,000). The lesion is much less common in the second and third trimesters (0.6 in 1,000) (12,103).

Etiology. The marked similarity to placental malaria suggests that monocyte-macrophages accumulate in the intervillous space secondary to the inappropriate expression of adhesion molecules on the syncytiotrophoblast. Possibly relevant is the experimentally demonstrated upregulation of the adhesion molecule ICAM-1 on the syncytiotrophoblast in response to gamma-interferon and other inflammatory cytokines (124).

Clinical Features. Chronic (histiocytic) intervillositis is associated with recurrent spontaneous abortion, FGR, and intrauterine fetal death. The overall perinatal mortality rate is extremely high (77 percent in one study) and only 18 percent of all pregnancies in affected mothers reach the third trimester (12). A relationship with maternal autoimmune disease and other immunoregulatory abnormalities has been suggested. Uncontrolled trials have reported positive results using immunosuppressive therapy (37).

Gross and Microscopic Findings. Placentas are often small for gestational age. Microscopically, the pathognomonic finding is a uniform intervillous infiltrate of histiocytic cells of monocyte-macrophage lineage (fig. 5-55). Virtually all of the infiltrating cells express CD68 (fig. 5-56) and a significant minority express

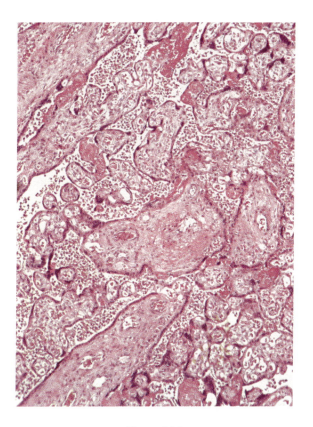

Figure 5-55

CHRONIC HISTIOCYTIC INTERVILLOSITIS (MASSIVE CHRONIC INTERVILLOSITIS)

Third trimester placenta with diffuse infiltration of the intervillous space by a uniform population of immature monocyte-macrophages in the absence of malarial pigment or chronic villitis.

Mac387, a marker for immature monocyte-macrophages (12). Cases with chronic villitis or a polymorphous intervillous inflammatory infiltrate are excluded from this category. Perivillous matrix-type fibrinoid with intermediate trophoblast is seen to a variable extent and is most common in the first trimester (fig. 5-57).

Chronic Chorioamnionitis

Definition. Chronic chorioamnionitis is the infiltration of the placental membranes by small lymphocytes and other chronic inflammatory cells with, at most, a minor component of neutrophils.

Incidence. Chronic chorioamnionitis is rare and overlaps with other inflammatory lesions. Two small series with a total of 48 cases have been reported (28,43).

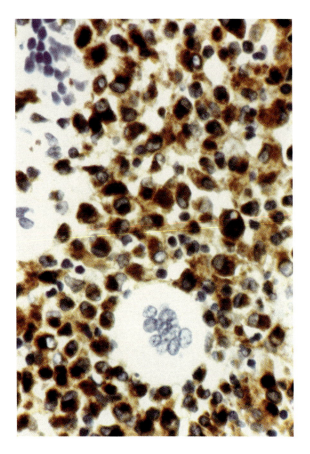

Figure 5-56

CHRONIC HISTIOCYTIC INTERVILLOSITIS (MASSIVE CHRONIC INTERVILLOSITIS), CD68 STAIN

Almost all intervillous inflammatory cells stain for CD68, a monocyte-macrophage marker.

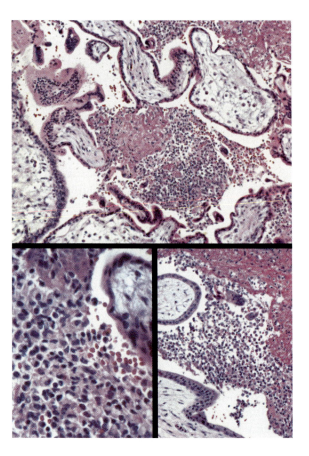

Figure 5-57

CHRONIC HISTIOCYTIC INTERVILLOSITIS (MASSIVE CHRONIC INTERVILLOSITIS)

Composite demonstrating the typical pattern of involvement in first trimester cases, which is generally accompanied by prominent perivillous fibrin deposition.

Etiology. The etiology is unknown, but the lesion is commonly found either in association with VUE (79 percent of cases) or with evidence of longstanding ascending infection (premature rupture of membranes, maternal fever, neutrophils, significant fetal vasculitis).

Clinical Features. In the limited number of reported cases, there are a variety of associated antenatal findings including hypertension, diabetes, hydrops, FGR, and oligohydramnios. Premature labor and delivery are common.

Gross and Microscopic Findings. No typical gross lesions have been described. Cases are separated into two groups. One is characterized by focal chronic inflammation of the membranes only. The second tends to have a more polymorphous inflammatory infiltrate, including neutrophils that involve other anatomic compartments such as amnion, chorionic plate, and fetal vessels (fig. 5-58). This latter pattern overlaps with subacute chorioamnionitis (described above).

Chronic Deciduitis

Definition. Chronic deciduitis is an accumulation of small lymphocytes, with or without plasma cells, in the decidualized endometrium of the basal plate (46).

Incidence. In our experience, an abnormal infiltrate of small lymphocytes in the decidua basalis is seen in 12 percent of spontaneous abortions, 11 percent of preterm deliveries, and 3 percent of term deliveries. Plasma cells are identified in 6 percent of spontaneous abortions, 8 percent of preterm deliveries, and 2

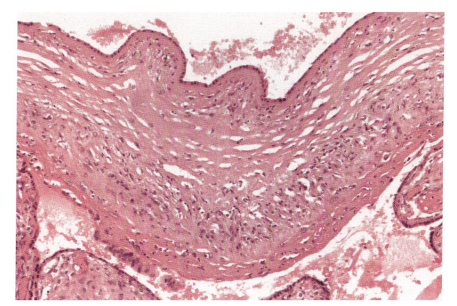

Figure 5-58

CHRONIC CHORIOAMNIONITIS

Chronic inflammation and fibrosis of the chorionic plate and overlying amnion.

percent of term births (Table 5-3) (103). Heavy infiltration of lymphocytes in the decidua basalis was reported in 1 to 2 percent of all third trimester placentas examined in the Collaborative Perinatal Project (77).

Etiology. Unlike many other mucosal organs, most leukocyte subsets (with the exception of natural killer cells) are not found in normal endometrium. Chronic inflammation, and particularly including plasma cells, is considered to be a sign of inappropriate antigenic stimulation (10,93). Chronic inflammatory responses may be directed against maternal autoantigens, fetal alloantigens, developmental oncofetal proteins, or microorganisms (56).

Clinical Features. Chronic deciduitis with plasma cells in the absence of other placental lesions is reported in 3 to 4 percent of placentas from very low birth weight infants and may be a distinct cause of preterm labor (114). Two other common placental lesions sometimes associated with chronic deciduitis are acute chorioamnionitis in preterm placentas and VUE at term. Subclinical bacterial endometritis has been suggested as a cause for the former and a local immune response to fetal antigens for the latter (94).

Gross and Microscopic Findings. No specific gross features accompany chronic deciduitis. Chronic deciduitis of the basal plate has been recently defined as either the presence of plasma cells (see fig. 5-48) or diffuse chronic inflammation without plasma cells (fig. 5-59). Focal or multifocal inflammation without plasma cells has been excluded from this category. The association of chronic deciduitis with plasma cells with VUE is strong, and the finding of even a single plasma cell should elicit a careful search for VUE in the overlying placenta.

Eosinophilic/T-Cell Vasculitis

Definition. This is a fetally-derived chronic inflammatory infiltrate composed of eosinophils and small lymphocytes within the muscular wall of chorionic and primary stem villous vessels, sometimes associated with mild luminal narrowing due to a subendothelial cellular proliferative reaction.

Incidence. In the one published study, the prevalence of this lesion was 1.97 in 1,000 examined placentas (26).

Etiology. This idiopathic lesion has the characteristics typical of a TH2 delayed-type hypersensitivity response (as opposed to a TH1 cell-mediated immune response) (91). Immune responses with this character are often dominated by the cytokines IL-4 and IL-5, a characteristic pattern in the fetus and neonate (87). Eosinophil-rich infiltrates have been linked to elevated IL-5 levels (19,68). While no specific clinical associations have been made, most of the reported cases had either maternal or fetal abnormalities.

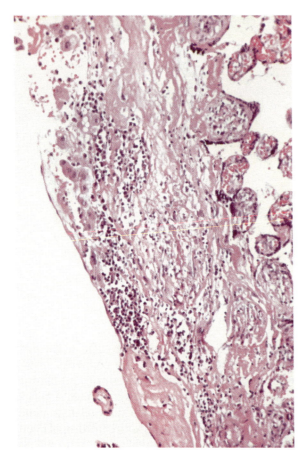

Figure 5-59

CHRONIC DECIDUITIS

Diffuse involvement of the decidua basalis by a lymphocytic infiltrate, with or without plasma cells.

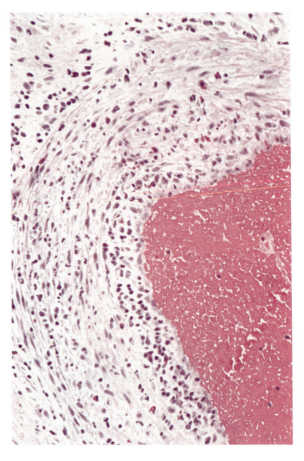

Figure 5-60

EOSINOPHILIC/T-CELL VASCULITIS

A fetal infiltrate composed of eosinophils and small lymphocytes in the muscular wall of a chorionic plate vessel. There is mild vessel narrowing and a subendothelial cellular proliferative reaction.

Gross and Microscopic Findings. No typical gross features have been described. Microscopic features are as described above and are illustrated in figure 5-60.

Chronic Decidual Periarteritis

A perivascular infiltrate of small lymphocytes and histiocytes surrounding small arteries in the membranes and basal plate is seen in placentas with evidence of maternal vascular underperfusion (fig. 5-61). This occurs particularly in those with a history of preeclampsia and idiopathic FGR (112).

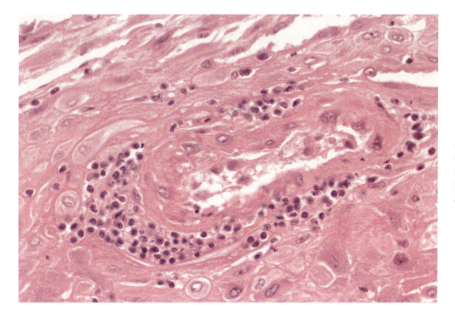

Figure 5-61

CHRONIC DECIDUAL PERIVASCULITIS

Maternal arterioles in the placental membranes have activated endothelial cells, an accentuated vessel wall matrix, and a periarterial infiltrate of large granular and small lymphocytes.

REFERENCES

1. Abramowsky C, Beyer-Patterson P, Cortinas E. Nonsyphilitic spirochetosis in second-trimester fetuses. Pediatr Pathol 1991;11:827–38.
2. Altemani AM. Decidual inflammation in villitis of unknown aetiology. Placenta 1992;13:89–98.
3. Altshuler G, Hyde SR. Fusobacteria. An important cause of chorioamnionitis. Arch Pathol Lab Med 1985;109:739–43.
4. Altshuler G, Russell P. The human placental villitides: a review of chronic intrauterine infection. Curr Top Pathol 1975;60:64–112.
5. Aquino TI, Zhang J, Kraus FT, et al. Subchorionic fibrin culture for bacteriologic study of the placenta. Am J Clin Pathol 1984;81:482–6.
6. Artlett CM, Ramos R, Jiminez SA, Patterson K, Miller FW, Rider LG. Chimeric cells of maternal origin in juvenile idiopathic inflammatory myopathies. Childhood Myositis Heterogeneity Collaborative Group. Lancet 2000;356:2155–6.
7. Baker C, Kasper D. Correlation of maternal antibody deficiency with susceptibility to neonatal group B streptococcal infection. N Engl J Med 1976;294:753–6.
8. Beer AE, Billingham RE. The immunobiology of mammalian reproduction. Englewood Cliffs, N.J.: Prentice Hall Inc.; 1976.
9. Bendon RW, Bornstein S, Faye-Petersen OM. Two fetal deaths associated with maternal sepsis and with thrombosis of the intervillous space of the placenta. Placenta 1998;19:385–9.
10. Bendon RW, Miller M. Routine pathological examination of placentae from abnormal pregnancies. Placenta 1990;11:369–70.
11. Blanc W. Pathology of the placenta and cord in ascending and haematogenous infections. In: Marshall W, ed. Perinatal infections, CIBA Foundation Symposium 77. London: Excerpta Medica; 1980:17–38.
12. Boyd TK, Redline RW. Chronic histiocytic intervillositis: a placental lesion associated with recurrent reproductive loss. Hum Pathol 2000;31:1389–96.
13. Burgess AM, Hutchins GM. Inflammation of the lungs, umbilical cord and placenta associated with meconium passage in utero. Review of 123 autopsied cases. Pathol Res Pract 1996;192:1121–8.
14. Caul EO, Usher MJ, Burton PA. Intrauterine infection with human parvovirus B19: a light and electron microscopy study. J Med Virol 1988;24:55–66.
15. Coid CR, Fox H. Short review: campylobacters as placental pathogens. Placenta 1983;4:295–305.
16. Cowles T, Gonik B. Perinatal infections. In: Fanaroff AA, Martin R, eds. Neonatal-perinatal medicine. St. Louis, MO: Mosby; 1997:327–49.
17. Dammann O, Durum S, Leviton A. Do white cells matter in white matter damage? Trends Neurosci 2001;24:320–4.
18. Dammann O, Leviton A. Maternal intrauterine infection, cytokines, and brain damage in the preterm newborn. Pediatr Res 1997;42:1–8.

19. Dent LA, Strath M, Mellor AL, Sanderson CJ. Eosinophilia in transgenic mice expressing interleukin 5. J Exp Med 1990;172:1425–31.
20. Dexter SC, Pinar H, Malee MP, Hogan J, Carpenter MW, Vohr BR. Outcome of very low birth weight infants with histopathologic chorioamnionitis. Obstet Gynecol 2000;96:172–7.
21. Diagne N, Rogier C, Sokhna C, et al. Increased susceptibility to malaria during the early postpartum period. N Engl J Med 2000;343:598–603.
22. Doss BJ, Greene MF, Hill J, et al. Massive chronic intervillositis associated with recurrent abortions. Hum Pathol 1995;26:1245–51.
23. Driscoll SG, Gorbach A, Feldman D. Congenital listeriosis: diagnosis from placental studies. Oncologia 1962;20:216–20.
24. Elliott WG. Placental toxoplasmosis. Report of a case. Am J Clin Pathol 1970;53:413–7.
25. Figueroa R, Bracero LA, Aguero-Rosenfeld M, Beneck D, Coleman J, Schwartz I. Confirmation of Borrelia burgdorferi spirochetes by polymerase chain reaction in placentas of women with reactive serology for Lyme antibodies. Gynecol Obstet Invest 1996;41:240–3.
26. Fraser RB, Wright JR. Eosinophilic/T-cell chorionic vasculitis. Pediatr Dev Pathol 2002;5:350–5.
27. Friedland JS, Jeffrey I, Griffin GE, Booker M, Courtenay-Evans R. Q fever and intrauterine death. Lancet 1994;343:288.
28. Gersell DJ, Phillips NJ, Beckerman K. Chronic chorioamnionitis: a clinicopathologic study of 17 cases. Int J Gynecol Pathol 1991;10:217–29.
29. Goldenberg R, Hauth J, Andrews W. Intrauterine infection and preterm delivery. N Engl J Med 2000;342:1500–7.
30. Gomez B, Romero R, Ghezzi F, Yoon BH, Mazor M, Berry SM. The fetal inflammatory response syndrome. Am J Obstet Gynecol 1998;179:194–202.
31. Greenough A. The TORCH screen and intrauterine infections. Arch Dis Child 1994;70:F163–5.
32. Guleria I, Pollard J. The trophoblast is a component of the innate immune system during pregnancy. Nat Med 2000;6:589–93.
33. Guyatt HL, Snow RW. Malaria in pregnancy as an indirect cause of infant mortality in sub-Saharan Africa. Trans R Soc Trop Med Hyg 2001;95:569–76.
34. Heifetz S, Bauman M. Necrotizing funisitis and herpes simplex infection of placental and decidual tissues. Hum Pathol 1994;25:715–22.
35. Henneke P, Takeuchi O, van Strijp JA, et al. Novel engagement of CD14 and multiple toll-like receptors by group B streptococci. J Immunol 2001;167:7069–76.
36. Hill GB. Preterm birth: associations with genital and possibly oral microflora. Ann Periodontol 1998;3:222–32.
37. Hill JA, Melling GC, Johnson PM. Immunohistochemical studies of human uteroplacental tissues from first-trimester spontaneous abortion. Am J Obstet Gynecol 1995;173:90–6.
38. Hillier SL, Martius J, Krohn M, Kiviat N, Holmes KK, Eschenbach DA. A case-control study of chorioamnionic infection and histologic chorioamnionitis in prematurity. N Engl J Med 1988;319:972–80.
39. Hood IC, DeSa DJ, Whyte RK. The inflammatory response in candidal chorioamnionitis. Hum Pathol 1983;14:984–90.
40. Hood M, Todd JM. Vibrio fetus—a cause of human abortion. Am J Obstet Gynecol 1960;80:506–11.
41. Hyde SR, Benirschke K. Gestational psittacosis: case report and literature review. Mod Pathol 1997;10:602–7.
42. Ismail MR, Ordi J, Menendez C, et al. Placental pathology in malaria: a histological, immunohistochemical and quantitative study. Hum Pathol 2000;31:85–93.
43. Jacques S, Qureshi F. Chronic chorioamnionitis: a clinicopathologic and immunohistochemical study. Hum Pathol 1998;29:1457–61.
44. Jacques SM, Qureshi F. Chronic intervillositis of the placenta. Arch Pathol Lab Med 1993;117:1032–5.
45. Keenan WJ, Steichen JJ, Mahmood K, Altshuler G. Placental pathology compared with clinical outcome. Am J Dis Child 1977;131:1224–7.
46. Khong TY, Bendon RW, Qureshi F, et al. Chronic deciduitis in the placental basal plate: definition and inter-observer reliability. Hum Pathol 2000;31:292–5.
47. Kida M, Abramowsky CR, Santoscoy C. Cryptococcosis of the placenta in a woman with acquired immunodeficiency syndrome. Hum Pathol 1989;20:920–1.
48. Kim CJ, Yoon BH, Romero R, et al. Umbilical arteritis and phlebitis mark different stages of the fetal inflammatory response. Am J Obstet Gynecol 2001;185:496–500.
49. Knowles S, Frost T. Umbilical cord sclerosis as an indicator of congenital syphilis. J Clin Pathol 1989;42:1157–9.
50. Knox WF, Fox H. Villitis of unknown aetiology: its incidence and significance in placentae from a British population. Placenta 1984;5:395–402.
51. Kundsin RB, Driscoll SG, Monson RR, Yeh C, Biano SA, Cochran WD. Association of ureaplasma urealyticum in the placenta with perinatal morbidity and mortality. N Engl J Med 1984;310:941–5.

52. Labarrere C, Mullen E. Fibrinoid and trophoblastic necrosis with massive chronic intervillositis: an extreme variant of villitis of unknown etiology. Am J Reprod Immunol Microbiol 1987;15:85–91.
53. Labarrere CA, Althabe O, Telenta M. Chronic villitis of unknown aetiology in placentae of idiopathic small for gestational age infants. Placenta 1982;3:309–18.
54. Labarrere CA, McIntyre JA, Page Faulk W. Immunohistologic evidence that villitis in human normal term placentas is an immunologic lesion. Am J Obstet Gynecol 1990;162:515–22.
55. Labarrere CA, Faulk W. Maternal cells in chorionic villi from placentae of normal and abnormal human pregnancies. Am J Reprod Immunol 1995;33:54–9.
56. Lachapelle MH, Miron P, Hemmings R, et al. Endometrial T, B, and NK cells in patients with recurrent spontaneous abortion. Altered profile and pregnancy outcome. J Immunol 1996;156:4027–34.
57. Langston C, Kaplan C, Macpherson T, et al. Practice guideline for examination of the placenta. Arch Pathol Lab Med 1997;121:449–76.
58. Lapointe N, Michaud J, Pekovic D, Chausseau JP, Dupuy JM. Transplacental transmission of HTLV-III virus. N Engl J Med 1985;312:1325–6.
59. Leviton A, Paneth N, Reuss ML, et al. Maternal infection, fetal inflammatory response, and brain damage in very low birth weight infants. Developmental Epidemiology Network Investigators. Pediatr Res 1999;46:566–75.
60. Lin H, Mosmann TR, Guilbert L, et al. Synthesis of T helper 2-type cytokines at the maternal-fetal interface. J Immunol 1993;151:4562.
61. Lin HH, Lee TY, Chen DS, et al. Transplacental leakage of HBeAg-positive maternal blood as the most likely route in causing intrauterine infection with hepatitis B virus. J Pediatr 1987;111:877–81.
62. Locksmith G, Clark P, Duff P. Maternal and neonatal infection rates with three different protocols for prevention of group B streptococcal disease. Am J Obstet Gynecol 1999;180:416–22.
63. MacGregor I. Epidemiology, malaria, and pregnancy. Am J Trop Med Hyg 1984;33:517–25.
64. Mascola L, Ewert D, Eller A. Listeriosis: a previously unreported medical complication in women with multiple gestations. Am J Obstet Gynecol 1994;170:1328–32.
65. Matsuda T, Nakajima T, Hattori S, et al. Necrotizing funisitis: clinical significance and association with chronic lung disease in premature infants. Am J Obstet Gynecol 1997;177:1402–7.
66. Maubert B, Guilbert LJ, Deloron P. Cytoadherence of Plasmodium falciparum to intercellular adhesion molecule 1 and chondroitin-4-sulfate expressed by the syncytiotrophoblast in the human placenta. Infect Immun 1997;65:1251–7.
67. McElrath T, Allred EN, Leviton A. Prolonged latency after premature rupture of membranes does not increase the risk of neonatal brain damage. Am J Obstet Gynecol 2002;187(Suppl):S66.
68. Mishra A, Hogan SP, Brandt EB, Rothenberg ME. IL-5 promotes eosinophil trafficking to the esophagus. J Immunol 2002;168:2464–9.
69. Miyano A, Miyamichi T, Nakayama M, Kitajima H, Shimizu A. Effect of chorioamnionitis on the levels of serum proteins in the cord blood of premature infants. Arch Pathol Lab Med 1996;120:245–8.
70. Morey AL, Keeling JW, Porter HJ, Fleming KA. Clinical and histopathological features of parvovirus B19 infection in the human fetus. Br J Obstet Gynaecol 1992;99:566–74.
71. Morgan B, Holmes C. Immunobiology of reproduction: protecting the placenta. Curr Biol 2000;10:R381–3.
72. Mostoufizadeh M, Lack EE, Gang DL, Perez-Atayde AR, Driscoll SG. Postmortem manifestations of echovirus 11 sepsis in five newborn infants. Hum Pathol 1983;14:818–23.
73. Mostoufi-zadeh M, Driscoll SG, Biano SA, Kundsin RB. Placental evidence of cytomegalovirus infection of the fetus and neonate. Arch Pathol Lab Med 1984;108:403–6.
74. Mueller-Heubach E, Rubinstein DN, Schwarz SS. Histologic chorioamnionitis and preterm delivery in different patient populations. Obstet Gynecol 1990;75:622–6.
75. Munn DH, Zhou M, Attwood JT, et al. Prevention of allogeneic fetal rejection by tryptophan metabolism. Science 1998;281:1191–3.
76. Naeye RL. Coitus and associated amniotic fluid infections. N Engl J Med 1979;301:1198–200.
77. Naeye RL. Functionally important disorders of the placenta, umbilical cord, and fetal membranes. Hum Pathol 1987;18:680–91.
78. Nelson KB, Dambrosia JM, Grether JK, Phillips TM. Neonatal cytokines and coagulation factors in children with cerebral palsy. Arch Neurol 1998;44:665–75.
79. Nijhuis EW, van Nort G. Clinicopathological correlations in chronic intervillositis. Pediatr Dev Pathol 1998;1:457.
80. Ohyama M, Fukui T, Tanaka Y, et al. Measles virus infection in the placenta of monozygotic twins. Mod Pathol 2001;14:1300–3.
81. Ohyama M, Itani Y, Yamanaka M, et al. Re-evaluation of chorioamnionitis and funisitis with a special reference to subacute chorioamnionitis. Hum Pathol 2002;33:183–90.

82. Ordi J, Ismail MR, Ventura PJ, et al. Massive chronic intervillositis of the placenta associated with malaria infection. Am J Surg Pathol 1998;22:1006–11.
83. Ornoy A, Dudai M, Sadovsky E. Placental and fetal pathology in infectious mononucleosis. Diagn Gynecol Obstet 1982;4:11–6.
84. Pankuch GA, Appelbaum PC, Lorenz RP, Botti JJ, Schachter J, Naeye RL. Placental microbiology and histology and the pathogenesis of chorioamnionitis. Obstet Gynecol 1984;64:802–6.
85. Piper J, Newton E, Berkus M, Peairs W. Meconium: a marker of peripartum infection. Obstet Gynecol 1998;91:741–5.
86. Pouvelle B, Buffet P, LePolard C, Scherf A, Gysin J. Cytoadhesion of Plasmodium falciparum ring-stage-infected erythrocytes. Nat Med 2000;6:1264–8.
87. Prescott SL, Macaubas C, Holt BJ, et al. Transplacental priming of the human immune system to environmental allergens: universal skewing of initial T cell responses toward the Th2 cytokine profile. J Immunol 1998;160:4730–7.
88. Qureshi F, Jacques S. Maternal varicella during pregnancy: correlation of maternal history and fetal outcome with placental histopathology. Hum Pathol 1996;27:191–5.
89. Qureshi F, Jacques SM, Benson RW, et al. Candida funisitis: a clinicopathologic study of 32 cases. Pediatr Dev Pathol 1998;1:118–24.
90. Qureshi F, Jacques SM, Reyes MP. Placental histopathology in syphilis. Hum Pathol 1993;24:779–84.
91. Redline R. Clinically and biologically relevant patterns of placental inflammation. Pediatr Dev Pathol 2002;5:326–8.
92. Redline RW. Recurrent villitis of bacterial etiology. Pediatr Pathol 1996;16:995–1002.
93. Redline RW. Role of uterine natural killer cells and interferon-gamma in placental development. J Exp Med 2000;192:F1–4.
94. Redline RW, Abramowsky CR. Clinical and pathologic aspects of recurrent placental villitis. Hum Pathol 1985;16:727–31.
95. Redline R, Faye-Peterson O, Heller D, Qureshi F, Savell V, Vogler C. Amniotic infection syndrome: nosology and reproducibility of placental reaction patterns. Pediatr Dev Pathol 2003;2003;6:435–48.
96. Redline RW, Lu CY. The role of local immunosuppression in murine fetoplacental listeriosis. J Clin Invest 1987;79:1234–41.
97. Redline RW, Lu CY. Specific defects in the antilisterial immune response in discrete regions of the murine uterus and placenta account for susceptibility to infection. J Immunol 1988;140:3947–55.
98. Redline RW, O'Riordan MA. Placental lesions associated with cerebral palsy and neurologic impairment following term birth. Arch Pathol Lab Med 2000;124:1785–91.
99. Redline RW, Patterson P. Patterns of placental injury: correlations with gestational age, placental weight, and clinical diagnosis. Arch Pathol Lab Med 1994;118:698–701.
100. Redline RW, Patterson P. Villitis of unknown etiology is associated with major infiltration of fetal tissue by maternal inflammatory cells. Am J Pathol 1993;143:473–9.
101. Redline RW, Wilson-Costello D, Borawski E, Fanaroff AA, Hack M. Placental lesions associated with neurologic impairment and cerebral palsy in very low birth weight infants. Arch Pathol Lab Med 1998;122:1091–8.
102. Redline R, Wilson-Costello D, Borawski E, Fanaroff A, Hack M. The relationship between placental and other perinatal risk factors for neurologic impairment in very low birth weight children. Pediatr Res 2000;47:721–6.
103. Redline RW, Zaragoza MV, Hassold T. Prevalence of developmental and inflammatory lesions in non-molar first trimester spontaneous abortions. Hum Pathol 1999;30:93–100.
104. Renaud R, Brettes P, Castanier C, Loubiere R. Placental bilharziasis. Int J Gynaecol Obstet 1972;10:24–30.
105. Ricci JM, Fojaco RM, O'Sullivan MJ. Congenital syphilis: The University of Miami/Jackson Memorial Medical Cente Experience, 1986-1988. Obstet Gynecol 1989;74:687–93.
106. Rogers BB, Alexander JM, Head J, McIntire D, Leveno KJ. Umbilical vein interleukin-6 levels correlate with the severity of placental inflammation and gestational age. Hum Pathol 2002;33:335–40.
107. Rogers BB, Rogers ZR, Timmons CF. Polymerase chain reaction amplification of archival material for parvovirus B19 in children with transient erythroblastopenia of childhood. Pediatr Pathol Lab Med 1996;16:471–8.
108. Rosenberg HS, Bernstein J. Perspectives in pediatric pathology, Vol. 6. Infectious diseases. New York: Masson Publ USA Inc.; 1981.
109. Russell P. Inflammatory lesions of the human placenta. Placenta 1980;1:227–44.
110. Russell P, Altshuler G. Placental abnormalities of congenital syphilis. Am J Dis Child 1974;128:160–3.
111. Russell P, Atkinson K, Krishnan L. Recurrent reproductive failure due to severe villitis of unknown etiology. J Reprod Med 1980;24:93–8.

112. Salafia C, Pezzullo J, Ghidini A, Lopez-Zeno J, Whittington S. Clinical correlations of patterns of placental pathology in preterm pre-eclampsia. Placenta 1998;19:67–72.
113. Salafia C, Silberman L, Herrera N, Mahoney M. Placental pathology at term associated with elevated midtrimester serum alpha-fetoprotein concentration. Am J Obstet Gynecol 1988;158:1064–6.
114. Salafia CM, Vogel CA, Vintzileos AM, Bantham KF, Pessulo J, Silberman L. Placental pathologic findings in preterm birth. Am J Obstet Gynecol 1991;165:934–8.
115. Seeliger H. Listeriosis. New York: Hafner; 1961.
116. Smulian JC, Shen-Schwarz S, Vintzileos AM, Lake MF, Ananth CV. Clinical chorioamnionitis and histologic placental inflammation. Obstet Gynecol 1999;94:1000–5.
117. Southwick F, Purich D. Intracellular pathogenesis of listeriosis. N Engl J Med 1996;334:770–6.
118. Uckan D, Steele A, Cherry B, et al. Trophoblasts express Fas ligand: a proposed mechanism for immune privilege in placenta and maternal invasion. Molec Hum Reprod 2000;3:655–62.
119. Valderrama E. Massive chronic intervillositis: report of three cases [Abstract]. Lab Invest 1992;66:10P.
120. Van Hoeven KH, Anyaegbunam A, Hochster H, et al. Clinical significance of increasing histologic severity of acute inflammation in the fetal membranes and umbilical cord. Pediatr Pathol Lab Med 1996;16:731–44.
121. Vawter GF. Perinatal listeriosis. Perspect Pediatr Pathol 1981;6:153–66.
122. Walter PR, Garin Y, Blot P. Placental pathologic changes in malaria. Am J Pathol 1982;109:330–42.
123. Watterberg KL, Demers L, Scott SM, Murphy S. Chorioamnionitis and early lung inflammation in infants in whom bronchopulmonary dysplasia develops. Pediatrics 1996;97:210–5.
124. Xiao J, Garcia LG, Winklerlowen B, et al. ICAM-1-mediated adhesion of peripheral blood monocytes to the maternal surface of placental syncytiotrophoblasts: implications for placental villitis. Am J Pathol 1997;150:1845–60.
125. Yoon BH, Jun JK, Romero R, et al. Amniotic fluid inflammatory cytokines (interleukin-6, interleukin-1 beta, and tumor necrosis factor-alpha), neonatal brain white matter lesions, and cerebral palsy. Am J Obstet Gynecol 1997;177:19–26.
126. Yoon BH, Romero R, Kim M, et al. Clinical implications of detection of Ureaplasma urealyticum in the amniotic cavity with the polymerase chain reaction. Am J Obstet Gynecol 2000;183:1130–7.
127. Yoon BH, Romero R, Yang SH, et al. Interleukin-6 concentrations in umbilical cord plasma are elevated in neonates with white matter lesions associated with periventricular leukomalacia. Am J Obstet Gynecol 1996;174:1433–40.
128. Zhang JM, Kraus FT, Aquino TI. Chorioamnionitis: a comparative histologic, bacteriologic, and clinical study. Int J Gynecol Pathol 1985;4:1–10.

6 CIRCULATORY PROBLEMS: THROMBI AND OTHER VASCULAR LESIONS

INTRODUCTION

Interruptions of the maternofetal circulatory exchange by extensive thrombi or vascular narrowing, affecting the vessels between the uterine arteries of the mother and the umbilical vascular branchings in the fetus, introduce the risk of reduced placental function. Decidual vasculopathy is included here because lesions of this type can initiate the process of thrombosis, resulting in placental ischemia and infarcts. In addition to their direct effects on blood flow, instances of vascular occlusion by thrombi of any size also indicate a predisposition to significant injury in either the mother, fetus, or both by somatic thrombi elsewhere in their circulations, secondary to a thrombophilic state.

A balance between factors that favor coagulation and fibrinolysis is necessary for homeostasis. Pregnancy itself tends to shift the balance toward thrombosis. Within the placenta, the expression of a phospholipid binding protein, annexin V, at the syncytiotrophoblast surface, normally inhibits clotting in the intervillous space (74). Pathologic states such as autoimmune diseases (74,75) and preeclampsia (104), which appear to interfere with this system, also promote clotting in the intervillous space. Clotting in the fetal circulation of the placenta may be the result of a local or systemic thrombophilic shift in the coagulation balance (5,52).

Most adults with thrombi secondary to thrombophilic states do not die of pulmonary emboli. Similarly, not all women with thrombophilias have pregnancies complicated by preeclampsia, abruption, miscarriage, or fetal growth restriction, nor do all of the newborns in this context have the placental lesions described below (65). However, there is a high prevalence of thrombotic lesions of all the types in the placentas of women with thrombophilias (70), especially in women whose thrombophilias have not been treated, and the number of injured fetuses without treatment is increased (5). The fact that some or even many fetuses are not injured does not reduce the importance of thrombi and thrombophilic states in fetuses that are affected permanently. More refined clinicopathologic studies will ultimately clarify the prevalence of fetal injuries in the context of placental thrombi and suggest clinical approaches to alleviate their devastating effects.

Circulatory Relationships in the Placenta and the Varied Effects of Intraplacental Clotting

The vascular anatomy of the placenta, with its double circulation (see chapter 1), is complex. Both the appearance and the deleterious effects of clots or fibrin deposition depend on whether they are located in the fetal or the maternal compartment. As an aid to understanding the descriptions that follow, the normal circulation of maternal blood from vessels in the uterus to and from the intervillous space, and fetal blood through the umbilical vessels, is displayed in figure 6-1. A magnified diagram of spiral arteries, comparing normal arteries with those that are focally narrowed, as in preeclampsia, is shown in figure 6-2.

Figures 6-3 and 6-4 illustrate the types of grossly evident distortion produced by the different types of hematoma referred to in the text that follows. Other forms of clotting in the intervillous space (infarct and perivillous fibrin deposit) and in thrombi in fetal vessels are represented and contrasted with the appearance of the hematomas in figure 6-5.

While the intervillous space is clearly not a blood vessel, it does bridge the gap between maternal blood flow into the placenta and maternal venous return from the placenta. For this reason, clots and other events within it are relevant in a vascular context and are therefore included here.

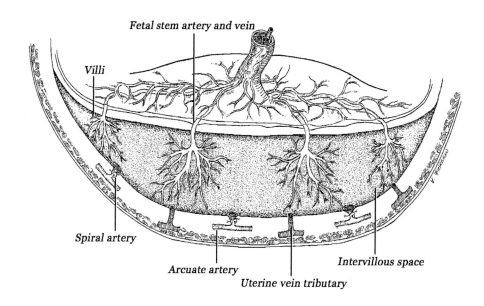

Figure 6-1

NORMAL FETAL AND MATERNAL CIRCULATORY RELATIONSHIPS

Fetal blood enters the placenta through umbilical arteries in the umbilical cord. These arteries branch and rebranch into capillaries in the villi and fetal blood returns through vein tributaries into the umbilical vein, which empties through the ductus venosus of the fetus into the fetal vena cava. Maternal arterial blood in the arcuate artery branches of the uterine artery enters the intervillous space of the placenta in spurts through approximately 60 to 70 spiral arteries distributed around the placental floor. Maternal blood then drains back into the maternal venous system through uterine vein tributaries distributed in a similar way in the placental floor.

MATERNAL CIRCULATION: THROMBI, HEMATOMAS, AND DECIDUAL VASCULAR LESIONS

Decidual Vasculopathy: Acute Atherosis and Spiral Artery Thrombi

Definition. Decidual vasculopathy describes a group of related pathologic changes in the spiral arteries of the maternal decidua, including failure to complete the physiologic change sequence, necrosis (acute atherosis), and thrombosis, either mural or occlusive.

Incidence. Acute atherosis, the main form of decidual vasculopathy, is associated with a failure of the physiologic sequences of spiral artery enlargement (see chapter 1) and is found in about half of placentas of women with preeclampsia. This probably underestimates its frequency, because spiral arteries are often difficult to find in the decidua attached to the membranes or placental floor even under normal conditions. Preeclampsia has a prevalence of 10 to 14 percent in primiparous (105) and 5 to 7 percent in multiparous pregnant women in a population of relatively high-risk women (106), but the frequency is somewhat less in the general population. The prevalence of thrombotic occlusion of normally developed spiral arteries is unknown, but occlusions of spiral arteries are more frequently observed in maternal thrombophilic states (76).

Clinical Features. Acute atherosis is one of the pathologic correlates of the poorly understood syndrome of preeclampsia, or toxemia of pregnancy (see chapter 3). This lesion may also occur in placentas of women with lupus erythematosus and scleroderma (25), the antiphospholipid antibody syndrome (55), and small for gestational age infants, with or without maternal hypertension (86). Thus, acute atherosis does not occur in all cases of preeclampsia, and all placentas with acute atherosis do not necessarily cause maternal hypertension.

Severe preeclampsia has been associated with a variety of maternal thrombophilic (38,54, 72,112,113,116) and antifibrinolytic (43) states.

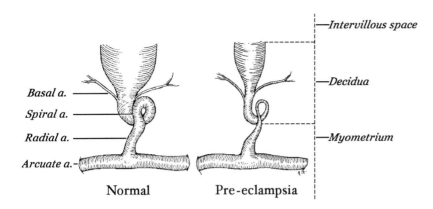

Figure 6-2

NORMAL FETAL AND MATERNAL CIRCULATORY RELATIONSHIPS

A magnified image of a normal spiral artery which has widened extensively into a funnel-shaped structure is at the left. Small basal arterioles supply the surrounding decidua. The narrow spiral artery at the right indicates the mechanical basis for the decreased maternal blood flow into the placental intervillous space that occurs in preeclampsia.

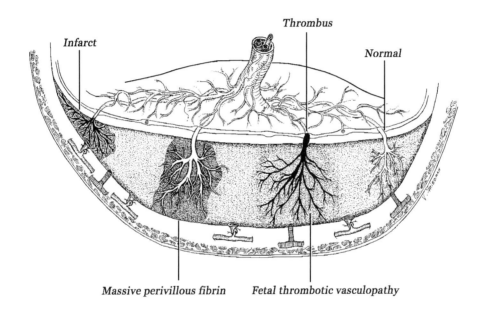

Figure 6-3

CIRCULATORY ALTERATIONS THAT OCCUR IN ASSOCIATION WITH DIFFERENT CLOTTING LESIONS

An infarct, at left, forms as a result of an occlusion or reduced flow through spiral arteries in the placental floor. The intervillous space usually collapses so that the villi are closer to each other, with a mixture of fibrin and red blood cells between them. Massive perivillous fibrin deposits, in contrast, actually appear to expand the intervillous space, which contains only masses of fibrin but no red blood cells. Thrombosis of a fetal stem vessel propagates or causes stasis throughout the fetal arterial branches or fetal venous tributaries peripheral to it. The intervillous space between the affected villi appears normal, and the villous trophoblast, still nourished by the maternal circulation, survives, while the villous capillaries disappear and the villous stroma becomes fibrotic.

A genetic predisposition appears to be transmitted, both paternally and maternally (71). The angiotensinogen gene, Thr235, may be involved in abnormal vascular remodeling of the spiral arteries (64). Maternal endothelial dysfunction, apparently based on oxidative stress, is commonly present (20), even in the nonpregnant state long after delivery (13), and can be reversed by the administration of ascorbic acid, an antioxidant (13). This endothelial dysfunction may be the result of a reduction in available vascular endothelial growth factor (VEGF) and placental growth factor (PlGF), caused by the up-regulation of soluble fms-like tyrosine kinase 1 (sFlt 1) (60).

Decidual vasculopathy causes a reduction in uteroplacental blood flow, as measured by the

Placental Pathology

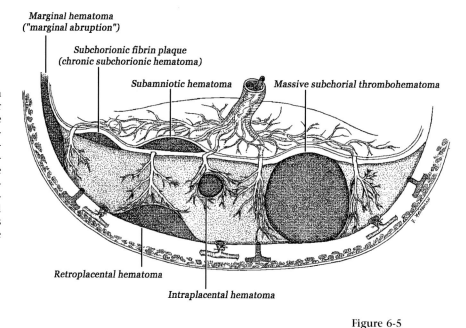

Figure 6-4

HEMATOMAS IN DIFFERENT LOCATIONS

The expanding hematoma compresses adjacent softer placental structures; the more rigid myometrium is not compressed locally by a retroplacental hematoma. Intraplacental hematomas are identified only by examination of cut surfaces of placental sections, and small lesions are not found unless the slices are reasonably close together (about 1.0 cm).

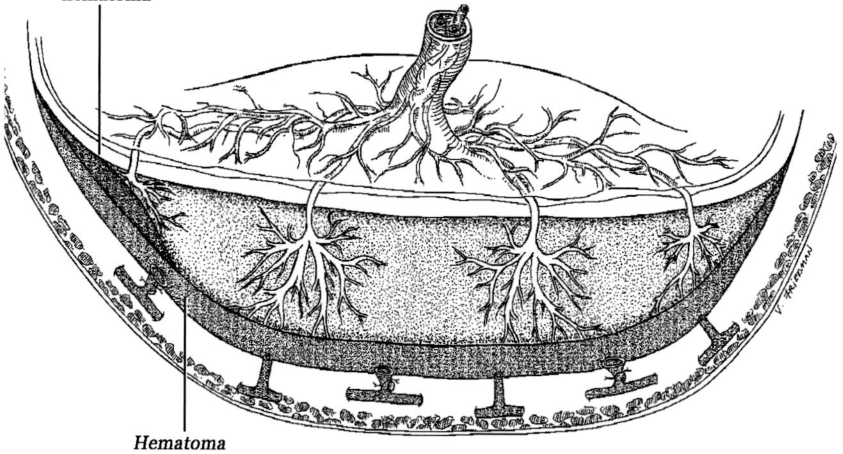

Figure 6-5

COMPLETE PLACENTAL SEPARATION

Complete placental separation is associated with a layer of recent clot covering the entire placental floor. The placenta itself has no localized deformity unless an older, usually marginal hematoma is present. While a marginal hematoma is not always evident, such a lesion is almost never visible on external inspection, and is easily overlooked. A complete abruption is always difficult and sometimes impossible to demonstrate unless the clot is provided to the pathologist. It is unlikely to be discovered by a pathologist who has not been informed of the clinical circumstances and is thereby prompted to look in the specimen for subtle abnormalities.

technique of Doppler velocimetry (59). The result is relative placental ischemia, causing the syndrome of preeclampsia, and, in some cases, fetal growth restriction (1). The preeclampsia syndrome (defined in chapter 3) occurs not only in the context of decidual vasculopathy, but also in patients with hydatidiform mole and other forms of a greatly enlarged placental mass, including multiple gestations, diabetes, and hydropic placentas (80).

Thrombosis in normally developed spiral arteries occurs in women with thrombophilic states (51,76). Significant infarction may occur in the regions of the placenta supplied by such occlusions.

Gross Findings. Placentas associated with acute atherosis and preeclampsia may be of normal size, but are often smaller than average, below the 10th percentile for placental weight, when the manifestations of the syndrome are severe. Infarcts (described below) are common, also somewhat in proportion to severity, producing multiple areas of nodular induration (fig. 6-6).

Microscopic Findings. An adequate blood supply to the growing placenta depends upon the normal physiologic widening that allows for ever increasing blood flow through the spiral arteries in the maternal decidua basalis. This evolution is incomplete in preeclampsia (35, 46,84), and as a result, the spiral arteries remain disproportionately narrow. Smooth muscle cells of the vascular media persist, and the enlarging placenta is underperfused (see fig. 6-2). The abnormal spiral arteries are predisposed to develop acute atherosis (fig. 6-7A,B), characterized by mural fibrinoid necrosis and the accumulation of large, foamy, lipid-filled macrophages and neutrophils (46,84,118). Occlusive and mural thrombi are common (fig. 6-7C). Ultrastructural studies of the placental bed vessels show endothelial injury (99).

In some cases of preeclampsia, diabetes, or idiopathic intrauterine growth retardation decidual arterioles show mural hypertrophy similar to the changes seen with renal arteriolosclerosis (fig. 6-8). These cases may represent abnormal vascular remodeling related to local renin-angiotensin imbalance. This was correlated with abnormal uterine artery Doppler studies in diabetics (6). The term *hypertrophic decidual vasculopathy,* or simply thick-walled decidual arterioles, may be used in this context. The expression decidual vasculopathy is intended to include all of the foregoing vascular abnormalities. In placentas with decidual vasculopathy there is often persistence of smooth muscle in the spiral arteries (absence of physiologic change) and an increase in the amount of immature, proliferating, intermediate trophoblast in the implantation site beneath the placenta (fig. 6-9) (80).

Distinctive alterations are common in the villi of placentas associated with maternal preeclampsia and other states of maternal vascular underperfusion. The syncytiotrophoblastic nuclei in preeclampsia often aggregate into tight clusters (fig. 6-10) called *trophoblastic,* or *syncytial, knots* (also known as *Tenney-Parker change.* The placental stem villi in preeclampsia are often slender with reduced branching, and terminal villi are very small, producing a stunted or atro-

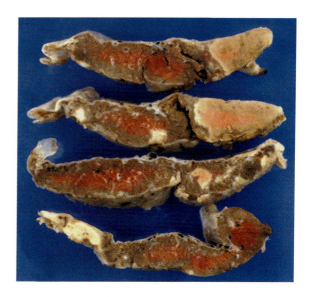

Figure 6-6

INFARCTS

Gross appearance of a placenta at 25 weeks with decidual vascular changes of acute atherosis. Placental weight is below the 10th percentile. The presence of multiple chronic infarcts, which are pale tan or gray-white firm areas, is common. The mother had severe preeclampsia. The light brown infarcts at the right in the upper two sections are of intermediate age, perhaps 7 to 10 days, while that at left in the lower cross section is old and completely depigmented, 2 to 3 weeks old, or more.

phic-appearing pathologic pattern. This combination of findings has been called *accelerated maturation* (fig. 6-11, compare with fig. 6-12).

A better term than accelerated maturation for the reduction in villous size and villous capillaries, which better describes the findings in recent detailed anatomic studies of preeclampsia with more severe growth restriction and absent or reversed end-diastolic flow, is *distal villous hypoplasia.* These villi are much smaller than normal mature villi in cross section, with reduced stroma, and capillaries are reduced in number. Prominent trophoblastic knots are most apparent when villous size and vascularity are closer to normal; this pattern is less likely to be associated with growth restriction, and may represent a form of adaptation (110). Ultrastructural studies of such villi confirm focal necrosis of syncytiotrophoblast with loss of microvilli and other degenerative changes attributable to ischemia (39).

Figure 6-7

ACUTE ATHEROSIS

A: Histologic appearance of a decidual spiral artery with multiple cross sections of the same vessel altered by changes of acute atherosis. The necrotic vessel walls have a dense eosinophilia. The lumen in some loops of the vessel is thrombosed.

B: Spiral artery in a section of membrane roll, with acute atherosis. The accumulations of large foamy macrophages and fibrin are also seen in C.

C: Acute atherosis in severe preeclampsia. The vessel wall is necrotic, and the lumen is nearly occluded by fibrin. There is a prominent accumulation of intermediate trophoblast cells at the lower right corner.

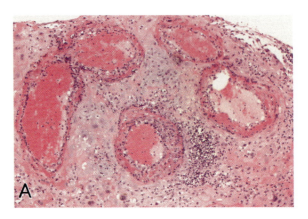

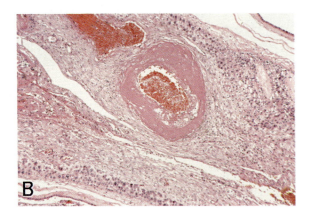

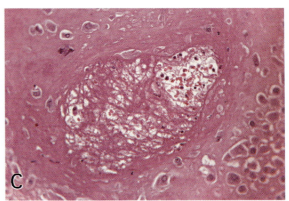

Figure 6-8

HYPERTROPHIC DECIDUAL VASCULOPATHY

This decidual spiral artery is very narrow. It presents multiple loops in cross section, and has a thick wall composed of smooth muscle cells which are normally absent at this stage (29th week) of pregnancy. The mother had severe preeclampsia and diabetes mellitus. The fetus had growth restriction and developed peri-ventricular leukomalacia. (Figs. 6-8 and 6-10 are from the same patient.)

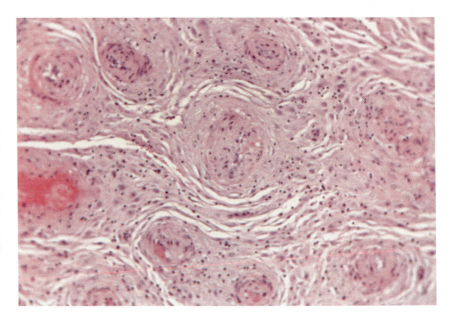

Villi just beneath the chorionic plate in a normal placenta usually have features similar to distal villous hypoplasia. For this reason, the terms distal villous hypoplasia and accelerated maturation should be reserved for changes located in the normally better perfused centrolobular regions and adjacent to the entrance of the spiral arteries from the decidual basalis.

Circulatory Problems: Thrombi and Other Vascular Lesions

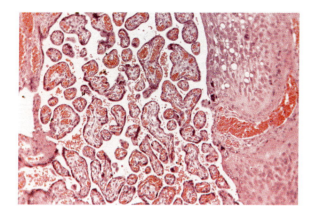

Figure 6-9

PREECLAMPSIA

Persistent smooth muscle in a narrow basal plate artery is seen at right. The superficial implantation site has increased immature intermediate trophoblast.

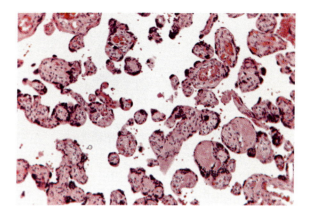

Figure 6-10

TROPHOBLASTIC KNOTS

Placental villi in preeclampsia shows trophoblastic knots, also called Tenney-Parker change. There is marked variation in villous diameters, with focal formation of tight adherent villous clusters.

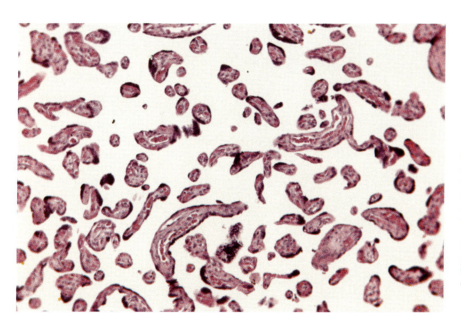

Figure 6-11

ACCELERATED MATURATION (DISTAL VILLOUS HYPOPLASIA, PERIPHERAL VILLOUS HYPOPLASIA)

Placental villi in severe preeclampsia at 30 weeks' gestation show an accelerated maturation pattern. Many terminal villi are extremely small, stem villi are slender with reduced branching, and trophoblast nuclei of many villi are clustered, forming trophoblastic knots. The weight of this placenta, 145 g, was well below the 10th percentile at 30 weeks. Compare with figure 6-12.

Differential Diagnosis. The inflammation associated with decidual infections may produce localized decidual vasculitis, with or without thrombosis, which may be confused with the milder inflammatory features of acute atherosis. The inflammatory infiltrate of infection is more heterogeneous and prominent, and includes plasma cells and larger numbers of neutrophils.

Prognosis. Pregnancy outcome depends on the clinical factors associated with the specific clinical diagnosis (see chapter 3).

Infarcts

Definition. A placental infarct is a localized region of ischemic necrosis of villi, which becomes surrounded by coagulated blood (see fig. 6-3). The term *villous infarct* is sometimes used (88).

Incidence. Small infarcts (less than 3 cm) are found in as many as one fourth of placentas from uncomplicated pregnancies. They are more frequent in placentas associated with maternal hypertension; for example, about two

Placental Pathology

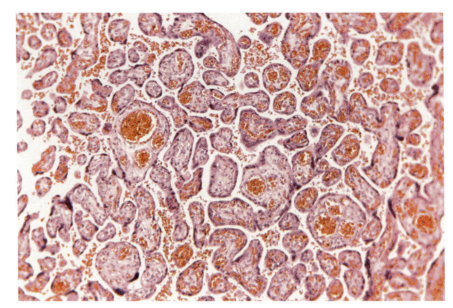

Figure 6-12

NORMAL VILLI AT 30 WEEKS

More normal-appearing immature villi at 30 weeks' gestation, for comparison with accelerated maturation in figure 6-11. Villous diameters are larger, stroma is more abundant, and syncytiotrophoblast nuclei are more evenly distributed.

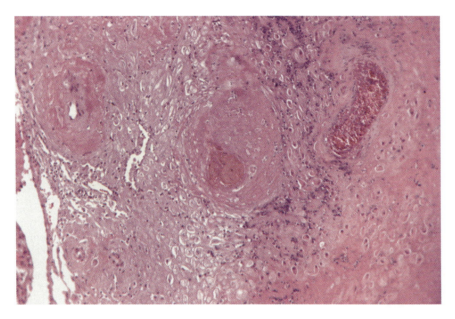

Figure 6-13

DECIDUAL SURFACE OF PLACENTA IN PREECLAMPSIA

The thrombosed spiral artery at the center is occluded by a recent thrombus. The adjacent placenta at right is infarcted.

thirds of placentas from preeclamptic women have infarcts.

Clinical Features. Placental infarcts occur when maternal blood flow through the spiral arteries is insufficient. Localized failure of uteroplacental blood flow may result from a reduction in perfusion pressure, especially in regions with spiral artery narrowing or occlusion (figs. 6-13–6-15). Multiple spiral arteries must usually be affected because there is often overlap in placental regions supplied by adjacent vessels. Occlusion of a small upstream uterine artery branch could also affect multiple spiral arteries in its area of distribution.

A small infarct of less than 3 cm in diameter near the placental margin is a common occurrence, and as an isolated finding has no clinical significance. In contrast, any more centrally located infarct in a placenta prior to term should be regarded as abnormal and potentially an indication of suboptimal placental function. Infarcts larger than 3 cm and multiple infarcts, especially in the context of gestational abnormalities, indicate a significant probability of an interruption

Circulatory Problems: Thrombi and Other Vascular Lesions

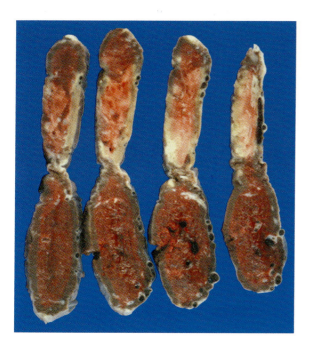

Figure 6-14

PLACENTAL INFARCTS, RECENT AND INTERMEDIATE

The lighter contracted region at top in all cross sections is a large, partly depigmented infarct of intermediate age, about 7 to 10 days. The ill-defined somewhat lighter red region around the dark red hematomas at bottom is a recent infarct, probably 3 to 5 days. The mother had severe preeclampsia. The placental weight was below the 10th percentile and the newborn was growth restricted.

in uteroplacental blood supply, and are unlikely to be the only pathologic lesions present. Infarcts involving as much as 50 percent of the placental mass cause a significant reduction of placental function, and may be enough to cause hypoxia and intrauterine fetal death. These adverse effects are further potentiated if the placenta is small, below the 10th percentile, for the gestational age. There is a consistent positive correlation between infarcts and maternal thrombophilias (57), and with intrauterine growth restriction, in both term (90) and preterm (88) infants.

Gross Findings. Infarcts are circumscribed and firmer than the adjacent placenta. They are dark red at first and become pale and indurated with age. Any estimation of the age of a placental infarct from its appearance is necessarily crude because there are no signs or symptoms to signal the time of its inception. Estimates such as recent (1 to 7 days), older (7 to 14 days), and old (2 weeks or more) infarcts are based upon analogy

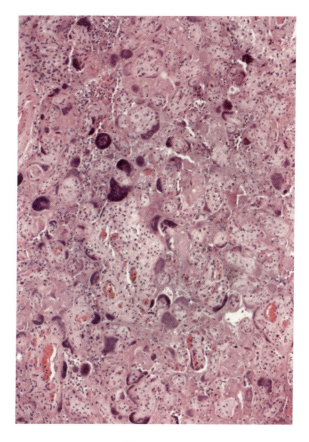

Figure 6-15

RECENT PLACENTAL INFARCT

The trophoblast nuclei are clustered (trophoblastic knots) and necrotic, with clumped, partly dispersed DNA; the intervillous space has collapsed; and the villi are adherent, glued together by strands of fibrin. The mother had severe preeclampsia.

or comparison with the evolution of changes in infarcts in somatic organs of adults. Recent infarcts are red and only slightly indurated, with a homogeneous or solid-appearing cut surface because the villi have become agglutinated by the thin layer of clot between them (figs. 6-6, 6-14). Because they closely resemble the normal placenta, even large recent infarcts are easily overlooked, but are somewhat easier to detect after partial fixation in formalin. Older infarcts are more indurated and demarcated, and become progressively brown, tan, and finally white as the hemoglobin within them is degraded (figs. 6-6, 6-14). The cut surface of infarcts at any stage of evolution is finely granular, reflecting the presence of villi, in contrast to hematomas, which have a more glassy, laminated cut surface.

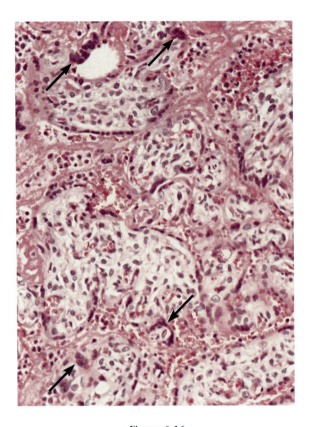

Figure 6-16

RECENT PLACENTAL INFARCT

In this recent infarct caused by retroplacental hematoma there are prominent trophoblastic knots (arrows) and minimal separation of villi by strands of fibrin and blood cells. The mother had a 10-year history of disseminated lupus erythematosus.

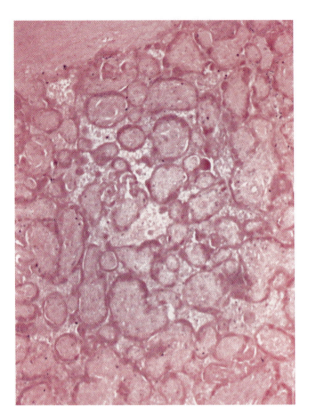

Figure 6-17

OLD CHRONIC PLACENTAL INFARCT

The intervillous space is collapsed, and the villi are crowded together, with virtual disappearance of nuclear DNA. This is consistent with a duration of 2 to 3 weeks or more.

Microscopic Findings. All of the affected tissues and cells in the infarcted zone become necrotic. Villi in an acute infarct are crowded together and attached to one another by strands of fibrin (figs. 6-15, 6-16). The extreme ischemia also produces prominent trophoblastic knots. The nuclear membranes of all trophoblast, stromal, and endothelial cells disappear and the chromatin progressively clumps into amorphous masses, eventually disappearing in old, chronic infarcts. Ultimately, all that remains is an acellular pink area in which the villous outlines are barely discernable (fig. 6-17). There is no fibroblastic ingrowth. Phagocytosis of necrotic cells, organization, and fibroblastic scarring, as observed in cardiac or splenic infarcts, do not occur.

Differential Diagnosis. The villi in an infarct are collapsed together, and all cellular and nuclear material disappears, while the villi in massive perivillous fibrin deposits are more widely separated by the fibrin matrix, which is consistently intermixed with living mononuclear extravillous (intermediate) trophoblast cells (see figs. 6-38–6-44). Intraplacental hematomas (intervillous thrombi) are composed only of blood clot, which has a laminated appearance and a smooth glassy cut surface, having expanded and pushed the villi apart (figs. 6-18–6-20).

Prognosis. Fetal injury caused by infarcts depends upon their size and number relative to the amount of functionally healthy placental tissue. Effects on the mother depend on the underlying medical problem responsible for the infarct, such as preeclampsia, coagulopathy, or collagen-vascular disease.

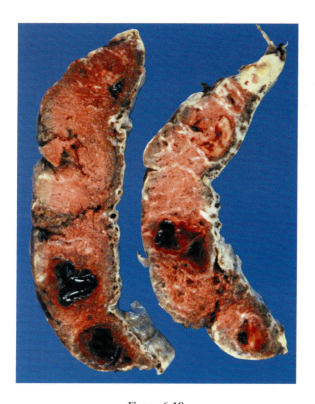

Figure 6-18

RECENT INTRAPLACENTAL HEMATOMAS

The dark red clots with glassy cut surfaces in the lower half of these placental slices have expanded and pushed the villi apart. The narrow strands of pale material toward the top in the slice on the right are perivillous fibrin. A small chronic infarct is present at the top margin of the slice on the right.

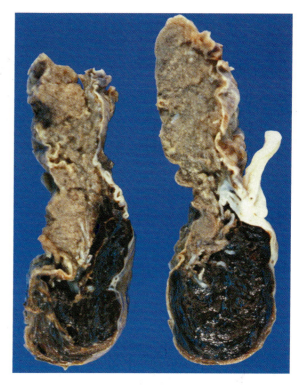

Figure 6-19

ACUTE MASSIVE SUBCHORIAL HEMATOMA

The clot extends from the chorionic plate to the placental floor. It more than doubled the placental mass. Sudden intrauterine fetal death occurred at 23 weeks.

Intraplacental Hematomas (Intervillous Thrombi) and Massive Subchorial Hematomas

Definition. Intraplacental hematomas are localized, circumscribed clots in the maternal intervillous space (see fig. 6-4). Fresh examples, as in figure 6-18, have sometimes been called *Kline's hemorrhages*, an unnecessary distinction with no specific significance.

Incidence. Small (1 to 2 cm) intraplacental hematomas are common, and identified in 36 (30) to 48 percent (115) of placentas.

Clinical Features. Hematomas of the intervillous space are usually innocuous when small and few in number. Although most of the blood in a hematoma is maternal, most hematomas appear to form at the site of a leak in the fetal circulation, which causes the adjacent maternal blood to form an expanding clot. When hematomas are numerous, they may be associated with significant fetal-maternal hemorrhage. Fetal anemia may result, leading to underperfusion in the fetal circulation and ultimately to end-organ damage, placentofetal hydrops, and stillbirth. Fetal-maternal hemorrhage can be evaluated quantitatively by the Kleihauer-Betke test (see below) or flow cytometry (18), and by demonstrating fetal erythrocytes in the hematomas (44).

Massive subchorial hematomas (formerly called *Breus mole*) produce a catastrophic reduction in placental function, resulting in abortion of early gestations or sudden intrauterine fetal death in the second and third trimesters (98). Heller et al. (41) have demonstrated an association between subchorionic hematomas and inherited thrombophilias.

Gross Findings. Recent intraplacental hematomas are dark red and may have a layered or laminated appearance (figs. 6-18, 6-19). Older lesions evolve through shades of brown to gray and white as the hemoglobin is degraded (fig. 6-20). Massive

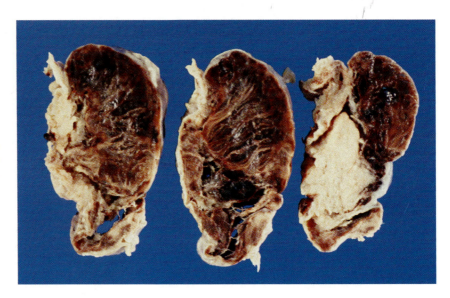

Figure 6-20

RECENT AND CHRONIC MASSIVE INTRAPLACENTAL HEMATOMA

The white area in the specimen at the right is an old chronic infarct. Intrauterine fetal death occurred about 1 week before delivery at 15 weeks. Note the layered appearance of the clot. The fetus was macerated.

subchorial hematomas are large, often laminated, clots which significantly distort the placental architecture by displacing the villi and forming an expansile mass, often extending from chorionic plate to the decidua basalis (figs. 6-19, 6-20).

Microscopic Findings. The clot pushes the villi apart, forming a cavity filled with blood and surrounded by villi (fig. 6-21A,B). Some clots have a layered appearance in which strata of erythrocytes alternate with platelets and fibrin. The adjacent villi are thrust aside and compressed by the expanding margins of the clot. Older clots become depigmented in time, as infarcts do. Fibroblastic organization does not occur. Infarction of surrounding villi is common. Most of the blood is of maternal origin. The presence of a component of fetal red blood cells may be demonstrated by immunohistochemical stains for fetal hemoglobin (44).

The Kleihauer-Betke test is employed to estimate the amount of fetal blood in the maternal circulation. It is based on the greater solubility of adult hemoglobin at pH 3.0. An air-dried smear of maternal blood is fixed in 80 percent alcohol, eluted by buffer at an appropriate pH, and stained with hematoxylin and eosin. The fetal red blood cells stain darkly, while the maternal red blood cells are pale (fig. 6-21C). Assuming an average maternal blood volume of 5,000 mL, maternal hematocrit of 35, and fetal hematocrit of 45, if one counts 40 fetal red blood cells per 1,000 maternal red blood cells, the estimated volume of fetal blood lost into the maternal circulation is $40/1{,}000 \times 35/45 \times 5{,}000 = 155$ mL. Various approaches to improving accuracy have been presented (8). Currently, the flow cytometry approach may prove superior (18).

Differential Diagnosis. Other nodular areas of induration with similar color changes and variations include infarcts, perivillous fibrin deposits, chorangiomas, and in rare instances, intraplacental choriocarcinomas. The presence of villi or other tissue within the lesion excludes hematomas, which are composed only of degenerating blood clot.

Prognosis. The impact of hematomas on the fetus depends upon their size, location, and effect on placental function. The possibility of significant of fetal blood loss should be considered, especially when multiple intraplacental hematomas cause fetomaternal hemorrhage and fetal anemia (fig. 6-21).

Retroplacental Hematomas, Marginal Hematomas, and Placental Abruption

Definition. Retroplacental hematomas are clots, recent or chronic, situated in the decidua between the placental floor and the muscular wall of the uterus (see fig. 6-4). Placental abruption refers to the clinically symptomatic state, in the mother, of premature placental separation, with pain, bleeding, and progressive accelerated uterine enlargement. Symptomatic placental separation may often be sudden and extensive, and even complete detachment may occur (see fig. 6-5). The two terms are often used interchange-

Circulatory Problems: Thrombi and Other Vascular Lesions

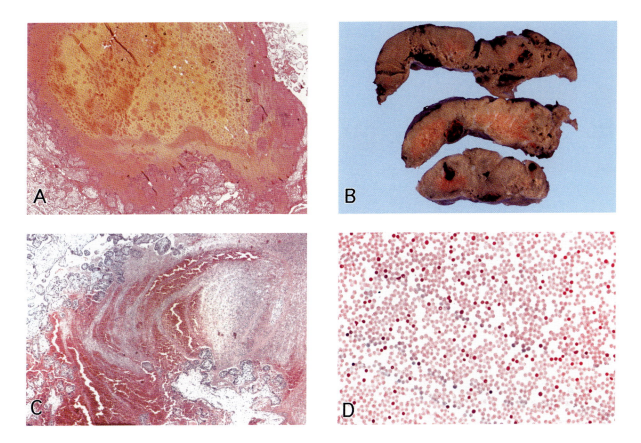

Figure 6-21

INTRAPLACENTAL HEMATOMA

A: Villi are spread apart by the expanding clot. Central lysis of red blood cells and degraded hemoglobin result in the yellow discolored center of the clot.

B: Multiple small intraplacental hematomas, more than 15, were present in this placenta associated with severe fetal-maternal hemorrhage and intrauterine fetal death.

C: Histologic appearance of an intraplacental hematoma. The villi, which were edematous, have been pushed to the left. Nucleated red blood cells were present in large numbers in fetal vessels. The Kleihauer-Betke test indicated a fetal-maternal hemorrhage of more than 150 mL. The fetus was stillborn and appeared pale.

D: Representative slide from a Kleihauer-Betke test. The fetal red blood cells stain darkly, while the maternal cells are pale, after elution with an acidic pH. See description of the technique in the text.

ably, an unfortunate practice that easily leads to confusion between a clinical diagnosis with grave implications and a demonstrated pathologic lesion that is less threatening when small.

Incidence. In 1987 the national rate of clinically symptomatic abruption was 11.5 in 1,000 live births (85). Incidence figures for all retroplacental hematomas of any size or location (central or marginal) relative to number of live births are not available; Fox (30) and Benirschke (8) found retroplacental hematomas of various sizes and ages in approximately 4 percent of placentas submitted for evaluation. This is probably an underestimate because many retroplacental hematomas are easily overlooked or not submitted for examination.

Clinical Features. Small hematomas in the decidual layer occur days or weeks prior to delivery, sometimes in association with a circumvallate placenta. Clinicians frequently refer to this clinical state as *chronic abruption*. Preterm vaginal bleeding and preterm delivery may result, sometimes in association with oligohydramnios (26).

Acute bleeding from a ruptured decidual artery spreads along the decidua between the placenta and the uterine wall, often resulting in complete detachment of the placenta. A retroplacental

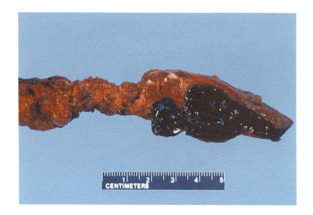

Figure 6-22

ACUTE MARGINAL HEMATOMA

An acute marginal hematoma has extended beneath the placental margin and produced a localized area of marginal abruption. This caused sudden onset of premature labor, but did not compromise the fetus.

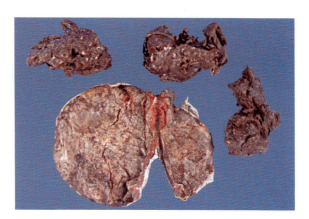

Figure 6-23

LARGE RETROPLACENTAL HEMATOMA

View of the maternal surface of a 30-week, 260-g placenta with a large area of partial separation. Detached portions of the clot (total weight of formed clot, 378 g), older than that in figure 6-22, are situated above and right. The area of separation involved approximately 65 percent of the maternal surface, resulting in intrauterine fetal death. The compressed placenta is appreciated best in the area sectioned. Villous stromal hemorrhage was also present microscopically, and there were numerous nucleated red blood cells in the fetal vessels.

clot, which is often larger than the placenta itself, forms. The clinical term for this calamity is placental abruption. The large formed clot may have the shape of a placenta and can be identifiable as such even after a vaginal delivery. The placenta, as seen at the time of cesarean section, appears to be floating within the uterine cavity. This observation establishes the diagnosis even without pathologic examination. The placenta does not, in these circumstances, become deformed by the clot, and once isolated from the uterus has no distinctive features sufficient for pathologic diagnosis. Predisposing factors for placental abruption include preeclampsia, essential hypertension, smoking, previous abruption, and chorioamnionitis (17). Cocaine abuse has been implicated, but no specific placental lesions are usually found (12). Important recent studies implicate thrombophilic states, such as the factor V Leiden mutation, resistance to activated protein C, protein S deficiency, and hyperhomocysteinemia (5,24,38,48,53,116), as risk factors for placental abruption. Abdominal trauma, usually in the form of an automobile accident, may also cause acute abruption (103).

Hemorrhage at the margin between the placenta and membranes is generally less forceful and may recur throughout gestation (acute and/or chronic peripheral separation). Clinically, this process may be correlated with vaginal bleeding in all three trimesters and in its most severe form has been termed the *chronic abruption-oligohydramnios sequence* (26). Clinical factors associated with chronic peripheral separation include advanced maternal age, multiparity, and smoking (82). It has been suggested that peripheral separations (or *marginal abruptions* as they are sometimes called) are due to uterine venous hemorrhages, as opposed to the more common nonperipheral uterine arteriolar hemorrhages associated with abruptio placenta.

Gross Findings. Smaller, more localized retroplacental hematomas are easily overlooked unless the placenta is sliced carefully, after 24 hours of formalin fixation. Recent clots are dark red, like the placenta (fig. 6-22), but the texture is more firm and solid. The region of the clot may not be apparent on the affected maternal surface, which is flat like the rest of the maternal surface, but cut sections show compression of the overlying placenta (figs. 6-22–6-25). Older retroplacental hematomas are firm, have a brownish color, and the overlying placenta is usually infarcted, especially if the hematoma is large (fig. 6-23). Old hematomas are gray or white.

Circulatory Problems: Thrombi and Other Vascular Lesions

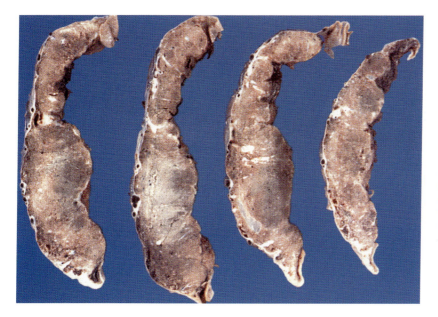

Figure 6-24

RETROPLACENTAL HEMATOMA

Specimens of a placenta with about 50 percent partial separation, clot removed. The compressed areas are at the top. The pale areas represent massive perivillous fibrin deposition, which further diminished placental function. The mother had preeclampsia. Intrapartum fetal monitoring appeared normal, but the newborn developed intractable respiratory failure shortly after birth, and died 2 1/2 hours postpartum.

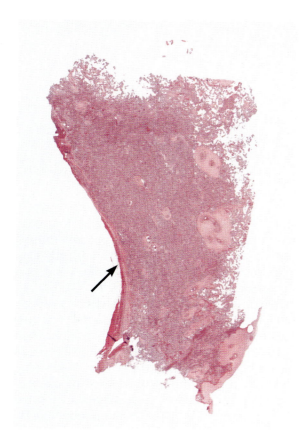

Figure 6-25

RETROPLACENTAL HEMATOMA

This histologic section of placenta is compressed by a recent clot. A thin rim of clot (arrow) remains on the concave maternal surface. The villi above are compacted together.

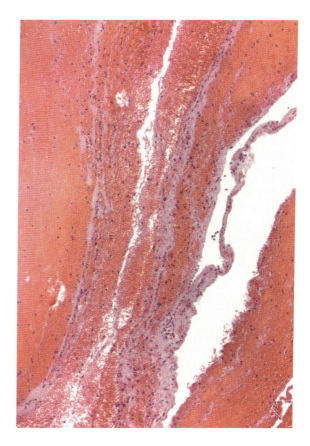

Figure 6-26

RETROPLACENTAL HEMATOMA

This portion of a clot from an acute complete separation shows alternate layers of fibrin and red blood cells. The clot in this case weighed 600 g.

Placental Pathology

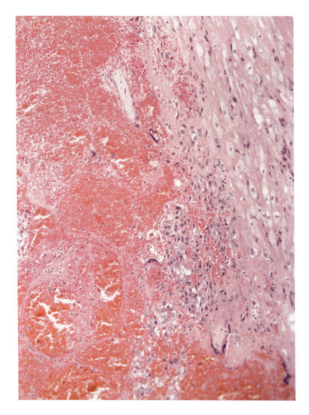

Figure 6-27

RETROPLACENTAL HEMATOMA

This retroplacental clot has dissected into the decidua. Note the layered appearance of fibrin in the clot.

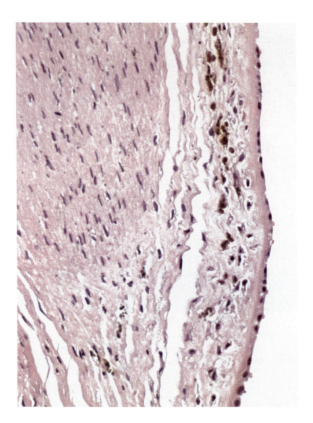

Figure 6-28

CHORIOAMNIONIC HEMOSIDERIN DEPOSITION

Dark golden brown refractile pigment in the amnionic and superficial chorionic connective tissue in a patient at 25 weeks' gestation, following first trimester bleeding and a history of two prior miscarriages.

Microscopic Findings. The red blood cells and fibrin have a compressed appearance, with strands of fibrin oriented parallel to the plane of the placental floor (fig. 6-26). Blood may dissect into or through the decidua, and clumps of decidua may become detached and intermixed with the clot (fig. 6-27). With the passage of time hemosiderin appears in macrophages at the margins of the clot (figs. 6-28, 6-29).

The clinical diagnosis of sudden complete abruption may not be demonstrated by gross examination of the placenta, although dissection of fresh blood into the decidual surfaces is suggestive of abruption. However, histologic examination of the clot may be extremely informative, especially if the separation occurs in stages. Histologic sections of the clot may confirm the appearance of layering and compression, and clumps of decidua are sometimes found within it (fig. 6-30). The most informative parts of the clot have a more defined smooth surface, with tiny strands or clumps of paler tissue near the surface. Clinicians should be encouraged to submit the clot with the placenta from a sudden acute abruption if documentation is expected.

Retroplacental hematomas that are large enough to cause adverse prenatal effects on the fetus may also produce secondary abnormalities in the placenta, such as focal villous stromal edema and hemorrhage (figs. 6-31, 6-32) (63). These changes are probably caused by sudden acute hypoxic damage or cytokine release from the injured decidua. Acute inflammation may be present; there is a definite association between preterm abruption and chorioamnionitis (17,49). Nucleated red blood cells may be abundant in cross sections of fetal vessels, and easily identified in the blood remaining in the larger vessels of the chorionic plate or umbilical cord.

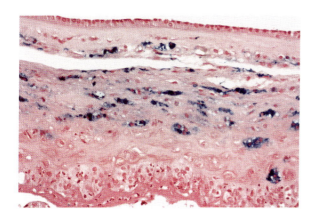

Figure 6-29

HEMOSIDERIN MACROPHAGES

Iron stain (Prussian blue) confirms the presence of hemosiderin in macrophages at the margin of an old hematoma.

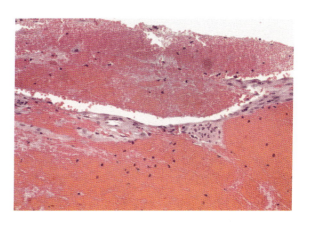

Figure 6-30

RETROPLACENTAL HEMATOMA

Small clumps of decidua are intermixed with fibrin strands in a recent clot from acute separation.

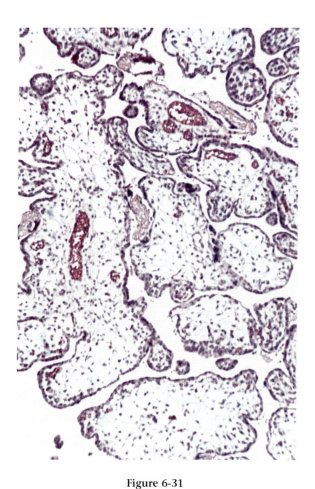

Figure 6-31

VILLOUS EDEMA

Villous edema is associated with acute abruption in a 23-week fetus. (Figs. 6-31 and 6-32 are from the same patient).

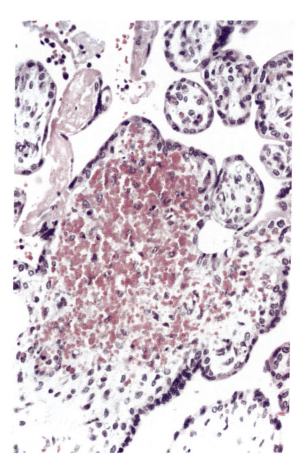

Figure 6-32

FOCAL VILLOUS STROMAL HEMORRHAGE

Villous stromal hemorrhage is associated with acute abruption.

Placental Pathology

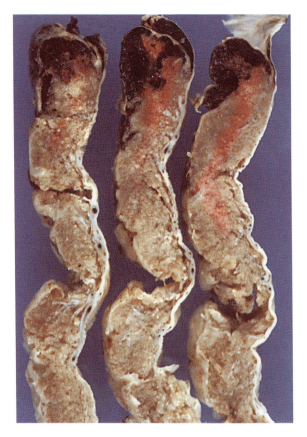

Figure 6-33

ACUTE MARGINAL HEMATOMA (MARGINAL SEPARATION)

Stage III acute chorioamnionitis was present, a relatively common association with acute marginal hematoma. Intrauterine fetal death, which occurred at 21 weeks, was more directly related to the infection than to the marginal hematoma.

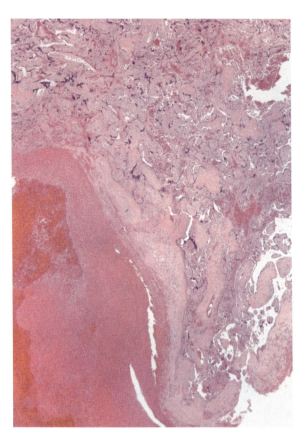

Figure 6-34

ACUTE AND CHRONIC MARGINAL HEMATOMA (MARGINAL SEPARATION)

There is a slight indentation of the placental margin at the left. Intrapartum hemorrhage was marked. This small lesion was not definitely identifiable on gross inspection.

Recent marginal hematomas may be associated with excessive vaginal bleeding in the peripartum period (figs. 6-33, 6-34). They may be associated with previous marginal hemorrhage (chronic peripheral separation, or chronic abruption). Features suggestive of chronic peripheral separation include chronic marginal hematomas, which appear brown (see fig. 6-23), and a circumvallate placenta characterized by a circumferential rim of degenerating clot (see chapter 3). Stainable hemosiderin (figs. 6-28, 6-29) may be seen focally, near areas of chronic hematoma or circumvallation, or diffusely distributed throughout the placental membranes (82). Hemosiderin-stained placentas may be green, which can be misinterpreted as meconium. There is a propensity to premature delivery and growth retardation in infants whose placentas have hemosiderin staining (82,87).

Differential Diagnosis. Sudden, complete, or substantial placental separation with a recently formed soft retroplacental hematoma is identifiable with certainty by direct observation of the detached placenta within the uterine cavity at the time of cesarean section. In contrast, smaller marginal or retroplacental clots that compress adjacent placenta sometimes resemble infarcts if the absence of villi is not apparent grossly. Histologic demonstration of compressed clot, absence of villi, and compressed adjacent placenta at one surface and decidua on the opposite surface is definitive for diagnosis.

Prognosis. Complete or extensive partial placental separation eliminates or markedly reduces the oxygen lifeline to the fetus. The most immediate effect is anoxia, which is fatal unless immediate cesarean section is possible. Smaller retroplacental clots may cause infarcts. The potential for injury varies with the size of the clot and the amount of placenta affected relative to the amount of remaining functional placenta, and increases when a small clot enlarges progressively. While small retroplacental hematomas may be insignificant, considerable intrapartum maternal blood loss may occur from the area of a marginal hematoma.

MATERNAL CIRCULATION: NONVASCULAR LESIONS

Massive Perivillous Fibrin Deposition (Gitterinfarcts) and Maternal Floor Infarct

While the maternal intervillous space is a blood-filled chamber, not a blood vessel in the usual sense, it does allow the afferent maternal blood flow to the placenta to connect to the efferent maternal venous system. More significantly, it also provides the proximity of maternal blood to fetal villi for transport of maternal-fetal interchange, so that obstruction within it has the effect of an interruption of the maternal-fetal vascular supply line.

Massive perivillous fibrin deposits and maternal floor infarcts are considered together because the distribution of the fibrin material in these two lesions is not distinctively different in many cases. Whether they represent variants of the same process or two separate processes is not settled. The pathologic features are similar except for the distribution of the fibrin, localized at the maternal floor of a floor infarct or more diffusely distributed as massive perivillous fibrin. The clinical correlations are also similar (114), although massive perivillous fibrin deposition may include more cases of intrauterine fetal growth restriction than maternal floor infarct (45).

Definitions. Both lesions are characterized by clumps and masses of amorphous, eosinophilic material called matrix-type fibrin which surround and entrap groups of villi (see fig. 6-3). The diagnostic criteria for maternal floor infarct at this time are necessarily arbitrary, but, as noted by Katzman and Genest (45), some quantitative limits are necessary to denote the extensive nature of clinically significant lesions. These authors defined a maternal floor infarct as those placentas in which the villi of the entire maternal floor are embedded in fibrin, to a thickness of at least 3 mm, evident on at least one slide. Massive perivillous fibrin deposition implies full thickness involvement of the placenta, entrapping at least 50 percent of the villi as seen on at least one slide (45). The fibrin aggregates are large enough to be grossly visible on cut section as pale gray areas of induration. Fibrin is generally intermixed with clusters of intermediate trophoblast cells (also known as X cells). Small clumps of fibrin, attached to one or two villi, and scattered focally throughout the placenta, are a common histologic finding in normal placentas, probably related to apoptosis of trophoblast (67). These foci are not pathologic lesions and are specifically excluded from this discussion of massive perivillous fibrin deposition.

The nature of placental fibrin, or fibrinoid, requires further study. The terms have been used in different ways for more than 100 years, a history reviewed well by Benirschke and Kaufmann (8). Currently, two types of material are identified: fibrin-type fibrinoid and matrix-type fibrinoid (33). Fibrin-type fibrinoid has immunohistochemical features of a blood clot product (fibrin and cellular fibronectin), and, as found in the placenta, without extravillous (intermediate) trophoblast cells. Matrix-type fibrinoid is composed of oncofetal fibronectin, collagen IV, laminin, and tenascin; rarely or never includes fibrin; and appears to be a product of extravillous trophoblast, with which it is consistently associated. The generic term fibrin is used throughout this text to refer to all amorphous eosinophilic deposits, except in specific studies that have characterized the content of the matrix.

Prevalence. Prevalence figures depend on the criteria for the minimum amounts of fibrin deposit regarded as significant. Small, grossly identifiable clumps of perivillous fibrin are common and usually innocuous. Fox (31) found them in 22 percent of full-term placentas. Accumulations sufficient to affect placental function are less common, usually centrally located, and involve about one fourth of the placental mass. Growth restriction may result in these cases (79). Andres et al. (3) found 30 maternal floor infarcts in a series of 32,182 placentas (0.09 percent), while Naeye (66) found 0.5 percent in the

Placental Pathology

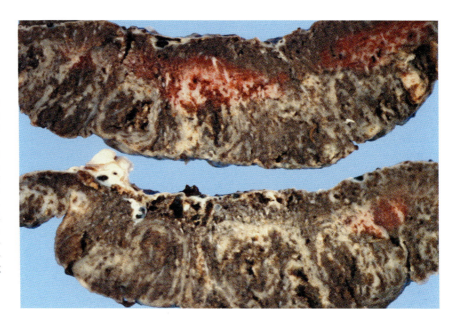

Figure 6-35

MASSIVE PERIVILLOUS FIBRIN DEPOSITS

This was the second pregnancy so affected. The mother had protein S and antithrombin III deficiencies, and is heterozygous for the *MTHFR C677T* gene mutation. Strands of firm, gray, amorphous material ramify throughout, producing a generalized woody, indurated consistency. The previous affected pregnancy ended fatally at term. This infant, delivered by cesarean section as soon as amniocentesis findings indicated lung maturation, survived.

Collaborative Perinatal Study. The combined prevalence of maternal floor infarct and massive fibrin deposition, as defined more restrictively by Katzman and Genest (45), was 0.005 percent.

Clinical Features. Both maternal floor infarct and massive perivillous fibrin deposition, when sufficiently extensive, are associated with sudden intrauterine fetal death late in the third trimester. A poor reproductive history with repeated spontaneous abortions is common. Perivillous fibrin deposition involving 40 to 50 percent of the placental mass is fortunately uncommon, but nearly always fatal. Maternal floor infarction generally has a smaller component of fibrin, which seems, in this location, to interfere materially with maternofetal perfusion and consistently causes intrauterine fetal growth restriction. Surviving fetuses are at risk for growth retardation or serious neurologic handicaps (3, 79). Both conditions may recur in subsequent pregnancies, and a poor maternal reproductive history is common.

The mothers in Naeye's report (see above) (66) had a greater frequency of phlebitis. Both massive perivillous fibrin deposition and maternal floor infarcts have been associated with instances of maternal thrombophilia in our experience (4) and others (56), but coagulopathy evaluations usually have not been performed. Three patients reported by Sebire et al. (96) had antiphospholipid antibodies and a history of repeated miscarriages. One instance of maternal floor infarct occurred in a child with long-chain 3-hydroxyacyl-CoA dehydrogenase (LCHAD) deficiency caused by two mutations in the gene, one inherited from each parent (58). Mild disseminated intravascular coagulation in two women with gestational sepsis was associated with extensive intervillous thrombosis that caused second trimester fetal death (7).

Gross Findings. Clumps of perivillous fibrin, 3 cm or more in diameter, affect many villi, and are visible as irregular strands and masses of pale gray induration on cut section (figs. 6-35, 6-36). In placentas with maternal floor infarct, the basal plate becomes thickened, stiff, and pale (fig. 6-37). The fibrin material and the entrapped villi resemble the pattern of perivillous fibrin deposits, except for the basal plate localization (fig. 6-38). Some placentas show both patterns (fig. 6-39).

Microscopic Findings. Groups of villi are enmeshed and separated by masses of matrix-type fibrin, or fibrinoid, material, a complex mixture of fibrin and other proteins, as defined above. The syncytiotrophoblast and capillary endothelium undergo necrosis and disappear. Mononuclear extravillous trophoblast cells resembling intermediate trophoblast cells appear to migrate into the fibrin matrix, while villous stromal cells and villous outlines persist (figs. 6-40–6-42). While by definition the fibrin material in maternal floor infarction is consistently located at the placental floor (figs. 6-43, 6-44), large clumps of perivillous fibrin may also be

Circulatory Problems: Thrombi and Other Vascular Lesions

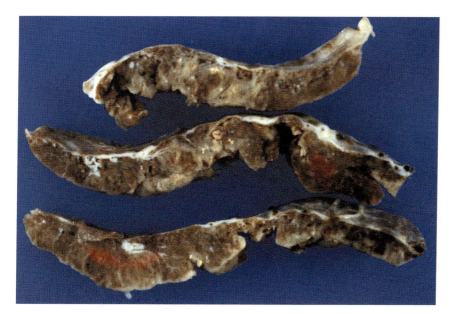

Figure 6-36

MATERNAL FLOOR INFARCT ASSOCIATED WITH MULTIFOCAL PERIVILLOUS FIBRIN DEPOSITS

The mother had gestational diabetes mellitus.

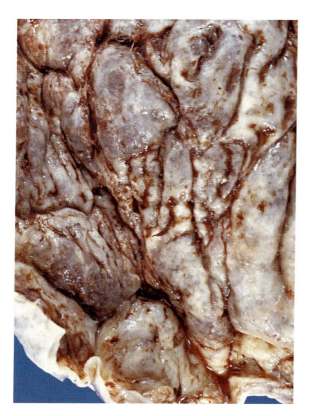

Figure 6-37

MATERNAL FLOOR INFARCT, BASAL (MATERNAL) PLATE SURFACE

The entire maternal surface is firm, stiff, convoluted, and pale gray. Gestational age is 39 weeks. Mother was gravida 10, para 5, abortus 5. (See cross section in fig. 6-38.)

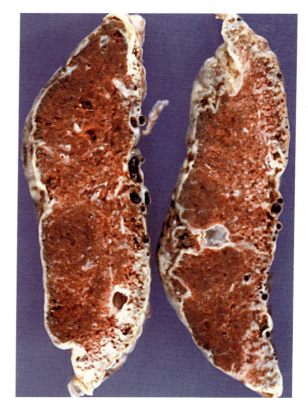

Figure 6-38

MATERNAL FLOOR INFARCT

A cross section of the placenta in figure 6-37 shows generally normal cut surfaces except for the thick rind of pale gray covering the maternal surface of each slice. The mother was gravida 10, para 5. Apgar scores were 3 and 8, and there were abnormal cardiac decelerations.

Placental Pathology

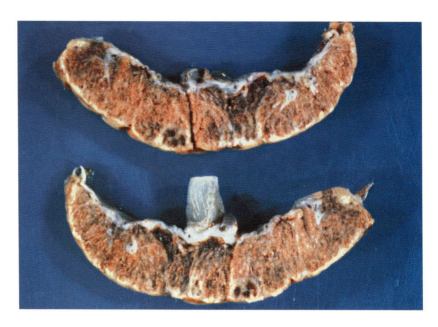

Figure 6-39

DIFFUSE BASAL PERIVILLOUS FIBRIN DEPOSITION (MATERNAL FLOOR INFARCT)

There is marked thickening of the entire basal plate with focal extension into the nearby placenta of a fetus with growth restriction.

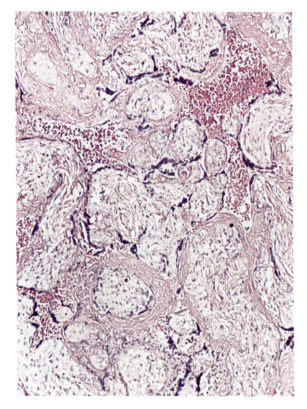

Figure 6-40

MASSIVE PERIVILLOUS FIBRIN DEPOSITS

The intervillous space is expanded and obliterated by wide bands of eosinophilic fibrin, which separate the villi. The villous capillaries have disappeared. Intrauterine fetal death occurred at 27 weeks' gestation. (Figs. 6-40 and 6-41 are from the same patient.)

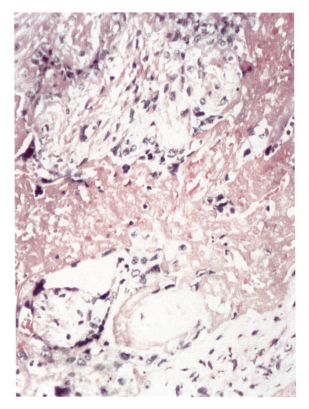

Figure 6-41

MASSIVE PERIVILLOUS FIBRIN DEPOSITS

Higher magnification of figure 6-40 shows the disappearance of the syncytiotrophoblast, with persistence of mononuclear intermediate trophoblast. The villi are widely separated by masses of fibrin, in contrast with the appearance of villous crowding seen in a conventional placental infarct.

Circulatory Problems: Thrombi and Other Vascular Lesions

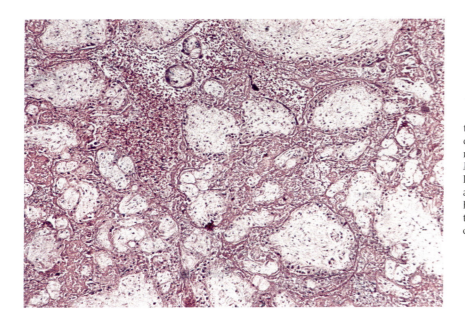

Figure 6-42

MASSIVE PERIVILLOUS FIBRIN DEPOSITS

Cellular components of all types have disappeared from this older, more chronic lesion. The mother was heterozygous for the *MTHFR* gene mutation, had low levels of activated protein C, and anticardiolipin antibodies. She had two prior fetal losses and two living children. This fetus died in utero.

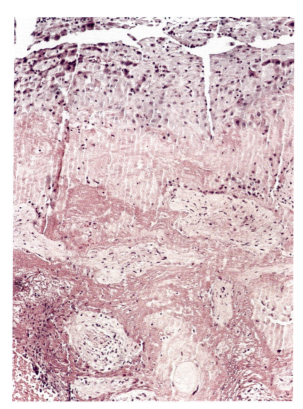

Figure 6-43

MATERNAL FLOOR INFARCT

Basal plate villi are encompassed by perivillous fibrin. There were three previous intrauterine fetal deaths. The mother had antithrombin III deficiency and was heterozygous for the *MTHFR* gene mutation. (Figs. 6-43 and 6-44 are from the same patient.)

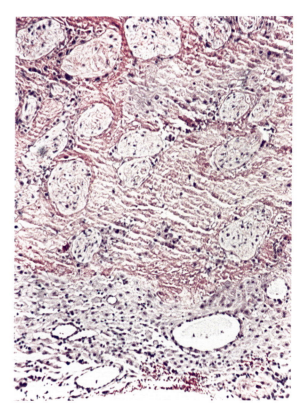

Figure 6-44

MATERNAL FLOOR INFARCT, RECURRENT

Recurrent, but less extensive, placental floor infarct in a subsequent pregnancy of the patient in figure 6-43. The mother was treated with anticoagulants and the infant delivered as soon as fetal lung maturity became adequate.

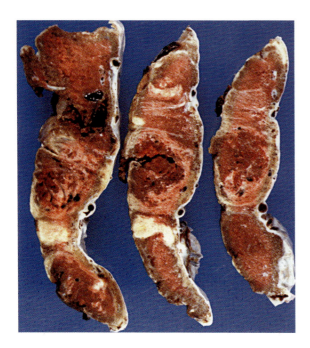

Figure 6-45

MASSIVE PERIVILLOUS FIBRIN DEPOSITS

Massive perivillous fibrin deposition is the dominant abnormality in the irregular, somewhat lighter areas. Focal fetal thrombotic vaculopathy (FTV) is also present near the bottom margin of the specimen at right. The large, central, dark red area in the center of the two slices at right is a recent infarct, and the small pale yellow wedge below center is an old infarct. Abnormal fetal heart tracings led to cesarean section. This mother, and her brother and father, all had low (below 50 percent) antithrombin III levels and a history of deep leg vein thrombosis. The mother was also heterozygous for *MTHFR* gene mutation. (Figs. 6-45 to 6-48 are from the same patient.)

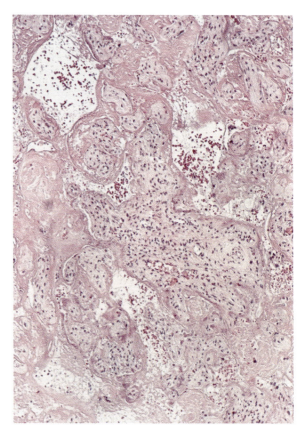

Figure 6-46

MASSIVE PERIVILLOUS FIBRIN DEPOSITS

Microscopic sections of the placenta shown in figure 6-45. (Figures 6-46–6-48 are from the same placenta.)

found scattered throughout the placenta, blurring the distinction between the two conditions.

In preterm placentas, the extent of the fibrin deposition may be less apparent grossly and require more comprehensive histologic evaluation to confirm the presence of massive involvement. Placentas with massive perivillous fibrin deposits may also be involved by fetal thrombotic vasculopathy (see below) and large infarcts of the more conventional type (figs. 6-45–6-48). The relationship of the fibrin to the mononuclear extravillous trophoblast is a consistent feature, except in some very old lesions. Major basic protein produced by intermediate trophoblast cells (trophoblastic X cells) may contribute to the formation of the fibrin deposits (114).

Differential Diagnosis. Older, massive perivillous fibrin deposits resemble chronic infarcts if they are confluent. Irregular-shaped lesions of chronic fetal thrombotic vasculopathy sometimes resemble massive perivillous fibrin deposits. Extensive lesions in preterm placentas are sometimes difficult to see or palpate on gross examination.

Prognosis. Perivillous fibrin deposits involving 40 percent of the placenta, and maternal floor infarcts that involve the entire placental floor, are often fatal to the fetus. Intrauterine fetal death may occur suddenly, without warning. In some cases, the mothers report decreased fetal movements, especially if they are tabulating kick counts. In a few instances, fetuses that survive, when delivered by immediate cesarean section because of fetal distress identified on fetal heart monitoring, later develop evidence of neurologic injury (2). Both lesions tend to recur in subsequent pregnancies.

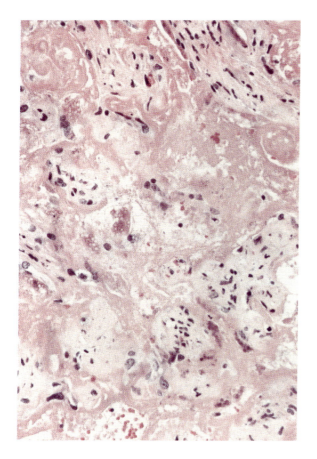

Figure 6-47

MASSIVE PERIVILLOUS FIBRIN DEPOSITS

Higher magnification of the perivillous fibrin deposits shown in figure 6-46.

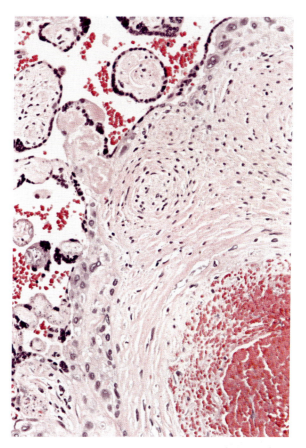

Figure 6-48

MASSIVE PERIVILLOUS FIBRIN DEPOSITS AND FETAL THROMBOTIC VASCULOPATHY

Fetal thrombotic vasculopathy was present in this placenta. A thrombosed stem vessel is at right, avascular fibrotic villi at left.

FETAL CIRCULATION: THROMBI AND HEMATOMAS

Fetal Stem Vessel (Large Vessel) Thrombi and Fetal Thrombotic Vasculopathy

Definition. Occlusive and mural thrombi in branches of the umbilical arteries, tributaries of the umbilical vein on the placental surface, and stem vessels within the placenta produce secondary regressive changes in fetal vessels peripheral to the thrombi (see fig. 6-3). Wedge-shaped areas of pale pink or gray-tan avascular villi are the result (figs. 6-49, 6-51). Both the large vessel lesions and the changes in the peripheral villi have been termed fetal thrombotic vasculopathy (FTV). Other terms for lesions closely resembling this type of vascular transformation include *avascular terminal villi* (89,90), *fetal stem artery thrombosis* (32), *fibrinous vasculosis* (95), *endothelial cushions* (21), and, in the opinion of some, *hemorrhagic endovasculitis* (93).

Incidence. Fox (32) reported fetal artery thrombosis in 4.5 percent of placentas from full-term pregnancies. In association with maternal diabetes mellitus, the frequency is 10 percent. Redline and Pappin (78) estimated a prevalence of 3 to 10 in 1,000 placentas from 9,316 consecutive deliveries.

Clinical Features. Lesions that are extensive grossly or are shown by thorough sampling to involve 40 to 60 percent of the placental mass usually cause sudden intrauterine or intrapartum fetal death. Those with smaller foci may be asymptomatic at birth, unless the fetus is growth-restricted, the placenta itself is small for gestational age, or thrombi are also present in somatic vessels of the newborn. The latter may take the form of prenatal cerebral infarcts (52, 108) and renal vessel thrombosis (52). FTV in the placenta may identify newborns at risk for inherited coagulopathies, including those with postnatal cerebral infarcts and other thromboembolic diseases (23). Doppler blood flow studies confirm a cessation or even reversal of diastolic blood flow in the fetal circulation (89). Fetal growth restriction may occur (86). There is also an association with maternal diabetes mellitus (32,111). Other less common conditions associated with FTV include perinatal liver disease (16) and discordant growth in twins (47,81).

Identification of thrombi in the fetal circulation of the placenta is important, because this observation identifies newborns at risk for prenatal injury caused by thrombi in the fetus or by reduced placental function caused by larger lesions. Thrombi that occur prenatally in the somatic vessels of the fetus may cause very destructive injuries, including massive systemic thrombosis (97), limb reduction (42), and infarcts in the heart (11) and brain (52,108). The lesions in the brain of newborns with FTV identified by ultrasound and magnetic resonance imaging may be dramatic (figs. 6-50, 6-52). The significance of FTV as a risk factor is further documented in twin gestations by the selective injury to the twin whose placenta contains this lesion (47,81).

FTV is associated with hypercoagulable states (4,51,57), although not all mothers tested have an identifiable coagulopathy. Placental and fetal somatic vessel thrombi are also associated with maternal diabetes mellitus, which happens to have a prominent multifactorial thrombophilic diathesis (14,111). The fetus may inherit the coagulopathy from either parent, or with extra bad luck, from both parents heterozygous for the same mutation, neither of whom necessarily has reported a thrombotic history (37,107). Neurologic injury is the most common problem in affected newborns (19,78); bowel involvement may cause some cases of meconium ileus (109); and thrombi in the vena cava and hepatic vein may result in the Budd-Chiari syndrome (16).

Some newborns with prominent placental FTV appear normal in the neonatal period, and the frequency with which later problems may develop remains unknown. Infants and children with homocystinuria, detected by urinalysis at birth, have a well-recognized thrombophilic tendency. We have not encountered a placenta known to be associated with the defect in cystathione synthase enzyme function. Homozygosity for the methylenetetrahydrofolate reductase *(MTHFR)* gene mutation may be an important factor in determining fetal brain injury (39). In two instances of dizygotic twins of parents heterozygous for the *MTHFR* gene mutation, the homozygous twin with placental FTV was either injured or stillborn, while the heterozygous twin was normal (47,107). The occurrence of placental venous thrombi in a monoamnionic twin placenta may destroy the balance between the two circulations, resulting in the rapid onset of severe twin-twin transfusion syndrome (68).

Autopsy studies (9,10,15) and perinatal ultrasonographic or radiographic imaging (101,102) indicate the prenatal timing of many instances of cerebral infarction in FTV (figs. 6-50G,H; 6-52E,F; 6-53C,D; 6-54B-D; 6-55). The risk for childhood stroke, though rare, remains in affected children who are normal during infancy (73). Whether identification of FTV in otherwise normal newborns can identify a group at increased risk for thrombotic disease remains to be determined. In some instances, coagulopathic states combine with other factors, such as vascular anomalies, local trauma or stasis in velamentous vessels, or amniotic fluid infection, to produce brain lesions that can result in cerebral palsy (76), and a complex of multiple abnormalities is common in the most severely affected infants (83).

FTV occurs in some placentas with chorangiomas and vascular malformations. Chorangiosis (see chapter 4) may occur in association with FTV. In one case report, maternal hemolytic uremic syndrome (thrombotic thrombocytopenic purpura) was associated with multiple old and recent lesions of FTV in the placenta (40), while in another case, a decidual thrombotic vasculopathy with infarcts occurred (117).

Gross Findings. Thrombi in large vessels of the chorionic plate may be grossly visible (fig. 6-49A). Occlusive lesions in stem vessels within the placenta are usually undetectable grossly. The villi in the distribution of occluded stem vessels are visible as a wedge-shaped pale region that is triangular on cut section (figs. 6-49A, 6-50A); in older lesions this is gray-white and firm (fig. 6-51A).

Circulatory Problems: Thrombi and Other Vascular Lesions

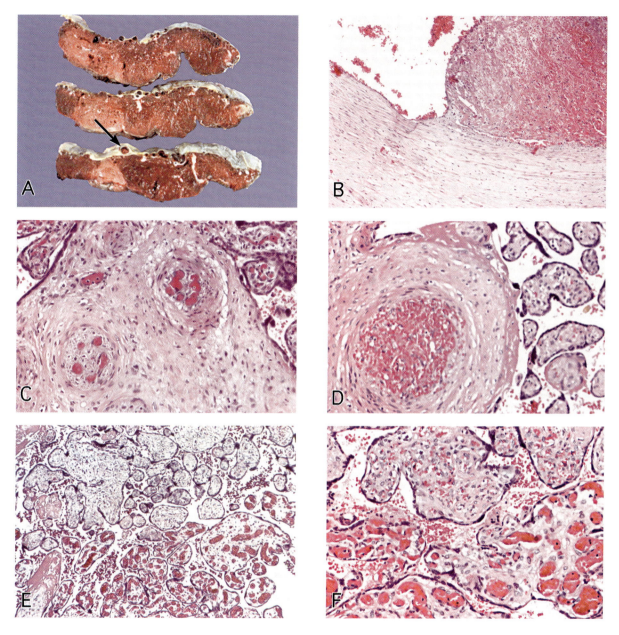

Figure 6-49

FETAL THROMBOTIC VASCULOPATHY

A: Gross appearance of FTV. Multiple wedge-shaped pale areas with a base at the placental floor are characteristic. There is a large thrombosed surface vessel in the lower section (arrow) of this placenta. Grossly visible thrombi in surface vessels or large stem vessels are not identifiable in most placentas with FTV, however.

B: Histologic appearance of the thrombus of the large surface vessel.

C: Two smaller fetal stem vessels show a pattern of partial organization, with multiple channels, called septation.

D: Partial organization in a larger stem vessel. Red blood cells at the margin have extravasated focally, and fibroblasts proliferate in from the margins.

E: The interface between normal villi at the bottom half and abnormal villi at the top half of the figure is shown. Degenerative changes in the villi at top, which are downstream from a recently occluded fetal vessel, include destruction of capillary endothelium, loss of villous capillaries, extravasation of red blood cells, and enlarged villous outlines. The intervillous space is open and trophoblastic epithelium persists.

F: Higher magnification of the interface between FTV in a more recent area (above) shows endothelial karyorrhexis (above) and normal villi (below).

Placental Pathology

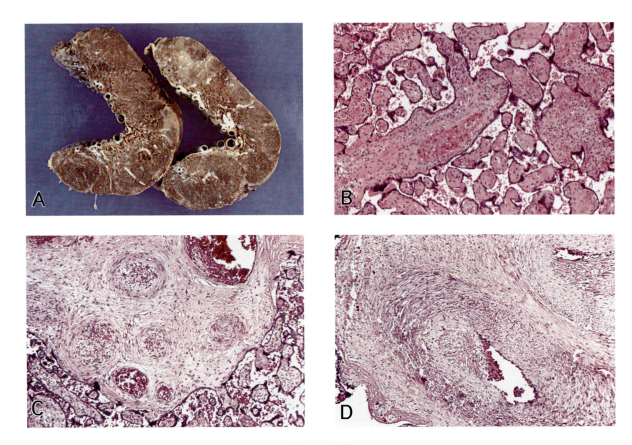

Figure 6-50

FETAL THROMBOTIC VASCULOPATHY

A: This newborn from a mother with gestational diabetes mellitus was flaccid at birth and developed periventricular leukomalacia, but responded to resuscitation and went home breathing and feeding adequately. Coagulation studies were not done. The gross abnormalities in this instance of very extensive FTV are subtle, even after fixation. The gross placental abnormality was not recognized at the time of first examination, and is only faintly apparent here after fixation as variegated, somewhat mottled areas of pale and darker gray.

B: Microscopic appearance of FTV. A thrombosed stem vessels (center) is surrounded by avascular fibrotic villi with some residual stromal cells.

C: Large thrombosed stem vessel at top right, smaller completely organized stem vessels at center, and fibrotic avascular villi at bottom.

D: Occlusive thrombus in a stem vessel at right, mural thrombus at center.

Fixation makes some of the larger avascular villous lesions more apparent, but the gross pathologic changes are often subtle (figs. 6-50A, 6-52A). In fact, the placenta may show surprisingly little gross evidence of any abnormality, even in areas with well-defined histologic abnormalities.

Microscopic Findings. Occlusive or mural thrombi have a histologic evolution comparable to intravascular thrombi in other locations. While the specific features of organization as in a myocardial infarct do not occur (phagocytosis of dead tissue by macrophages, ingrowth of fibroblasts, and endstage contracted scar), there is a recognizable progression of change in a fetal vessel occluded by thrombus. Recent thrombi expand the vessel, are clearly attached to the vessel wall, and may have a layered appearance (figs. 6-49B,D; 6-52B). The endothelial cells beneath the clot lyse and disappear, and spindle-shaped cells that resemble fibroblasts appear within the thrombus (figs. 6-49D, 6-52B). As erythrocytes degenerate, a pattern of multilocular fibroblastic septation, resembling recanalization, occurs (fig. 6-49C). Eventually the vessel becomes obliterated and fibrotic so that only an indistinct outline remains

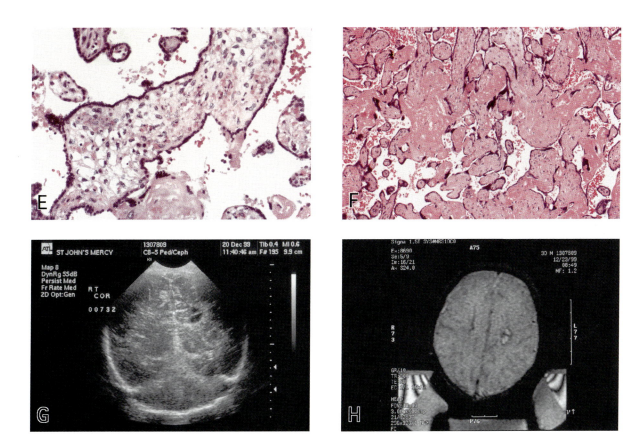

Figure 6-50 (Continued)

E: Higher magnification of avascular villi. Most capillaries have disappeared. A few stromal cells with karyorrhexis and scattered red blood cells persist. The intervillous space and trophoblast are preserved.

F: Older area of more fibrotic FTV.

G: Cerebral ultrasound image of this infant on the day of birth shows a focal lesion consistent with prenatal cystic encephalomalacia or infarct in the patient's left cerebrum (right).

H: Magnetic resonance image (MRI) of the same infant's brain 3 days later shows a focal lesion consistent with evolving infarct in patient's left cerebrum (right). (Courtesy of Dr. Thomas Applewhite, St. Louis, MO.)

(figs. 6-50C, 6-51B, 6-54A). There is often some degree of fibroblastic reaction in the vessel wall, and the wall may eventually become calcified. It may be difficult or impossible to determine whether an occluded stem vessel was an artery or a vein after these marked alterations.

Distinctive alterations occur in the villi and villous capillaries rendered nonfunctional by occluded stem vessels. Two patterns may be seen. One, found in earlier lesions, is characterized by fragmentation of capillary endothelial cell nuclei, red blood cell extravasation, and stromal karyorrhexis. Iron deposits commonly appear in the basement membranes beneath the syncytiotrophoblast (fig. 6-55) (41,61). Similar findings occur diffusely throughout the vessels in the placentas of stillborns who die 1 to 2 days before delivery. Much of the appearance of FTV is related to villous vascular stasis, probably caused by downstream venous obstruction (fig. 6-50E). Iron-calcific deposits in the trophoblastic basement membrane also occur in cases of fetal Bartter's syndrome (27). The second, probably older, pattern of villous alteration is characterized by bland fibrosis and loss of capillaries, which may represent upstream arterial occlusion with devascularization of the dependent villous tree (figs. 6-50F, 6-51 right, 6-54A).

These two patterns may represent sequential phases of the same process. The avascular villi with either pattern form either large confluent clusters with a segmental distribution (fig. 6-51), usually attributable to chorionic plate or large stem vessel thrombi, or are grouped in

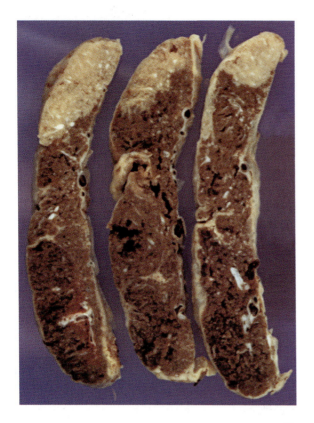 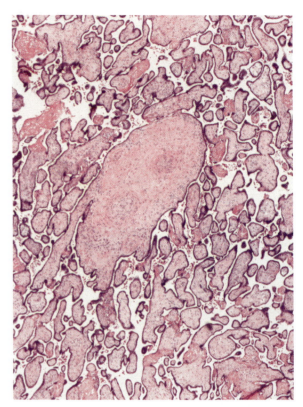

Figure 6-51

FETAL THROMBOTIC VASCULOPATHY

Left: This large, firm, very pale tan single focus of FTV has the appearance of an older, more chronic lesion (see right figure). The gestational age is 38 weeks. The newborn was growth restricted, amnionic fluid volume was low, and the placenta was small (320 g). The nuchal cord was tightly wrapped around the body.

Right: Microscopically, the villi are completely fibrotic, but the syncytiotrophoblast covering remains viable and the patency of the intervillous space is maintained.

small clusters (multifocal), related to thrombi, often of the platelet-fibrin type, forming in smaller arteries and arterioles. Only the fibrotic pattern is detectable by gross examination. Redline and Pappin (78) found thrombi in about one third of cases with extensive segmental or multifocal avascular villi. Avascular villi in the absence of thrombi may also be classified as FTV if other potential nonthrombotic causes such as chronic villitis and perivillous fibrin deposition are not present in the affected areas.

The minimum number of avascular villi required to make a diagnosis of FTV has not been established. In one study, only placentas with 10 or more small foci (3 to 5 villi) or 45 or more total avascular villi were more prevalent in infants with cerebral palsy or other forms of neurologic impairment (77). The authors propose that small foci be defined as a grouping of 3 to 5 fibrotic villi, intermediate-sized foci as a cluster of 6 to 19 villi, and large foci as more than 20 villi in one plane of section (fig. 6-56). We regard lesions estimated to involve 25 to 50 percent of the placental mass as "massive."

Differential Diagnosis. In areas of chronic villitis, the villous capillaries also disappear and the villous stroma also becomes fibrotic, but in FTV there is no chronic inflammatory infiltrate and agglutination of the villi by strands of fibrin (see chapter 5). In contrast to FTV, where the villi are normally separated, the intervillous space in areas of infarct or perivillous fibrin deposition is obliterated and the syncytiotrophoblast layer disappears.

Lesions with histologic features overlapping with those of large vessel thromboses, designated

Circulatory Problems: Thrombi and Other Vascular Lesions

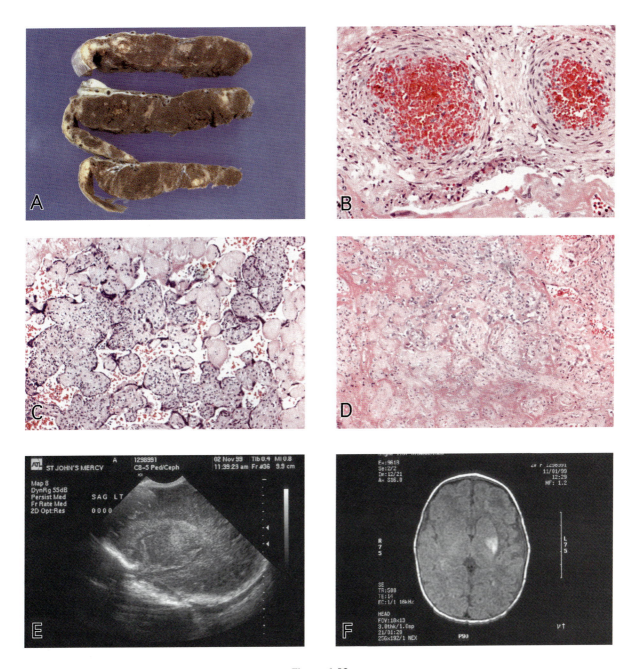

Figure 6-52

FETAL THROMBOTIC VASCULOPATHY

The FTV was focal, perivillous fibrin (PVF) was extensive, and chronic villitis was present. The growth-retarded newborn, delivered at 39 weeks, was thrombocytopenic at birth, then had seizures at age 12 hours. The mother has lupus anticoagulant.

A: Gross appearance of the placenta, which was small at 298 g, less than the 10th percentile for weight at 39 weeks' gestation. The pale areas represent perivillous fibrin deposits and foci of chronic villitis. FTV was not identified grossly.

B: Focal area of FTV; two stem vessels contain partly organized thrombi.

C: Extensive areas of chronic villitis are also present. The villi are avascular and fibrotic, as in FTV, but are adherent to one another (unlike FTV), and there is fibrin deposition, with a mild mononuclear inflammatory cell infiltrate.

D: Perivillous fibrin deposits are also present, suggesting the potential for an accumulative effect from multiple placental lesions.

E: Ultrasound images of the brain of the neonate were interpreted as infarct in the basal ganglia.

F: MRI at age 14 days confirms an infarct in the left basal ganglia. (E and F courtesy of Dr. Thomas Applewhite, St. Louis, MO.)

Placental Pathology

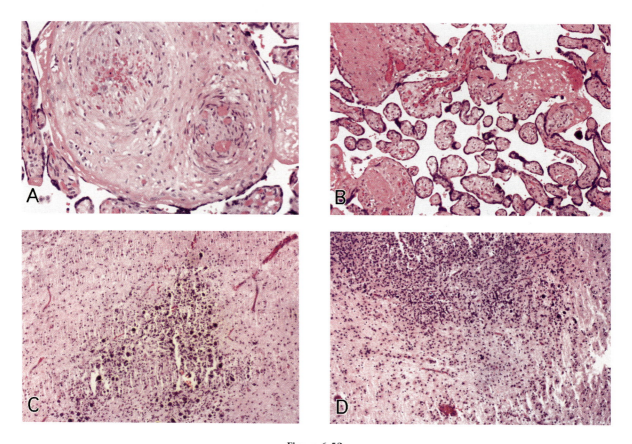

Figure 6-53

FETAL THROMBOTIC VASCULOPATHY

This newborn survived 2 1/2 hours. The mother had a history of deep vein thrombosis; coagulation testing was normal, however.
A: Two stem vessels with FTV, partly organized with septation, are shown.
B: Multiple foci of clustered fibrotic avascular villi (chronic FTV) are present.
C,D: Sections of neonatal brain from the autopsy show foci of prenatal, focally calcified cerebral infarcts.

intimal fibrin cushions and fibrinous vasculosis (see below), may be seen alone or with other features of FTV. An intimal fibrin cushion consists of laminated subendothelial fibrin, generally located within the wall of a chorionic or large stem villous vein. Fibrinous vasculosis is also a thrombotic process, associated with edema in the vascular wall. Increased intravascular pressure secondary to obstruction or thrombosis of the umbilical fetal circulation has been invoked as an etiology. With time, these fibrin deposits may undergo calcification. In some cases, intimal fibrin cushions may represent thrombi that have undergone reendothelialization after incorporation into the vessel wall.

Prognosis. The fate of infants with FTV depends upon the extent of the condition and whether additional thrombi occur in the somatic circulation and, if so, what organs are affected. Some fetuses with placental FTV are born with central nervous system (CNS) injury (figs. 6-50G,H; 6-52E,F) (50,52,77,78). Extensive FTV leads to stillbirth from failure of placental function (19). In instances of stillbirth or neonatal death, autopsy studies may demonstrate prenatal thrombi in the somatic circulation of the fetus and cerebral infarcts in some cases (figs. 6-53, 6-54) (9,52). The risks of prenatal injury are compounded by the presence of other placental lesions, including infection, chronic villitis, and thrombi or infarcts in the maternal circulation (77). Some infants born with relatively small CNS lesions associated with placental FTV are symptomatic at birth, but eventually grow and develop normally, because of the capacity of the immature brain for

Circulatory Problems: Thrombi and Other Vascular Lesions

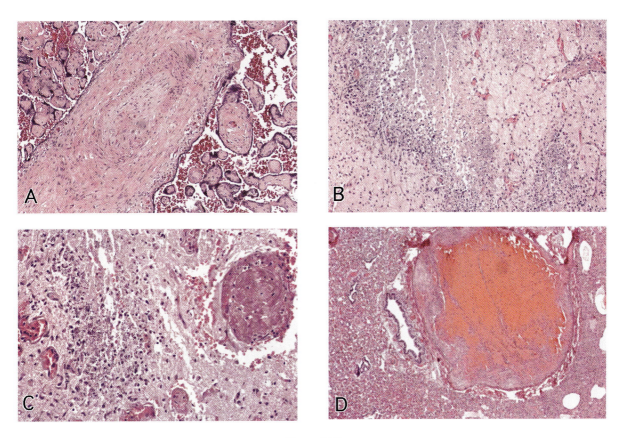

Figure 6-54

FETAL THROMBOTIC VASCULOPATHY

The newborn survived 24 hours. No maternal coagulation testing was done.
A: There is a chronic stem vessel occlusion with adjacent fibrotic villi.
B,C: Sections of the autopsied brain show areas of infarct, with gliosis and Gitter cell infiltrate. A small cerebral vessel in C is distended by thrombus.
D: A fetal pulmonary artery is occluded by a recent thrombus.

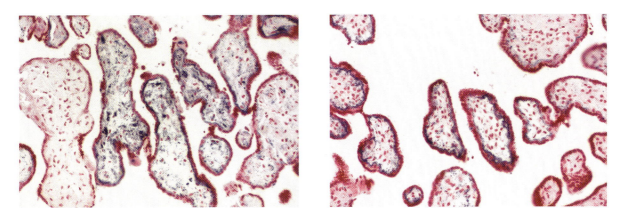

Figure 6-55

FETAL THROMBOTIC VASCULOPATHY

Left: Hemosiderosis in macrophages and basement membranes of villi in a chronic lesion of FTV. The villous stromal component suggests that a component of villous stromal hemorrhage was present in the acute lesion.
Right: Hemosiderin is localized to the basement membrane (Prussian blue iron stain).

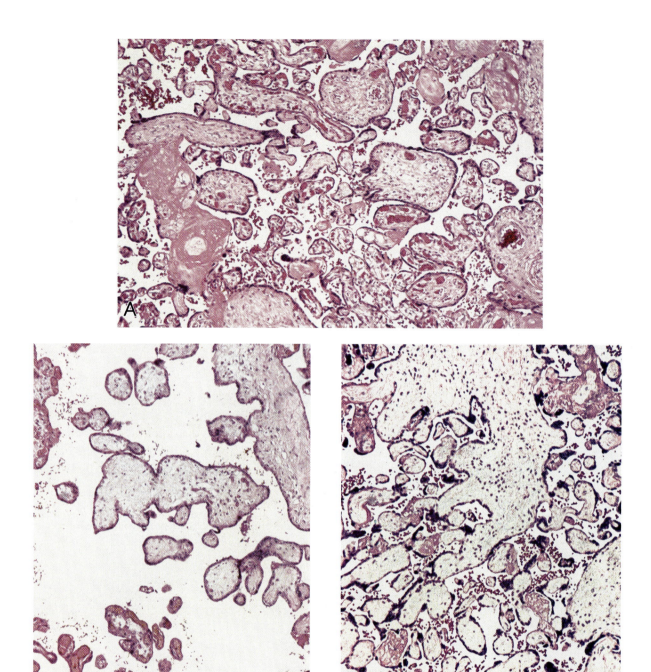

Figure 6-56

FETAL THROMBOTIC VASCULOPATHY

A: Avascular villi (FTV), small focus (2 to 5 terminal villi) just above center. A small cluster of terminal villi lack fetal capillaries and show bland dense collagenization of the villous stroma in the placenta of a 40-week newborn with low Apgar scores.

B: Avascular villi (FTV), intermediate focus (6 to 19 terminal villi). Tertiary stem villi and dependent terminal villi lack fetal vessels and show bland dense collagenization of villous stroma, associated with meconium-stained fluid at 40 weeks. Villous chorangiosis was also present. Normal villi are at lower left.

C: Avascular villi (FTV), large focus (greater than 20 terminal villi). Secondary and tertiary stem villi, plus dependent terminal villi, lack fetal vessels and show bland dense collagenization of villous stroma at 34 weeks' gestation in the placenta of a newborn with intrauterine growth restriction.

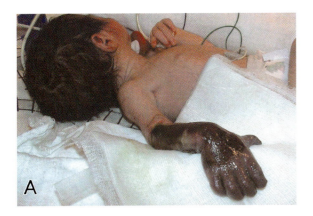

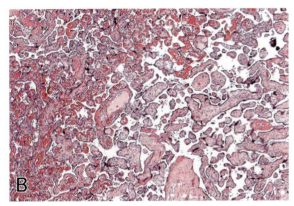

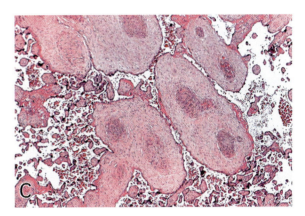

Figure 6-57

FETAL THROMBOTIC VASCULOPATHY

This delivery was complicated by growth restriction and oligohydramnios. The newborn was delivered at 38 weeks with a birth weight of 2,070 g. In a previous ultrasound at 30 weeks the fetus had appeared normal. (All figures are from the same case and courtesy of Drs. Ilana Ariel and R. Ravel, Jerusalem, Israel.)

A: Necrosis (gangrene) of the right arm. The newborn survived, but the arm had to be amputated.

B: Fetal thrombotic vasculopathy (extensive avascular villi), at right, affecting downstream villi.

C: Multiple fetal stem vessels were occluded by thrombi.

repair and healing (fig. 6-58). Thrombotic occlusion of major vessels to limbs, a rare complication of FTV, can result in gangrene, which may lead to amputation (fig. 6-57).

Fetal Vascular Narrowing and Increased Umbilical Vascular Resistance

A form of fetal vessel narrowing, identified by morphometric studies (28,62), appears to correlate directly with marked resistance or obstruction to fetal blood flow, as determined by Doppler velocimetry. The villous abnormalities illustrated in one of these studies (28) resembled the villous pattern of FTV. Small fetal stem arteries had thickened walls and either obliterated or markedly narrowed lumens based on detailed morphometric analysis. Stem vessel thrombi also occurred in both studies. The placental and neonatal birth weights were abnormally low in comparison to controls. A comparable example from our experience is illustrated in figures 6-58–6-60. It is not clear whether these reports identify a subset of placentas with FTV or an additional related process. This lesion may overlap with the thickened stem arteries occasionally seen in normal pregnancies, which may be related to postdelivery processing artefacts. Fetal vascular narrowing should probably be diagnosed only in morphometrically studied placentas with the appropriate clinical context: marked intrauterine growth restriction and abnormal pulsed flow Doppler results.

Hemorrhagic Endovasculitis

Definition. A vasodisruptive process that affects fetal vessels, from larger stem vessels to villous capillaries, hemorrhagic endovasculitis (HEV) is characterized by endothelial injury, hemorrhage, erythrocyte fragmentation, and extravasation of red blood cells, often fragmented and deformed, into the surrounding stroma (93). Lesions causing vessel necrosis are regarded as vasodestructive. HEV is considered by Sander (93) to be a distinct lesion of uncertain pathogenesis, while a very strong association with placental fetal vessel thrombi and villous fibrosis is recognized. In the opinion of the authors, there appears to be significant overlap between cases of HEV and FTV. The existence of HEV as a separate entity is regarded as controversial by some (8,30).

Placental Pathology

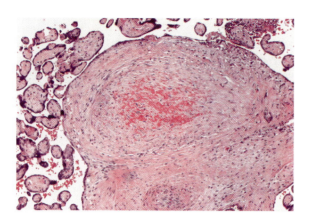
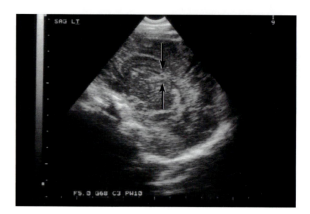

Figure 6-58

FETAL THROMBOTIC VASCULOPATHY

Left: FTV in a stem vessel and fibrotic villi were associated with focal chronic villitis (top right). The newborn had delay in development of feeding and respiratory function, but by age 5 years was developing normally. The mother was later found to have protein S deficiency.

Right: Brain ultrasound examination at birth showed a small cystic lesion (arrows), which eventually disappeared in later studies.

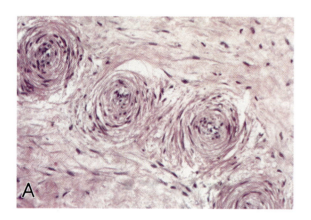
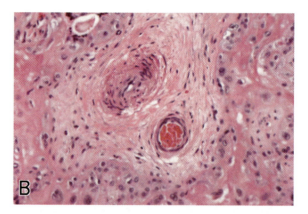
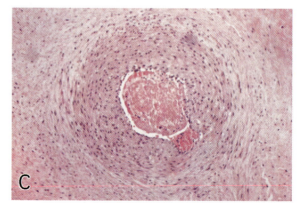

Figure 6-59

INTRAUTERINE GROWTH RESTRICTION

A,B: The stem vessel is narrow and tortuous, and appears disproportionately small and very thick-walled for its location and the size of the stem villus.

B: A thick-walled, partly hyalinized stem artery is next to a normal-appearing vein.

C: Another large stem vessel is occluded by a degenerating thrombus. Abnormal Doppler umbilical blood flow studies indicated absent end-diastolic blood flow, presumably caused by increased fetal vascular resistance.

Incidence. Shen-Schwartz et al. (100) identified 13 cases of HEV in a series of 1,938 consecutive unselected singleton pregnancies (0.67 percent). Based upon the finding of three placentas with HEV among 53 consecutive pregnancies examined under the detailed Michigan Placental Tissue Registry protocol, Sander (92) concluded that the prevalence in the pregnant population at large is between 5 and 6 percent. Among the 10,820 placentas (most from complicated

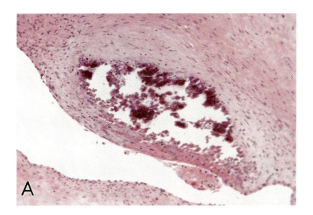
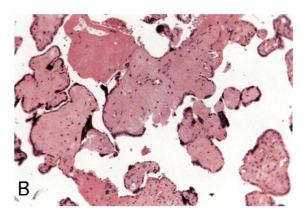
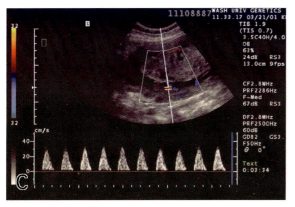

Figure 6-60

INTRAUTERINE GROWTH RESTRICTION

A: One of several stem vessels has a markedly reduced lumen caused by large mural thrombi, which in some cases were calcified.

B: Multiple foci of avascular villi with stromal fibrosis (chronic FTV).

C: The umbilical artery flow velocity waveform, measured prior to delivery, demonstrates absent end-diastolic flow in the placenta shown in A and B. This fetus also had intrauterine growth restriction and multiple malformations. The fetal karyotype was trisomy 13. (Doppler image and interpretation courtesy of Dr. Jeffrey M. Dicke, St Louis, MO.)

pregnancies) referred to the Michigan Placenta Tissue Registry between January 1, 1990 and December 31, 1996, Sander found HEV in 11.1 percent of liveborn infants and 30 percent of stillborn infants (93). The number of sections examined may explain some of the apparent discrepancy between these figures, and there may be some variation in the sensitivity of different observers to the diagnosis.

Clinical Features. Sander (94) found statistically significant correlations with stillbirth, intrauterine growth restriction, and neurologic injury among survivors with HEV placentas at age 5 years. Neurologic injury was also noted by Foley et al. (29). A smaller group of placentas with HEV was associated with nonimmune hydrops (69). The severity of perinatal complications increased with increasing severity of the placental HEV (29,93).

In contrast, Shen-Schwartz et al. (100) found no association with stillbirth or intrauterine growth restriction. One of 13 newborns had neonatal seizures and some persistent neurologic problems at 2 years of age. There was an association with nuchal cord, pregnancy-induced hypertension, and post-term gestation.

HEV is thought to be an inflammatory process, as suggested by the name. Attempts to detect an infectious etiology have produced suggestive results (94), but no definitive proof.

Gross Findings. The placentas originally examined by Sander (91) were smaller than controls, and more frequently stained by meconium. Intravascular thrombi were sometimes present, and nuchal cord or other umbilical cord entanglements were more common. Larger areas of acute villous stromal hemorrhage appear dark red in comparison with normal adjacent placental villi.

Microscopic Findings. The most dramatic feature is the presence of vessel wall injury, with hemorrhage into the stroma of villi and vessel walls (figs. 6-61A,B; 6-62A,B). At early stages, the integrity of vessel walls and villous capillaries is lost, and irregular, clustered basophilic fragments of degenerating nuclei accumulate focally. Masses of extravasated fragmented red blood cells pour out into the villous stroma, still contained within the intact villous outlines. The villous stroma later becomes fibrotic after proximal vascular occlusion, still with a scattering of fragmented red blood cells in the vessel walls (fig. 6-

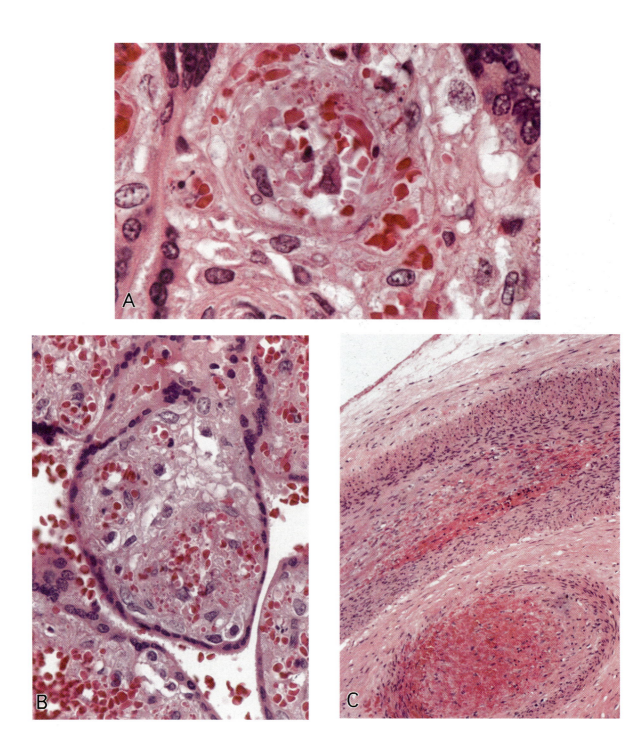

Figure 6-61

HEMORRHAGIC ENDOVASCULITIS

A: A muscular chorionic vessel affected by the active-vasodestructive form of hemorrhagic endovasculitis (HEV) shows a disrupted vessel wall with numerous erythrocyte fragments near the top. (A and B are figs. 1 and 3 from Sander CM, Gilliland D, Akers C, McGrath A, Bismar TA, Swart-Hills LA. Livebirths with placental hemorrhagic endovasculitis: interlesional relationships and perinatal outcomes. Arch Pathol Lab Med 2002;126:157–64.)

B: Terminal villus with totally disrupted intravillous capillaries at right and hypercellular stromal response.

C: Bland form of HEV involves a stem vessel, with partially preserved vessel wall and mural hemorrhage. The mother was gravida 7, para 2, with two abortions and two previous pregnancies complicated by abruption causing fetal death.

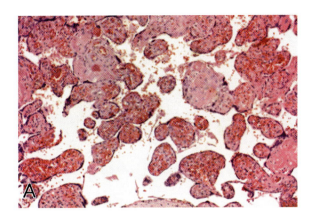
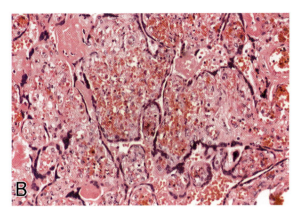
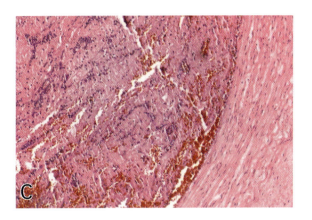

Figure 6-62

HEMORRHAGIC ENDOVASCULITIS

Villi in A and B are typical of hemorrhagic endovasculitis. A large segment of this placenta had this appearance, and was recognizable as a blotchy dark red area grossly (not shown). This area corresponded to the region drained by a large tributary of the umbilical vein, which was occluded by a recent thrombus (C) that extended into the adjacent umbilical vein at the insertion of the umbilical cord. Gestational age was 40 weeks; the mother had gestational diabetes mellitus. Protein A, protein C, and antithrombin III levels were normal. Intrauterine fetal death occurred 24 hours prior to delivery. The thrombi were consistently more than 24 hours old. At autopsy, a renal artery was occluded by a thrombus causing a renal infarct (D). Other placental sections showed multiple foci with the appearance of typical chronic FTV (E).

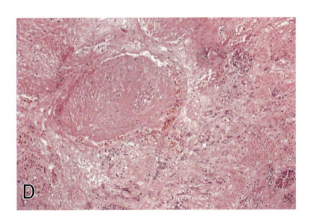
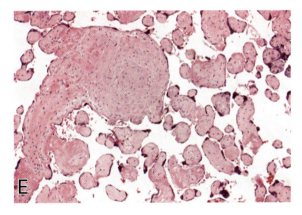

62E). In some placentas, we have found villous stromal hemorrhage associated with a thrombosed vein draining the affected villous sector (fig. 6-62). These histologic features overlap with those described for FTV, especially in the venous occlusive pattern of FTV. As with cases of FTV, it is necessary to distinguish HEV, a localized lesion, from the very similar but diffuse changes associated with intrauterine fetal death, which are well documented in the sequential studies reported by Genest (34). Obviously, it is important that a pathologist interpreting such a placenta know whether the fetus was or was not alive at birth.

Differential Diagnosis. The appearance of the stem vessel with HEV is always disruptive and often destructive as compared to many instances of FTV, in which mural or occlusive thrombi adhere to an intact vessel wall, not always in association with evident vascular injury. The intervillous space typically remains open, as in

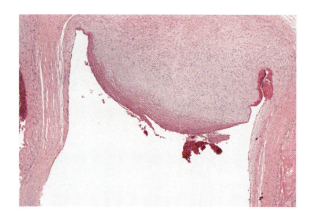 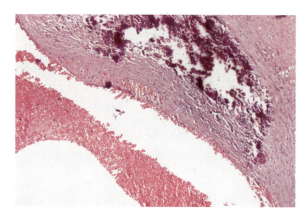

Figure 6-63

ENDOTHELIAL CUSHION

Left: An intraluminal fibroblastic mass (one of many) covered by a layer of fibrin thrombus protrudes from the vessel wall at top. Edema and mild degenerative changes were present in the adjacent vascular media. FTV was also present. The fetus died in utero a few hours before delivery.

Right: Endothelial cushion associated with calcification in the vessel wall and organizing fibrin clot replacing the endothelial surface.

FTV, but unlike the intervillous space within infarcts, acute or chronic villitis, and perivillous fibrin deposit. A distinctive morphologic feature of HEV is the hemorrhage into the villous stroma and extravasation of erythrocytes around thrombosed stem vessels, both of which also occur, though perhaps less dramatically, in FTV. Whether this is truly specific for a primary lesion or a manifestation of FTV, with secondary changes in villi and smaller stem vessels located upstream from a thrombosed fetal vein (fig. 6-62), is not settled.

Prognosis. In a series of 97 placentas (80 from infants who were stillborn) from the Michigan Placental Tissue Registry for which placentas from subsequent deliveries of the same women were examined, Sander et al. (62) found that HEV recurred in 28 placentas (28.9 percent). Of these, 18 of the infants were stillborn. Although there is a definite selection bias in these cases, HEV identifies women at risk for reproductive failure in future pregnancies. Risk factors for recurrence include a higher incidence of chronic villitis, a higher incidence of hypertensive placental lesions, and a history of toxemia or hypertension. Severe neurologic sequelae were more prevalent among liveborn infants with placental HEV than controls in a series of patients with follow-up data from the Michigan Placental Tissue Registry (29).

Endothelial Cushions and Fibrinous Vasculosis

Da Sa (21) described localized, protuberant mural lesions composed of proliferating fibroblasts intermixed with fibrin and erythrocytes in the walls of large placental veins. These "cushions" (fig. 6-63, left) are attributed to local vascular injury and necrosis, with the formation of thrombi. Older lesions are sometimes calcified (fig. 6-63, right). Elevated placental venous pressure is hypothesized as the injurious factor, in some cases resulting in rupture (22). The possibility of a hypercoagulable state is rejected because injury to the vessel wall seems to be the earliest manifestation of the process. An association with disseminated capillary thrombi elsewhere is attributed to emboli from the larger venous lesions.

Clinical features include low birth weight, abruption, maternal hypertension or toxemia, and unexplained intrapartum anoxia. In autopsied stillbirth cases (21), 70 percent showed pulmonary emboli, 35 percent had portal venous thrombi, and 61 percent had disseminated capillary thrombi. Experience with Doppler flow measurements has shown increased vascular resistance, apparently due to vascular obstruction or obliteration in comparable cases (28,36).

Based upon a morphologic analogy with somatic vascular lesions in malignant hypertension in adults, Scott (95) described very similar placental

Circulatory Problems: Thrombi and Other Vascular Lesions

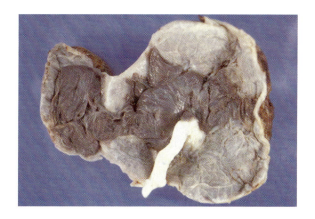

Figure 6-64

SUBAMNIONIC HEMATOMA

The pregnancy, delivery, newborn, and placenta were normal in other respects. Extravasation of blood may have occurred after delivery of the newborn, produced by manipulation of the placenta in the course of delivering it.

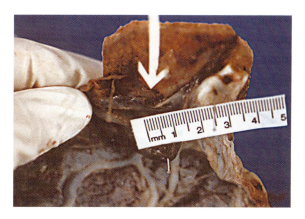

Figure 6-65

SUBAMNIONIC HEMATOMA

Injury to a velamentous vessel by an intrauterine pressure catheter caused this subamnionic hematoma.

lesions under the designation of fibrinous vasculosis, but emphasized edema in the walls of peripheral stem branch vessels. Fetal distress and asphyxia were common, and 40 percent were stillborn. Evidence of a coagulopathy was seen in 46 percent of the surviving newborns.

There is clearly a correlation between objective measurements of intraplacental fetal vascular resistance; obliterative, apparently thrombotic fetal vascular lesions in the placenta; and serious prenatal injury. Whether the primary factor is pressure elevation, intravascular thrombosis, some other local vascular injury, or a combination of factors remains to be determined.

FETAL CIRCULATION: OTHER LESIONS

Subamnionic Hematoma

Definition. Subamnionic hematoma is an accumulation of clotted blood just beneath the amnion and superficial to the chorionic plate (see fig. 6-4). The blood virtually always originates from a fetal vessel.

Incidence. Subamnionic hematomas presenting as well-formed clots just beneath the amnion are rare. Most accumulations of blood between the amnion and chorionic plate are an artifact of the delivery process, formed during or after delivery of the infant. The blood may be mixed with squamous cells from the amniotic fluid and may not have clotted. Significant subamnionic hematomas may follow rupture of a fetal vessel in the chorionic plate caused by injury from procedures such as placement of an intrauterine pressure catheter, amniocentesis, or placement of a fetal scalp electrode.

Gross Findings. Recent subamnionic hematomas are dark red, soft, usually fluctuant accumulations of blood just beneath the very thin amnionic membrane (figs. 6-64, 6-65).

Microscopic Findings. The relationship of the blood to the amnion is apparent in histologic sections. In cases in which significant fetal bleeding has occurred, nucleated red blood cells are sometimes identified.

Differential Diagnosis. The relationship of a hematoma to the amnion and chorionic plate sometimes requires histologic confirmation, especially if the hematoma is recent and the placenta is immature.

Prognosis. As most subamnionic hematomas probably occur after the delivery of the newborn, they are rarely clinically significant. However, instances of subamnionic hematoma caused by intrapartum instrumentation that has ruptured a chorionic plate vessel have caused fatal perinatal exsanguinating hemorrhage.

Stasis Problems

Thrombosis in chorangiomas (hemangiomas) and vascular malformations are discussed in chapter 4. See chapter 4 as well for details on chorangiosis in placentas with FTV.

REFERENCES

1. Aardema MW, Oosterhof H, Timmer A, van Rooy I, Aarnoudse JG. Uterine artery Doppler flow and uteroplacental vascular pathology in normal pregnancies and pregnancies complicated by pre-eclampsia and small for gestational age fetuses. Placenta 2001;22:405–11.
2. Adams-Chapman I, Vaucher YE, Mannino FL, Bejar R, Benirschke K. Association of maternal floor infarction of the placenta with adverse neurodevelopmental outcome [Abstract]. Pediatr Res 1998;43:204A.
3. Andres RL, Kuyper W, Resnik R, Piacquadio KM, Benirschke K. The association of maternal floor infarction of the placenta with adverse perinatal outcome. Am J Obstet Gynecol 1990;163:935–8.
4. Arias F, Romero R, Joist H, Kraus FT. Thrombophilia: a mechanism of disease in women with adverse pregnancy outcome and thrombotic lesions in the placenta. J Matern Fetal Med 1998;7:277–86.
5. Baergen RN, Chacko SA, Edersheim T, Etingin O, Hutson JM, Pirog E. The placenta in thrombophilias: a clinicopathologic study [Abstract]. Mod Pathol 2001;14:213A.
6. Barth WH Jr, Genest DR, Riley LE, Frigoletto FD Jr, Benacerraf BR, Greene MF. Uterine arcuate artery Doppler and decidual microvascular pathology in pregnancies complicated by type I diabetes mellitus. Ultrasound Obstet Gynecol 1996;8:98–103.
7. Bendon RW, Bornstein S, Faye-Peterson OM. Two fetal deaths associated with maternal sepsis and with thrombosis of the intervillous space of the placenta. Placenta 1998;19:385–9.
8. Benirschke K, Kaufmann P. Pathology of the human placenta, 4th ed. New York: Springer; 2000:196–200, 383–4, 551.
9. Burke CJ, Tannenberg AE. Prenatal brain damage and placental infarction—an autopsy study. Devel Med Child Neurol 1995;37:555–62.
10. Burke CJ, Tannenberg AE, Payton DJ. Ischaemic cerebral injury, intrauterine growth retardation, and placental infarction. Devel Med Child Neurol 1997;39:726–30.
11. Byard RW. Idiopathic arterial calcification and unexpected infant death. Pediatr Pathol Lab Med 1996;16:985–94.
12. Cejtin HE, Young SA, Ungaretti J, et al. Effects of cocaine on the placenta. Pediatr Dev Pathol 1999;2:143–7.
13. Chambers JC, Fusi L, Malik IS, Haskard DO, De Swiet M, Kooner JS. Association of maternal endothelial dysfunction with preeclampsia. JAMA 2001;285:1607–12.
14. Colwell JA, Jokl R. Vascular thrombosis in diabetes. In: Porte D, Sherwin S, eds. Ellenberg and Rifkin's diabetes mellitus, 5th ed. Stamford, Connecticut: Appleton Lange; 1997:207–16.
15. Cook V, Weeks J, Brown J, Bendon RW. Umbilical artery occlusion and fetoplacental thromboembolism. Obstet Gynecol 1995;85:870–2.
16. Dahms BB, Boyd T, Redline RW. Severe perinatal liver disease associated with fetal thrombotic vasculopathy. Pediatr Dev Pathol 2002;5:80–5.
17. Darby MJ, Caritis SN, Shen-Schwarz S. Placental abruption in the preterm gestation: an association with chorioamnionitis. Obstet Gynecol 1989;74:88–92.
18. Davis BH, Olsen S, Bigelow NC, Chen JC. Detection of fetal red cells in fetomaternal hemorrhage using a fetal hemoglobin monoclonal antibody by flow cytometry. Transfusion 1998;38:749–56.
19. Debus O, Koch HG, Kurlemann G, et al. Factor V Leiden and genetic defects of thrombophilia in childhood porencephaly. Arch Dis Child Fetal Neonatal Ed 1998;78:F121–4.
20. Dekker GA, Sibai BM. Etiology and pathogenesis of preeclampsia: current concepts. Am J Obstet Gynecol 1998;179:1359–75.
21. DeSa DJ. Intimal cushions in foetal placental veins. J Pathol 1973;110:347–52.
22. DeSa DJ. Rupture of fetal vessels on placental surface. Arch Dis Child 1971;46:495–501.
23. DeVeber G, Monagle P, Chan A, et al. Prothrombotic disorders in infants and children with cerebral thromboembolism. Arch Neurol 1998;55:1539–43.
24. deVries JI, Dekker GA, Huijens PC, Jakobs C, Blomberg BM, van Geijn HP. Hyperhomocysteinaemia and protein S deficiency in complicated pregnancies. Brit J Obstet Gynaecol 1997;104:1248–54.
25. Doss BJ, Jacques SM, Mayes MD, Qureshi F. Maternal scleroderma: placenta findings and perinatal outcome. Hum Pathol 1998;28:1524–30.
26. Elliott JP, Gilpin B, Strong TH Jr, Finberg HJ. Chronic abruption-oligohydramnios sequence. J Reprod Med 1998;43:418–22.
27. Ernst LM, Parkash V. Placental pathology in fetal Bartter syndrome. Pediatr Dev Pathol 2002;5:76–9.
28. Fok RY, Pavlova Z, Benirschke K, Paul RH, Platt LD. The correlation of arterial lesions with umbilical artery Doppler velocimetry in the placentas of small-for-dates pregnancies. Obstet Gynecol 1990;75:578–83.

29. Foley KM, McGrath A, Sander CM. Neurologic sequelae in liveborn infants with placental hemorrhagic endovasculitis [Abstract]. Mod Pathol 2002;15:311A.
30. Fox H. Pathology of the placenta, 2nd ed. Philadelphia: WB Saunders; 1997:122–7, 179.
31. Fox H. Perivillous fibrin deposition in the human placenta. Am J Obstet Gynecol 1967;98:245–5l.
32. Fox H. Thrombosis of the foetal arteries in the human placenta. J Obstet Gynaecol Br Commonw 1966;73:961–5.
33. Frank HG, Malekzadeh F, Kertschanska S, et al. Immunohistochemistry of two different types of placental fibrinoid. Acta Anat 1994;150:55–68.
34. Genest DR. Estimating the time of death in stillborn fetuses. II. Histologic evaluation of the placenta; a study of 71 stillborns. Obstet Gynecol 1992;80:585–92.
35. Gerretsen G, Huisjes HJ, Elema JD. Morphological changes in the spiral arteries in the placental bed in relation to pre-eclampsia and fetal growth retardation. Brit J Obstet Gynaecol 1981;88:876–81.
36. Giles WB, Trudinger BJ, Baird PJ. Fetal umbilical artery flow velocity waveforms and placental resistance: pathological correlation. Brit J Obstet Gynaecol 1985;92:31–8.
37. Giordano P, Laforgia N, Di Giulio G, Storelli S, Mautone A, Iolascon A. Renal vein thrombosis in a newborn with prothrombotic genetic risk factors. J Perinat Med 2001;29:163–7.
38. Goddijn-Wessel TA, Wouters MG, van de Molen EF, et al. Hyperhomocysteinemia: a risk factor for placental abruption and infarction. Eur J Obstet Gynecol Reprod Biol 1996;66:23–9.
39. Grow JL, Fliman PJ, Pipe SW. Neonatal sinovenous thrombosis associated with homozygous thermolabile methylenetetrahydrofolate reductase in both mother and infant. J Perinatol 2002;22:175–8.
40. Hebisch G, Bernasconi MT, Gmuer J, Huch A, Stallmach T. Pregnancy-associated recurrent hemolytic uremic syndrome with fetal thrombotic vasculopathy in the placenta. Am J Obstet Gynecol 2001;185:1265–6.
41. Heller DS, Rush DS, Baergen RN. Subchorionic hematoma associated with thrombophilia. Pediatr Dev Pathol 2003;6:261–4.
42. Hoyme HE, Jones KL, Van Allen MI, Saunders BS, Benirschke K. Vascular pathogenesis of transverse limb reduction defects. J Pediatr 1982;101:839–43.
43. Kanfer A, Bruch JF, Nguyen G, et al. Increased placental antifibrinolytic potential and fibrin deposits in pregnancy-induced hypertension and preeclampsia. Lab Invest 1996;74:253–8.
44. Kaplan C, Blanc WA, Elias J. Identification of erythrocytes in intervillous thrombi: a study using immunoperoxidase identification of hemoglobins. Hum Pathol 1982;13:554–7.
45. Katzman PJ, Genest DR. Maternal floor infarction and massive perivillous fibrin deposition: histological definitions, association with intrauterine fetal growth restriction, and risk of recurrence. Pediatr Dev Pathol 2002;5:159–64.
46. Khong TY. Acute atherosis in pregnancies complicated by hypertension, small for gestational age infants, and diabetes mellitus. Arch Pathol Lab Med 1991;115:722–5.
47. Khong TY, Hague WM. Biparental contribution to fetal thrombophilia in discordant twin intrauterine growth restriction. Am J Obstet Gynecol 2001;185:244–5.
48. Khong TY, Hague WM. The placenta in maternal hyperhomocysteinaemia. Br J Obstet Gynaecol 1999;106:273–8.
49. Kramer MS, Usher RH, Pollack R, Boyd M, Usher S. Etiologic determinants of abruptio placentae. Obstet Gynecol 1997;89:221–6.
50. Kraus FT. Cerebral palsy and thrombi in placental vessels of the fetus: insights from litigation. Hum Pathol 1997;28:246–8.
51. Kraus FT. Placental thrombi and related problems. Semin Diag Pathol 1993;10:275–83.
52. Kraus FT, Acheen VI. Fetal thrombotic vasculopathy in the placenta: cerebral thrombi and infarcts, coagulopathies, and cerebral palsy. Hum Pathol 1999;30:759–69.
53. Kupferminc MJ, Eldor A, Steinman N, et al. Increased frequency of genetic thrombophilia in women with complications of pregnancy. N Engl J Med 1999;340:9–13.
54. Kupferminc MJ, Fait G, Many A, Gordon D, Eldor A, Lessing JB. Severe preeclampsia and high frequency of genetic thrombophilia. Obstet Gynecol 2000;96:45–9.
55. Magid MS, Kaplan C, Sammaritano LR, Peterson M, Druzin ML, Lockshin MD. Placental pathology in systemic lupus erythematosus: a prospective study. Amer J Obstet Gynecol 1998;179:226–36.
56. Mandsager NT, Bendon R, Mostello D, Rosenn B, Miodovnik M, Siddiqui TA. Maternal floor infarction of the placenta: prenatal diagnosis and clinical significance. Obstet Gynecol 1994;83:750–4.
57. Many A, Schreiber L, Rosner S, Lessing JB, Eldor A, Kupferminc MJ. Pathologic features of the placenta in women with severe pregnancy complications and thrombophilia. Obstet Gynecol 2001;98:1041–4.

58. Matern D, Schehata BM, Shekhawa P, Strauss AW, Bennett MJ, Rinaldo P. Placental floor infarction complicating the pregnancy of a fetus with long-chain 3-hydroxyacyl-CoA dehydrogenase (LCHAD) deficiency. Mol Genet Metab 2001;72:265–8.
59. Matijevic R, Johnston T. In vivo assessment of failed trophoblastic invasion of the spiral arteries in pre-eclampsia. Br J Obstet Gynaecol 1999;106:78–82.
60. Maynard S, Min JY, Merchan J, et al. Excess placental soluble fms-like tyrosine kinase 1 (sFlt1) may contribute to endothelial dysfunction, hypertension, and proteinuria in preeclampsia. J Clin Invest 2003;111:649–58.
61. McDermott M, Gillan JE. Trophoblast basement membrane hemosiderosis in the placental lesion of fetal artery thrombosis: a marker for disturbance of maternofetal transfer? Placenta 1995;16:171–8.
62. Mitra SC, Seshan SV, Riachi LE. Placental vessel morphometry in growth retardation and increased resistance of the umbilical artery Doppler flow. J Matern Fetal Med 2000;9:282–6.
63. Mooney EE, al Shunnar A, O'Regan M, Gillan JE. Chorionic villous hemorrhage is associated with retroplacental hemorrhage. Br J Obstet Gynecol 1994;101:965–9.
64. Morgan T, Craven C, Lalouel JM, Ward K. Angiotensinogen Thr235 variant is associated with abnormal physiologic change of the uterine spiral arteries in first trimester decidua. Am J Obstet Gynecol 1999;180:95–102.
65. Mousa HA, Alfirevicl Z. Do placental lesions reflect thrombophilic state in women with adverse pregnancy outcome? Hum Reprod 2000;15:1830–3.
66. Naeye RL. Maternal floor infarction. Hum Pathol 1985;16:823–8.
67. Nelson DM. Apoptotic changes occur in syncytiotrophoblast of human placental villi where fibrin type fibrinoid is deposited in discontinuities in the villous trophoblast. Placenta 1996;17:387–91.
68. Nikkels PG, van Gemert MJ, Sollie-Szarynska KM, Mollendijk H, Timmer B, Machin GA. Rapid onset of severe twin-twin transfusion syndrome caused by placental venous thrombosis. Pediatr Dev Pathol 2002;5:310–4.
69. Novak PM, Sander CM, Yang SS, von Oeyen PT. Report of fourteen cases of nonimmune hydrops fetalis in association with hemorrhagic endovasculitis of the placenta. Am J Obstet Gynecol 1991;165:945–50.
70. Ogueh O, Chen MF, Spurll G, Benjamin A. Outcome of pregnancy in women with hereditary thrombophilia. Int J Gynaecol Obstet 2001;74:247–53.
71. Pipkin FB. Risk factors for preeclampsia (Editorial). N Eng J Med 2001;344:925–6.
72. Powers RW, Evans RW, Majors AK, et al. Plasma homocysteine concentration is increased in preeclampsia and is associated with evidence of endothelial activation. Am J Obstet Gynecol 1998;179:1605–11.
73. Prengler M, Sturt N, Flanagan M. Krywawych S, Liesner R, Kirkham F. The homozygous thermolabile variant of the methylene tetrahydrofolate reductase gene: a risk factor for cerebrovascular disease and stroke in childhood. Dev Med Child Neurol 1998;40 (Supp 79):10–11.
74. Rand JH. Antiphospholipid antibody-mediated disruption of the annexin-V antithrombotic shield: a thrombogenic mechanism for the antiphospholipid syndrome. J Autoimmun 2000;15:107–11.
75. Rand JH, Wu XX, Andree HA, et al. Pregnancy loss in the antiphospholipid-antibody syndrome—a possible thrombogenic mechanism. N Eng J Med 1997;337:154–60.
76. Rayne SC, Kraus FT. Placental thrombi and other vascular lesions. Classification, morphology, and clinical correlations. Path Res Pract 1993;189:2–17.
77. Redline RW, O' Riordan MA. Placental lesions associated with cerebral palsy and neurologic impairment following term birth. Arch Pathol Lab Med 2000;124:1785–91.
78. Redline RW, Pappin A. Fetal thrombotic vasculopathy: the clinical significance of extensive avascular villi. Hum Pathol 1995;26:80–5.
79. Redline RW, Patterson P. Patterns of placental injury. Correlations with gestational age, placental weight, and clinical diagnoses. Arch Pathol Lab Med 1994;118:698–701.
80. Redline RW, Patterson P. Pre-eclampsia is associated with an excess of proliferative immature intermediate trophoblast. Hum Pathol 1995;26:594–600.
81. Redline RW, Shah D, Saker H, Schluchter M, Salvator A. Placental lesions associated with abnormal growth in twins. Pediatr Dev Pathol 2001;4:473–81.
82. Redline RW, Wilson-Costello D. Chronic peripheral separation of placenta. The significance of diffuse chorionic hemosiderosis. Am J Clin Pathol 1999;111:804–10.
83. Redline RW, Wilson-Costello D, Borawski E, Fanaroff AA, Hack M. The relationship between placental and other perinatal risk factors for neurologic impairment in very low birth weight children. Pediatric Research 2000;47:721–6.

84. Robertson WB, Brosens I, Dixon HG. The pathological response of vessels of the placental bed to hypertensive pregnancy. J Pathol Bacteriol 1967;93:581–92.
85. Saftlas AF, Olson DR, Atrash HK, Rochat R, Rowley D. National trends in the incidence of abruptio placentae, 1979-1987. Obstet Gynecol 1991;78:1081–6.
86. Salafia CM. Placental pathology of fetal growth restriction. Clin Obstet Gynaecol 1997;40:740–9.
87. Salafia CM, Lopez-Zeno JA, Sherer DM, Whittington SS, Minior VK, Vintzileos AM. Histologic evidence of old intrauterine bleeding is more frequent in prematurity. Am J Obstet Gynecol 1995;173:1065–70.
88. Salafia CM, Minior VK, Pezzullo JC, Popek EJ, Rosenkrantz TS, Vintzileos AM. Intrauterine growth restriction in infants of less than thirty-two weeks gestation: associated placental pathologic features. Am J Obstet Gynecol 1995;173:1049–57.
89. Salafia CM, Pezzullo JC, Minior VK, Divon MY. Placental pathology of absent and reversed end-diastolic flow in growth-restricted fetuses. Obstet Gynecol 1997;90:830–6.
90. Salafia CM, Vintzileos AM, Silberman L, Bantham KF, Vogel CA. Placental pathology of idiopathic intrauterine growth retardation at term. Am J Perinatol 1992;9:179–84.
91. Sander CH. Hemorrhagic endovasculitis and hemorrhagic villitis of the placenta. Arch Pathol Lab Med 1980;104:371–3.
92. Sander CM. Hemorrhagic endovasculitis in the placenta. Am J Obstet Gynecol 1992;167:1483.
93. Sander CM, Gilliand D, Akers C, McGrath A, Bismar TA, Swart-Hills LA. Livebirths with placental hemorrhagic endovasculitis: interlesional relationships and perinatal outcomes. Arch Pathol Lab Med 2002;126:157–64.
94. Sander CH, Kinnane L, Stevens NG, Echt R. Haemorrhagic endovasculitis of the placenta: a review with clinical correlation. Placenta 1986;7:551–74.
95. Scott JM. Fibrinous vasculosis in the human placenta. Placenta 1983;4:87–99.
96. Sebire NJ, Backos M, Goldin RD, Regan L. Placental massive perivillous fibrin deposition associated with antiphospholipid antibody syndrome. BJOG 2002;109:570–3.
97. Seligsohn U, Berger A, Abend M, et al. Homozygous protein C deficiency manifested by massive venous thrombosis in the newborn. N Engl J Med 1984;310:559–62.
98. Shanklin DR, Scott JS. Massive subchorial thrombohaematoma (Breus' mole). Br J Obstet Gynaecol 1975;82:476–87.
99. Shanklin DR, Sibai BM. Ultrastructural aspects of preeclampsia. I. Placental bed and uterine boundary vessels. Am J Obstet Gynecol 1989;161:735–41.
100. Scher MS, Belfar H, Martin J, Painter MJ. Destructive brain lesions of presumed fetal onset: antepartum causes of cerebral palsy. Pediatrics 1991;88:898–906.
101. Shen-Schwarz S, Macpherson TA, Mueller-Heubach E. The clinical significance of hemorrhagic endovasculitis of the placenta. Am J Obstet Gynecol 1988;159:48–51.
102. Sherer DM, Anyaegbunam A, Onyeije C. Antepartum fetal intracranial hemorrhage, predisposing factors and prenatal sonography: a review. Am J Perinatol 1998;15:431–41.
103. Sherer DM, Schenker JG. Accidental injury during pregnancy. Obstet Gynecol Surv 1989;44:330–8.
104. Shu F, Sugimura M, Kanayama N, Kobayashi H, Kobayashi T, Terao T. Immunohistochemical study of annexin V expression in placentae of preeclampsia. Gynecol Obstet Invest 2000;49:17–23.
105. Sibai BM, Gordon T, Thom E, et al. Risk factors for preeclampsia in healthy nulliparous women: a prospective multicenter study. The National Institute of Child Health and Human Development Network of Maternal-Fetal Medicine Units. Am J Obstet Gynecol 1995;172:642–8.
106. Sibai BM, Ramadan MK, Usta I, Salama M, Mercer BM, Friedman SA. Maternal morbidity and mortality in 442 pregnancies with hemolysis, elevated liver enzymes, and low platlets (HELLP syndrome). Am J Obstet Gynecol 1993;169:1000–6.
107. Stanek J, Bove KE, Bofinger M, et al. Premature closure of foramen ovale and renal vein thrombosis in a stillborn twin homozygous for methylene tetrahydrofolate reductase gene polymorphism: a clinicopathologic study. J Perinat Med 2000;28:61–8.
108. Thorarensen O, Ryan S, Hunter J, Younkin DP. Factor V Leiden 19 mutations: an unrecognized cause of hemiplegic cerebral palsy, neonatal stroke, and placental thrombosis. Ann Neurol 1997;42:372–5.
109. Tibboel D, Gaillard JL, Molenaar JC. The importance of mesenteric vascular insufficiency in meconium peritonitis. Hum Pathol 1986;17:411–6.
110. Todros T, Sciarrone A, Piccoli E, Guiot C, Kaufmann P, Kingdom J. Umbilical Doppler waveforms and placental villous angiogenesis in pregnancies complicated by fetal growth restriction. Obstet Gynecol 1999;93:499–503.
111. van Allen MI, Jackson JC, Knopp RH, Cone R. In utero thrombosis and neonatal gangrene in an infant of a diabetic mother. Am J Med Genet 1989;33:323–7.

112. van der Molen EF, Verbruggen B, Novakova I, Eskes TK, Monnens LA, Blom HJ. Hyperhomocysteinemia and other thrombotic risk factors in women with placental vasculopathy. BJOG 2000;107:785–91.
113. van Pampus MG, Dekker GA, Wolf H, et al. High prevalence of hemostatic abnormalities in women with a history of preeclampsia. Am J Obstet Gynecol 1999;180:1146–50.
114. Vernof KK, Benirschke K, Kephart GM, Wasmoen TL, Gleich GJ. Maternal floor infarction: relationship to X cells, major basic protein, and adverse perinatal outcome. Am J Obstet Gynecol 1992;167:1355–63.
115. Wentworth P. The incidence and significance of intervillous thrombi in the human placenta. J Obstet Gynaecol Br Commonw 1964;71:894–8.
116. Wiener-Megnagi Z, Ben-Schlomo I, Goldberg Y, Shalev E. Resistance to activated protein C and the Leiden mutation: high prevalence of patients with abruptio placenta. Am J Obstet Gynecol 1998;179:1565–7.
117. Wurtzei JM. TTP lesions in placenta but not fetus. N Eng J Med 1979;301:503–4.
118. Zeek PM, Assali NS. Vascular changes in the decidua associated with eclamptogenic toxemia of pregnancy. Am J Clin Pathol 1950;20:1099–109.

7 NORMAL STRUCTURE AND PATHOLOGY OF THE MEMBRANES

The placental membranes, in continuity with the placenta, form a saccular "bag of waters" in which the growing fetus floats. They form a barrier to keep infectious agents out, and to keep the amnionic fluid in. This barrier is a dynamic interface, with important physical and metabolic properties.

ANATOMY AND PHYSIOLOGY

The innermost layer of the placenta is fetally derived. It is composed of the amniotic membrane with its basement membrane, and a thin stratum of connective tissue beneath. Next, loosely attached, is the chorion laeve, also fetally derived and composed of a second, thicker connective tissue stratum and a layer of trophoblast cells. In this region may be found scattered atrophic remnants of chorionic villi. The outermost component of the membranes is the maternally derived decidua capsularis, which interdigitates somewhat with the overlying trophoblast layer (fig. 7-1).

The amnionic epithelium is composed of cuboidal or columnar cells, which co-express cytokeratin, desmoplakin, and vimentin intermediate filaments, suggesting both epithelial and mesenchymal characteristics. Enzymes involved in prostaglandin synthesis (8), carbonic anhydrase isoforms (28), nitric oxide synthase (19), and matrix metalloproteinases (48) are all expressed by amnion cells. The variety of molecules indicates that the amnion actively supports intrauterine homeostasis and modulates events related to the onset of labor, whether normal or premature.

The amnionic epithelium also produces its basement membrane (type IV collagen) and the underlying, thin, compact stromal layer of amnionic mesoderm. Deep to this is an ill-defined plane (called the spongy layer) through which the amnion easily becomes detached. Next in sequence is the thicker chorionic mesodermal layer (fig. 7-1), which includes a cellular component of fibroblasts and macrophages.

Both the amnionic and chorionic mesoderm layers are composed of a dense, tough matrix of different collagen types (mainly I and III) and sizes, as well as fibronectins and laminins (7,25). The amnionic epithelium and the mesenchymal fibroblasts produce the collagen matrix, a process that is enhanced by adequate vitamin C (3).

Degradation of the collagen matrix during labor is accomplished by a large family of matrix metalloproteinase (MMP) enzymes and their activators, whose actions are enhanced by relaxin, and modulated by a group of inhibitors (20). The presence of amnionic fluid MMP-8, which is secreted by neutrophils during inflammatory conditions in the amnionic fluid, is an indication of a significant fetal inflammatory response to infection (amnionic fluid neutrophils appear to originate from the fetus [38, 40]), resulting in preterm delivery and adverse

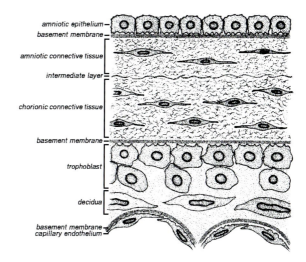

Figure 7-1

EXTRAPLACENTAL MEMBRANE HISTOLOGY

Diagram of exraplacental membrane histology in cross section. The tissues above the intermediate layer (which is actually a potential space through which the amnion strips from the chorionic tissue), chorionic tissue, and trophoblast are of fetal origin. The decidua and capillary vessels are maternal. (Modified from fig. 17 from reference 39.)

neonatal outcome (26,31). Exotoxins, lipopolysaccharide endotoxins, and MMP enzymes are also released directly by several of the more prominent bacterial species that cause chorioamnionitis, resulting in prostaglandin and cytokine release, thereby initiating the process of labor prematurely (47).

The chorionic trophoblast layer (fig. 7-1) is composed of a specific form of mononuclear trophoblast, which has been designated *chorionic-type intermediate trophoblast* (41). This name reflects a phenotype that has an immunostaining profile identical to the cell type of the placental site nodule. Between the trophoblast cells are small clumps of an amorphous eosinophilic material that is identical to matrix-type fibrinoid (14), which is predominantly a trophoblast secretion product, not a derivative of the blood clotting system. These chorionic-type intermediate trophoblast cells produce renin, for which a specific gestational function has not yet been identified (34).

MECONIUM STAINING

Prevalence. Meconium staining of the placenta is common and has long been perceived to be a nonspecific indicator of perinatal morbidity. The reported prevalence of meconium staining ranges from 7 to 25 percent (33). In one large study of term deliveries, the prevalence was 19 percent (29). Meconium is unlikely to be present before 30 weeks' gestation, but it is especially common in post-term placentas, of which 31 percent may be affected (46).

Clinical Features. A study of 8,136 newborns with meconium-stained amnionic fluid found that 8 percent had some form of morbidity (29). Neonatal morbidity occurred in only 2.5 percent of 34,573 newborn controls with clear fluid. Meconium in the amnionic fluid was significantly associated with neonatal morbidity of all kinds, when compared to the deliveries with clear fluid. Distinctions between "thick" and "thin" meconium-stained fluid are arbitrary, but important. Thick meconium, characterized as "viscous, tenacious, opaque, containing large amounts of particulate material" is associated with a three-fold increase in risk for adverse neonatal outcome independent of fetal heart rate abnormalities and maternal risk factors (6).

In the authors' experience with perinatal injury, meconium staining is usually not the only, or even the more significant, pathologic lesion in the placenta. Chorioamnionitis is an especially common association, and may be the major injurious factor in instances of neonatal morbidity when it accompanies meconium staining (11,33,37). The growth of group B *Streptococcus* is enhanced by the presence of meconium (13). Meconium staining was present in nearly half of the cases in a series of perinatal deaths attributed to fetal thrombotic vasculopathy (24). The probability of neonatal morbidity is significantly increased in the presence of other placental lesions (23). The role of meconium as the primary factor contributing to the so-called *meconium aspiration syndrome* is also controversial (15). Meconium may become more toxic in the presence of fetal acidosis (35). Autopsy studies indicates that the meconium aspiration syndrome appears to have chronic prenatal origins in most cases, related especially to intrauterine infection or chronic intrauterine hypoxia (15,44).

In vitro studies of the rate of diffusion and phagocytosis of meconium in the placental membranes indicate that meconium appears in the superficial amnion within 1 hour of exposure and in deeper chorionic macrophages within 3 hours (27). Meconium applied in vitro causes contraction of umbilical vein smooth muscle (2,17). Cytokines and meconium products have been demonstrated in macrophages in the walls of fetal vessels of meconium-stained placentas from miscarriages (42). It seems unlikely that meconium passage uncomplicated by any other problem could have caused the abortion or premature labor in these cases, which were not described in detail. The absence of appropriate microbial culture data lessens the credibility of meconium as a cause of chorioamnionitis without infection (9).

Gross Findings. The fetal surface of the placenta, the membranes, and the cord typically are dark green. The intensity of the color varies, becoming more intense and darker with the passage of time. The membranes are commonly edematous, with a slimy consistency (figs. 7-2, 7-3).

Microscopic Findings. Meconium is identifiable as irregular, brown cytoplasmic granules in macrophages (figs. 7-4, 7-5). The brown color fades with exposure to light, perhaps, in some

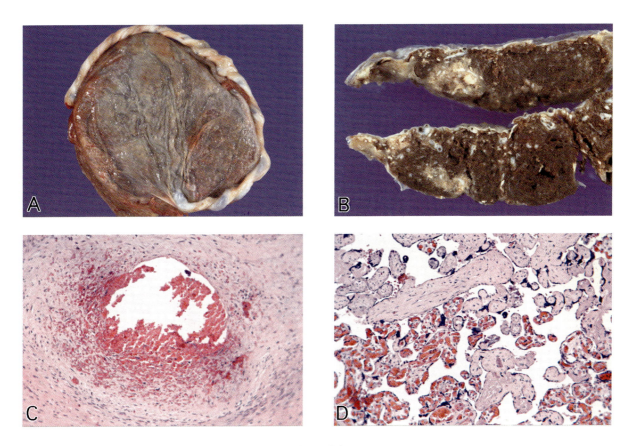

Figure 7-2

MECONIUM STAINING OF A TERM PLACENTA

A: There was a tight nuchal cord. The amnionic fluid contained "thick" meconium. Tracheal suction was required, with minor amounts below the vocal cords, followed by normal respirations subsequently. Histologic pigmentation was light.

B: The presence of extensive fetal thrombotic vasculopathy was the most significant gross and microscopic lesion in the placenta depicted in A, and this represents the basic cause of fetal distress in this case. Mild chorioamnionitis (stage I) was also present.

C: Features of fetal thrombotic vasculopathy included multiple occluded stem vessels.

D: Avascular fibrotic villi (top) contrast with normal villi (bottom). This lesion was responsible for the meconium discharge.

cases, as the slides sit upon the trays in the histology laboratory prior to pathologic evaluation (4). The amnionic epithelium may become vacuolated and ultimately necrotic (fig. 7-6). After prolonged periods of exposure, Altshuler et al. (1) found necrosis in the vascular smooth muscle of the cord and chorionic vessels in 10 of 1,100 meconium-stained placentas (fig. 7-7). Five of the 10 placentas in this study had chronic ischemic placental changes and 4 had chorangiosis, indicative of a possible contribution to the fetal injury by other, more chronic lesions as factors causing the meconium release. In another study, meconium-associated vascular necrosis was significantly increased in infants with cerebral palsy compared to a control group with meconium staining alone (36).

It is important to distinguish between meconium stain in the membranes and the stain produced by degraded blood products that diffuse out of hematomas within or adjacent to the placenta (fig. 7-8). The latter stain is easily mistaken for meconium, which is more common, and such a mistake is more likely when the possibility of hematoma is not even considered. Distinguishing true meconium from hematoma may be difficult because both pigments are forms of altered or degraded hemoglobin and the colors change with the passage of time. Degenerating blood products usually are brown or red-brown,

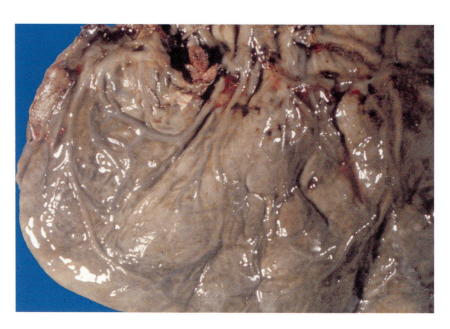

Figure 7-3
MECONIUM STAINING OF A POST-TERM PLACENTA

The dark green-brown coloring indicates prolonged exposure to meconium, comparable to the histology of the macrophages seen in figure 7-6. The opaque appearance is due to chorioamnionitis, which may have contributed to the severity of the meconium discharge. Cesarean section was done for fetal distress. Marked edema of the membranes produced a slimy consistency.

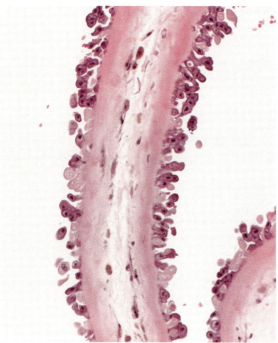

Figure 7-4
MECONIUM STAINING

The amnionic epithelium and macrophages contain brown pigment. The amnionic epithelial cells are vacuolated, piled up, and beginning to desquamate. Cesarean section was performed for fetal distress at term. The occurrence of multifocal chronic villitis and extensive fetal thrombotic vasculopathy in this placenta (not shown) contributed significantly to the fetal distress as well as to the expulsion of the meconium. Apgar scores were 1 at 1 minute and 8 at 5 minutes. (Figs. 7-4 and 7-5 are from the same patient.)

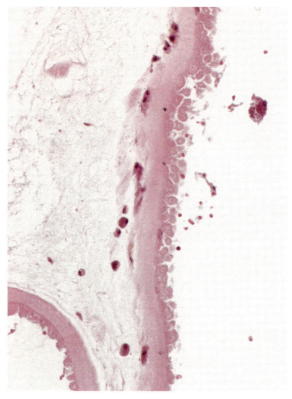

Figure 7-5
MECONIUM STAINING

Progressive necrosis of amnionic epithelial cells, which have lost nuclear staining, suggests prolonged exposure to the meconium. The subamnionic connective tissue matrix is edematous and contains meconium-stained macrophages.

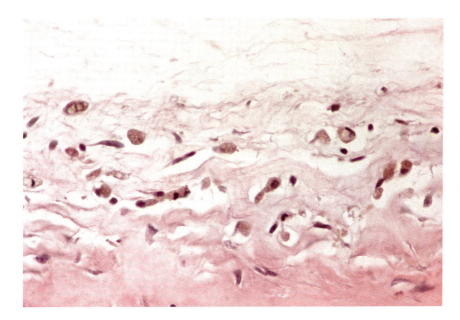

Figure 7-6
MECONIUM STAINING
Pronounced pigmentation of numerous macrophages, edema, and degenerative changes in the deeper matrix of the chorionic plate suggest prolonged meconium exposure.

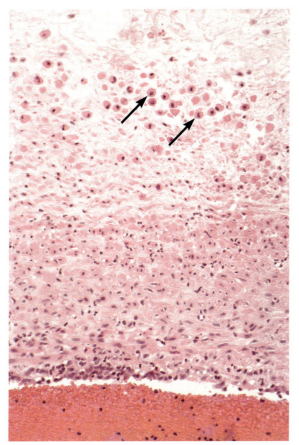
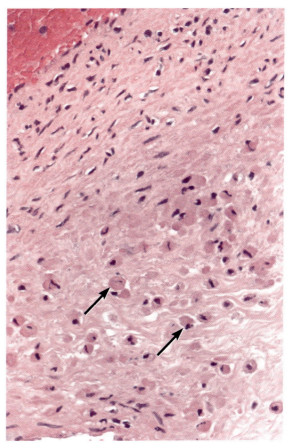

Figure 7-7
VASCULAR CHANGES IN PROLONGED MECONIUM STAINING
This umbilical artery from a meconium-stained placenta shows necrosis of the outer layer of vascular smooth muscle (arrows). The nuclei are pyknotic and the cytoplasm has a dense, eosinophilic, smudged appearance.

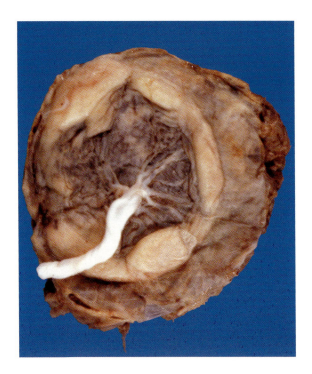

Figure 7-8

HEMOSIDERIN STAINING

Degraded hemoglobin from an old clot at the margins of a circumvallate placenta produces various shades of tan, yellow, and brown.

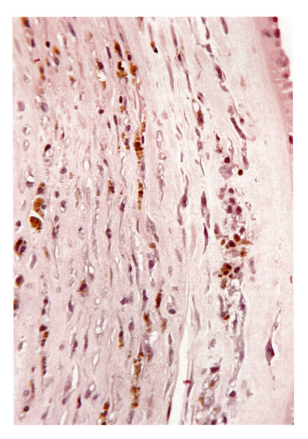

Figure 7-9

HEMOSIDERIN IN MACROPHAGES

Hemosiderin in macrophages in the amnion of this placenta occurred because of breakdown of old retroplacental clots (chronic abruption, not shown). Compare the golden particulate appearance of hemosiderin to the more amorphous brown meconium pigment in figures 7-4 to 7-6. (Figs. 7-9 and 7-10 are from the same patient.)

which may evolve into orange-brown or yellow. Hemosiderin granules in macrophages have a more crystalline, refractile gold to yellow-brown appearance (fig. 7-9; also see chapter 4, fig. 4-5). An iron stain should help make the distinction in ambiguous cases (fig. 7-10; also see fig. 4-6). Old, degenerating brown clot at the margin of a circumvallate placenta is common, and commonly overlooked (see figs. 4-2–4-4).

INFLAMMATION

The important topics of chorioamnionitis and related inflammatory conditions in the membranes are the subject of chapter 5.

SQUAMOUS METAPLASIA

Definition. Focal small patches of mature keratinizing squamous epithelium are frequently present on the amnionic surface of the cord, and are common on the fetal surface of the placenta as well. This is not a true metaplasia, as the normal amnion is a less mature form of squamous epithelium.

Prevalence. Small foci may be found in 60 percent of term placentas (5), but infrequently, if at all, in premature placentas.

Clinical Features. Squamous metaplasia is generally limited to the area near the cord insertion and may be related to mechanical stress as the fetus moves in utero. There are no adverse correlations.

Gross Findings. Squamous metaplasia has the appearance of small, opaque, shiny, gray or pale tan plaques, usually no more than 1 or 2 mm in diameter (fig. 7-11). These are to be distinguished from amnion nodosum and the focal keratin granulomas found on the denuded chorionic surfaces after amnionic rupture, with or without the amnionic band syndrome.

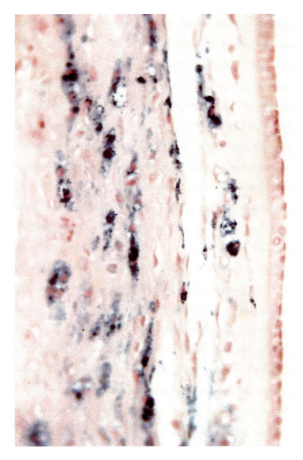

Figure 7-10

HEMOSIDERIN IN MACROPHAGES

Prussian blue stain confirms that the golden brown material in figure 7-9 is iron.

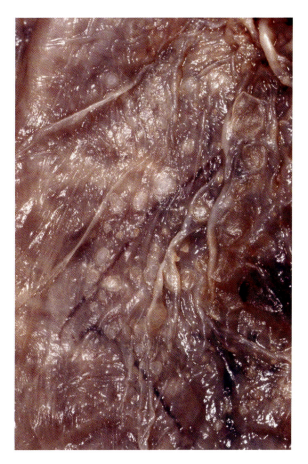

Figure 7-11

SQUAMOUS METAPLASIA

Squamous metaplasia of the amnion forms tiny, pale gray, opaque plaques, most prominent near the cord insertion at the upper right.

Microscopic Findings. The pattern is identical to keratinized squamous epithelium in other locations, such as skin, but without any skin appendages (fig. 7-12).

AMNION NODOSUM

Definition. Amnion nodosum are small granules that adhere to the amnionic surface of the placenta.

Prevalence. These are rare, except in association with severe oligohydramnios, where they are common. Amnion nodosum is rare before 20 weeks even in the presence of severe oligohydramnios.

Clinical Features. Severe oligohydramnios is especially common in fetuses with renal agenesis and sirenomelia, in which the fetal urine cannot contribute to the amnionic fluid. Severe oligohydramnios is also a feature of the amnion of the "stuck twin" donor partner in the monochorionic twin-twin transfusion syndrome, in which the small anemic donor is oliguric while the large plethoric recipient has polyhydramnios. Other causes include prolonged rupture of membranes and marked uteroplacental underperfusion.

Gross Findings. These small nodular structures have a rough, tan or yellow-brown surface (figs. 7-13, 7-14).

Microscopic Findings. A circumscribed heterogeneous granular matrix of eosinophilic debris replaces the amnion, and adheres to the chorionic matrix. Amnionic epithelium may partly cover some margins. Vernix squames and fragments of lanugo hair can be identified (figs. 7-15, 7-16).

Figure 7-12
SQUAMOUS METAPLASIA
Squamous metaplasia is composed of maturing keratinocytes with anucleate squames at the surface.

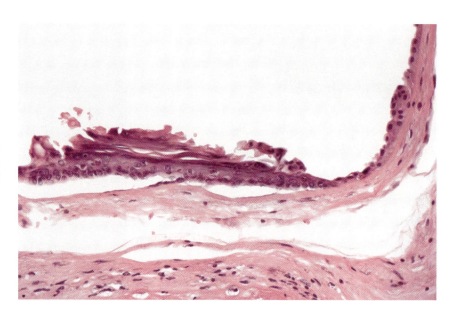

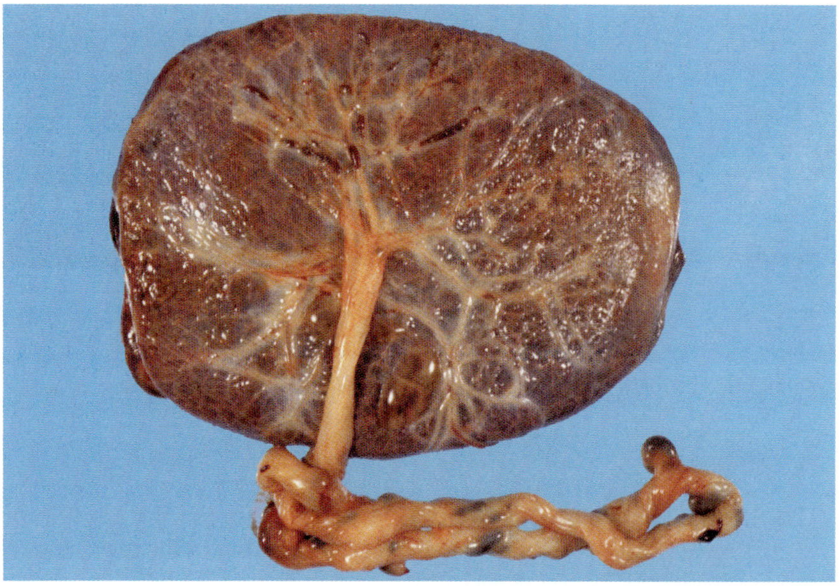

Figure 7-13
AMNION NODOSUM
Numerous small tan papules cover the amnionic surface of the placenta. The newborn had renal agenesis, resulting in severe oligohydramnios and pulmonary hypoplasia.

Figure 7-14
AMNION NODOSUM
Close-up view of the placenta in figure 7-13. The papules appear smooth and opaque.

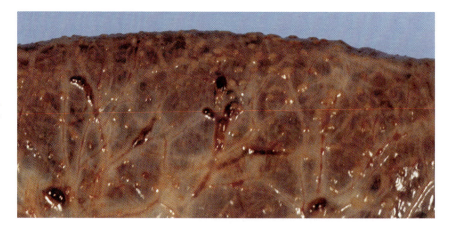

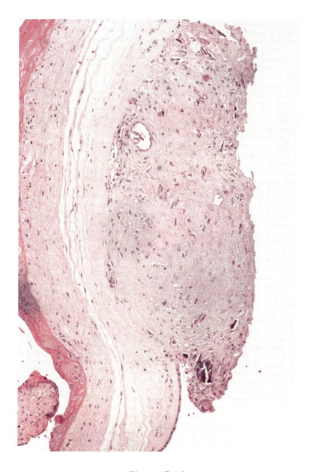

Figure 7-15

AMNION NODOSUM

At low magnification, there is a pale, eosinophilic, granular appearance, with scattered cells and debris intermixed with an amorphous matrix. The amnionic epithelium is obliterated.

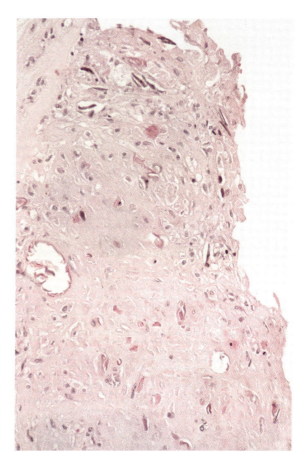

Figure 7-16

AMNION NODOSUM

Under higher magnification, amnion nodosum contains scattered squames, hair fragments, and other unidentifiable detritus.

AMNIONIC BANDS

Definition. Amnionic bands are strips of detached amnion that may entwine and constrict fetal appendages, resulting in amputations. Larger strips or sheets of amnion may lead to dramatic distortions of the head and trunk, including the limb-body wall complex. Synonyms include the *ADAM (amnionic deformity, adhesion, mutilation) complex, amnionic band disruption complex, amnion rupture sequence, amnionic adhesion malformation syndrome,* and *limb-body wall complex.*

Prevalence. The bands cause more problems early in pregnancy and are identified as a cause of fetal death for nearly 2 percent of previable aborted fetuses (22). Estimates for term occurrence range from 1 in 2,500 to 1 in 10,000 deliveries (5).

Clinical Features and Pathogenesis. Simple entanglements lead to loss of tissue distal to a constriction. Some massive deformities expose and distort the brain, or thoracic or abdominal contents, with facial clefts that do not follow any developmental pattern. A direct relationship between a constricting strip of detached amnion and atrophy or deformity of a limb distal to the constriction seems intuitively reasonable. The more massive and dramatic deformities are harder to explain on a purely mechanical or entrapment basis. Benirschke (5) has made a thorough review of the various theories advanced in this debate.

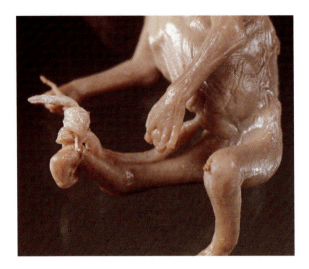

Figure 7-17

AMNIONIC BANDS

Amnionic bands attach and deform the right hand and foot as well as the umbilical cord of this macerated aborted fetus.

Gross Findings. Adherent strands of amnion that are associated with deformities in extremities are the most common (figs. 7-17, 7-18). Extensive, irrational, asymmetric disruptions of body cavities with extrusion of deformed organs represent the extreme complex end of the spectrum (figs. 7-19, 7-20). The fetal surface of the placenta loses the smooth shiny appearance of intact amnion, but the loss of light reflex and foci of roughened surface are often subtle and easily overlooked (fig. 7-21). Residual strands of amnion are often inconspicuous, attached near the insertion of the umbilical cord (fig. 7-22).

Microscopic Findings. Histologic examination of the strips of membranous tissue confirms its identity as amnion (fig. 7-23). In addition to the absence of an amnionic surface, the exposed chorionic plate may show clumps of adherent vernix. Squames of vernix origin may become incorporated into the tissues of the chorionic plate to produce ill-defined foci of fibrosis, which are called *vernix granulomas* (figs. 7-24, 7-25) (49).

EXTRAMEMBRANOUS PREGNANCY

Definition. Rupture of the full thickness of both the amnionic and chorionic layers of the membranes occurs, so that the fetus becomes situated in the endometrial cavity.

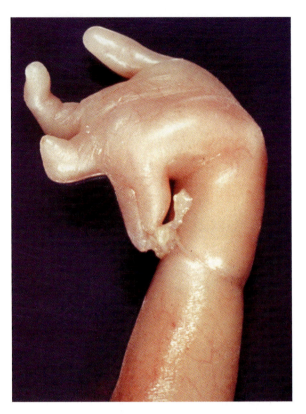

Figure 7-18

AMNIONIC BANDS

A fetal hand is deformed by an adherent amnionic band.

Prevalence. This condition is rare; information about it comes mainly from compilations of individual case reports.

Clinical Features. There are frequent episodes of amniorrhea, and episodic vaginal bleeding may also occur. The fetus may have pulmonary hypoplasia due to the scant amnionic fluid. Death commonly occurs from pulmonary insufficiency in the first few hours of life, but some infants survive (32). Compression deformities of the fetus, comparable to those associated with oligohydramnios, may occur.

Gross Findings. The placentas are consistently circumvallate, with old clot at the margins. Hemosiderin stain discolors the residual membranous surfaces. The opening in the residual membranes, through which the cord passes, is very small, suggesting that rupture occurred early in the gestation. Amnion nodosum may be present. The umbilical cord is short. In an instance of extramembranous

Normal Structure and Pathology of the Membranes

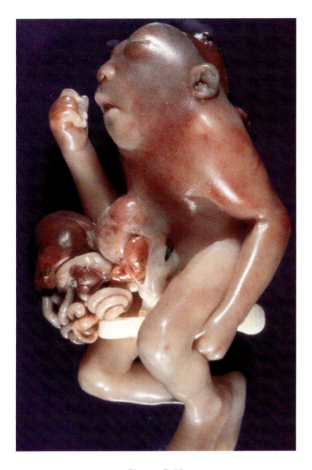

Figure 7-19

AMNIONIC BANDS

Massive gross deformities are associated with the limb-body wall complex.

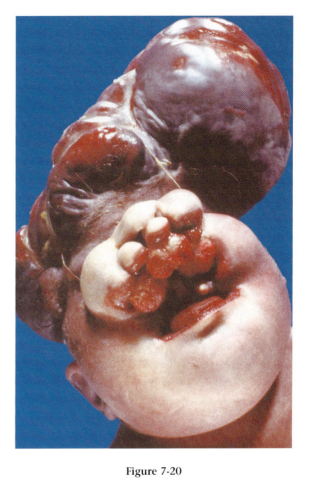

Figure 7-20

AMNIONIC BANDS

Marked asymmetric head and cerebral deformities in the limb-body wall complex, possibly a form of the amniotic band syndrome.

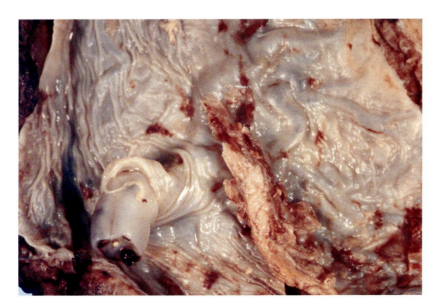

Figure 7-21

AMNIONIC BAND SYNDROME

The entire amnion has become chronically detached from the placenta except for a small strand of amnion attached to the cord insertion at left. The surface appears dull, with scattered clumps of brown debris. The incision at the upper right is an artifact.

Placental Pathology

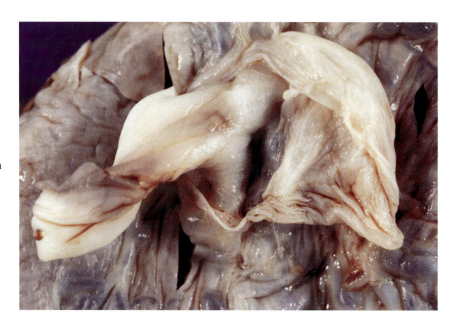

Figure 7-22

AMNIONIC BAND SYNDROME

A collar of residual amnion surrounds the cord insertion.

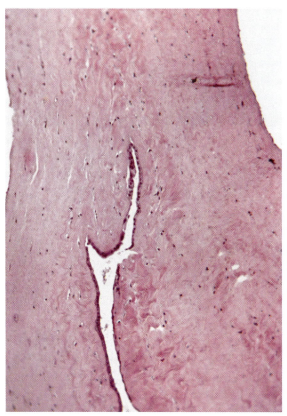

Figure 7-23

AMNIONIC BANDS

Amnionic bands are composed of a sparsely cellular, collagenous, connective tissue matrix with a partial covering of residual amnionic epithelium.

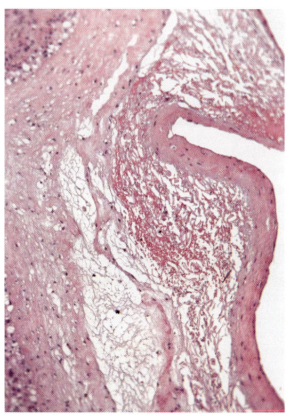

Figure 7-24

AMNIONIC BAND SYNDROME

The surface of the chorionic plate is composed of a bare, variably fibrotic or edematous connective tissue matrix, intermixed with patchy foci of buried squames and degenerating blood.

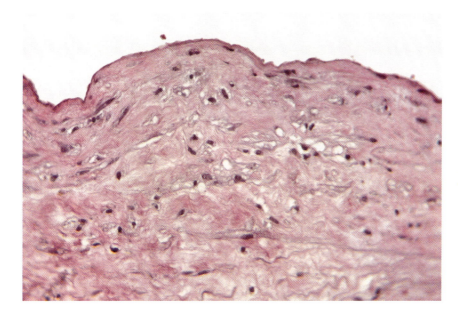

Figure 7-25

AMNIONIC BAND SYNDROME

At higher magnification, the chorionic plate may include foci of fibrosis, forming a bland reaction to buried squames.

pregnancy involving one of a set of dichorionic twins, the affected twin expressed the full clinical-pathologic spectrum of abnormalities, while the other, twin appeared normal and survived (30).

Microscopic Findings. Foci of amnion nodosum are present (see figs. 7-15, 7-16). Macrophages in the membranes or other placental and inner uterine surfaces contain hemosiderin.

GASTROSCHISIS

Definition. Gastroschisis is the result of a paraumbilical abdominal wall opening through which loops of bowel protrude. It is to be distinguished from omphalocele, in which the defect is at the cord insertion and the bowel loops are covered by a saccular membrane composed of peritoneum and amnion.

Incidence. A population study of 265,858 consecutive births in France (43) found that gastroschisis occurred in 1.76 in 10,000 births, and omphalocele in 2.18 in 10,000 births. There are significant geographic variations, and the incidence appears to be increasing (12).

Clinical Features. Other bowel anomalies occur in about one third of newborns with gastroschisis, but the high prevalence (up to 70 percent) of chromosomal anomalies associated with omphaloceles does not occur with gastroschisis. Surgical correction is usually possible. More than 90 percent of infants survive, and the long-term prognosis is excellent (12).

Gross Findings. Prior to the 30th week the loops of bowel are covered only by the normal serosa, but after that time a marked progressive fibrous serosal thickening occurs (45).

Microscopic Findings. The amnionic epithelial cells become enlarged and develop a distinctive vacuolated appearance due to the accumulation of fat droplets (fig. 7-26), which ultrastructurally are not membrane bound (16). The nature and origin of the lipid are unknown. This amnionic alteration is specific for gastroschisis, and does not occur the presence of omphaloceles.

The serosal fibrosis on the surface of the bowel appears to be a reaction to the amniotic fluid. Fragments of lanugo hair and squames are intermixed with granulation tissue. The timing of this reactive sequence is apparently related to changes in the composition of the fetal urine after 30 weeks (45).

Etiology and Pathogenesis. Early ablation of the omphalomesenteric artery has been proposed as a likely cause of gastroschisis (18). One recent study found an increased prevalence of thrombophilic mutations associated with gastroschisis (10), but another (21) did not.

CYSTS (SUBAMNIONIC FIBRIN CYSTS)

Definition. Subamnionic fibrin cysts are rounded, elevated, soft or fluctuant, fluid-filled spaces superficial to the chorionic plate that bulge

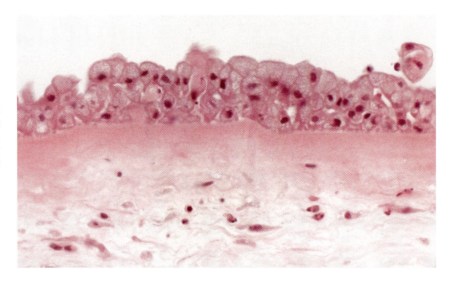

Figure 7-26

GASTROSCHISIS

The amnionic epithelium from the placenta of a newborn with gastroschisis has a unique, disorganized, multilayered pattern composed of enlarged distinctive vacuolated cells.

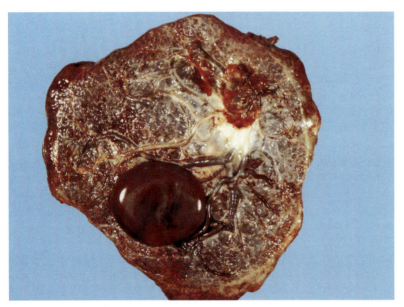

Figure 7-27

SUBAMNIONIC FIBRIN CYST

This dark red or red-brown subamnionic fibrin cyst bulges into the amnionic cavity. It contains liquefied bloody fluid, suggestive of an old hematoma that formed within the superficial layers of the chorionic plate.

into the amnionic cavity. These cysts are sometimes called chorionic fibrin cysts, a misnomer. Such cysts are not rare, and are found in approximately 1 in every 100 to 200 placentas.

Clinical Features. No adverse clinical correlations have been attributed to subamnionic cysts.

Gross Findings. Beneath a smooth and shiny thin-walled membranous surface is an accumulation of watery fluid, which is often blood-tinged or brown. Sometimes this fluid is more viscous, resembling a liquefied clot (fig. 7-27).

Microscopic Findings. There is usually no epithelial lining. Benirschke and Kaufmann (5) illustrated an unusual amnionic cyst lined by keratinized squamous epithelium.

Pathogenesis. Some cysts may represent localized edema in the amnionic or chorionic connective tissue. Others probably originate as a clot from a ruptured vessel of the chorionic plate.

REFERENCES

1. Altshuler G, Arizawa M, Molnar-Nadasdy G. Meconium-induced umbilical cord vascular necrosis and ulceration: a potential link between placenta and poor pregnancy outcome. Obstet Gynecol 1992;79:760–6.
2. Altshuler G, Hyde S. Meconium-induced vasocontraction: a potential cause of cerebral and other fetal hypoperfusion and of poor pregnancy outcome. J Child Neurol 1989;4:137–42.
3. Aplin JD, Campbell S, Donnai P, Bard JB, Allen TD. The importance of vitamin C in maintenance of the normal amnion: an experimental study. Placenta 1986;7:377–89.
4. Baergen RN, Morhaime JL, Park K, Benirschke K. Disappearance of meconium pigment in placental specimens on exposure to light [Abstract]. Mod Pathol 2002;15:310A.
5. Benirschke K, Kaufmann P. Pathology of the human placenta, 4th ed. New York: Springer; 2000.
6. Berkus MD, Langer O, Samueloff A, Xenakis EM, Field NT, Ridgeway LE. Meconium-stained amniotic fluid: increased risk for adverse neonatal outcome. Obstet Gynecol 1994;84:115–20.
7. Bryant-Greenwood GD. The extracellular matrix of the human fetal membranes: structure and function. Placenta 1998;19:1–11.
8. Bryant-Greenwood GD, Rees MC, Turnbull AC. Immunohistochemical localization of relaxin, prolactin and prostaglandin synthase in human amnion, chorion and decidua. J Endocrinol 1987;114:491–6.
9. Burgess AM, Hutchins GM. Inflammation of the lungs, umbilical cord and placenta associated with meconium passage in utero. Review of 123 autopsied cases. Path Res Pract 1996;192:1121–8.
10. Cardonick E, Kaufmann M, Reddy U, Wapner R. Thromboembolic mutations in neonates with gastroschisis: a possible etiology [Abstract]. Am J Obstet Gynecol 2001;184:S135.
11. Coughtrey H, Jeffery HE, Henderson-Smart DJ, Storey B, Poulos V. Possible causes linking asphyxia, thick meconium and respiratory distress. Aust N Z J Obstet Gynaecol 1991;31:97–102.
12. Curry JI, McKinney P, Thornton JG, Stringer MD. The aetiology of gastroschisis. BJOG 2000;107:1339–46.
13. Eidelman AI, Nevet A, Rudensky B, et al. The effect of meconium staining of amniotic fluid on the growth of Escherichia coli and Group B Streptococcus. J Perinatol 2002;22:467–71.
14. Frank HG, Malekzadeh F, Kertschanska S, et al. Immunohistochemistry of two different types of placental fibrinoid. Acta Anat 1994;150:55–68.
15. Ghidini A, Spong CY. Severe meconium aspiration syndrome is not caused by aspiration of meconium. Am J Obstet Gynecol 2001;185:931–8.
16. Grafe MR, Benirschke K. Ultrastructural study of the amniotic epithelium in a case of gastroschisis. Pediatr Pathol 1990;10:95–101.
17. Holcberg G, Huleihel M, Katz M, et al. Vasoconstrictive activity of meconium stained amniotic fluid in the human placental vasculature. Eur J Obstet Gynecol Reprod Biol 1999;87:147–50.
18. Hoyme HE, Higginbottom MC, Jones KL. The vascular pathogenesis of gastroschisis: intrauterine interruption of the omphalomesenteric artery. J Pediatr 1981;98:228–36.
19. Hsu CD, Meaddough E, Lu LC, et al. Immunohistochemical localization of inducible nitric oxide synthase on human fetal amnion in intra-amniotic infection. Am J Obstet Gynecol 1998;179:1271–4.
20. Hulboy DL, Rudolph LA, Matrisian LM. Matrix metalloproteinases as mediators of reproductive function. Molec Hum Reprod 1997;3:27–45.
21. James A, Howard T, Whorton M, et al. Analysis of thromboembolic polymorphisms in association with gastroschisis [Abstract]. Am J Obstet Gynecol 2001;184:s135.
22. Kalousek DK, Fitch N, Paradice BA. Pathology of the human embryo and previable fetus: an atlas. New York: Springer Verlag; 1990.
23. Kaspar HG, Abu-Musa A, Hannoun A, et al. The placenta in meconium staining: lesions and early neonatal outcome. Clin Exp Obstet Gynecol 2000;27:63–6.
24. Kraus FT, Acheen VI. Fetal thrombotic vasculopathy in the placenta: cerebral thrombi and infarcts, coagulopathies, and cerebral palsy. Hum Pathol 1999;30:759–69.
25. Malak TM, Ockleford CD, Bell SC, Dalgleish R, Bright N, MacVicar J. Confocal immunofluorescence localization of collagen types I, III, IV, V, and VI and their ultrastructural organization in term human fetal membranes. Placenta 1993;14:385–406.
26. Maymon E, Romero R, Chaiworapongsa T, et al. Amniotic fluid matrix metalloproteinase-8 in preterm labor with intact membranes. Am J Obstet Gynecol 2001;185:1149–55.
27. Miller PW, Coen RW, Benirschke K. Dating the time interval from meconium passage to birth. Obstet Gynecol 1985;66:459–62.

28. Muhlhauser J, Crescimanno C, Rajaniemi H, et al. Immunohistochemistry of carbonic anhydrase in the human placenta and fetal membranes. Histochemistry 1994;101:91–8.
29. Nathan L, Leveno KJ, Carmody TJ 3rd, Kelly MA, Sherman ML. Meconium: a 1990s perspective on an old obstetric hazard. Obstet Gynecol 1994;83:329–32.
30. Panayiotis G, Grunstein S. Extramembranous pregnancy in twin gestation. Obstet Gynecol 1979;53:34S–6S.
31. Park JS, Romero R, Yoon BH, Moon JB, Oh SY, Ko EM. The relationship between amniotic fluid matrix metalloproteinase-8 and funisitis. Am J Obstet Gynecol 2001;185:1156–61.
32. Perlman M, Tennenbaum A, Menashi M, Ron M, Ornoy A. Extramembranous pregnancy: maternal, placental, and perinatal complications. Obstet Gynecol 1980;55:34S–7S.
33. Piper JM, Newton ER, Berkus MD, Peairs WA. Meconium: a marker for peripartum infection. Obstet Gynecol 1998;91:741–5.
34. Poisner AM, Wood GW, Poisner R, Inagami T. Localization of renin in trophoblasts in human chorion laeve at term pregnancy. Endocrinology 1981;109:1150–5.
35. Ramin KD, Leveno KJ, Kelly MA, Carmody TJ. Amnionic fluid meconium: a fetal environmental hazard. Obstet Gynecol 1996;87:181–4.
36. Redline RW, O'Riordan MA. Placental lesions associated with cerebral palsy and neurologic impairment following term birth. Arch Pathol Lab Med 2000;124:1785–91.
37. Romero R, Hanaoka S, Mazor M, et al. Meconium-stained amniotic fluid: a risk factor for microbial invasion of the amniotic cavity. Am J Obstet Gynecol 1991;164:859–62.
38. Sampson JE, Theve RP, Blatman RN, et al. Fetal origin of amniotic fluid polymorphonuclear leukocytes. Am J Obstet Gynecol 1997;176:77–81.
39. Schmidt W. The amniotic fluid compartment: the fetal habitat. Adv Anat Embryol Cell Biol 1992;127:1–100.
40. Scott RJ, Peat D, Rhodes CA. Investigation of the fetal pulmonary inflammatory reaction in chorioamnionitis, using an in situ Y chromosome marker. Pediatr Pathol 1994;14:997–1003.
41. Shih IM, Seidman JD, Kurman RJ. Placental site nodule and characterization of distinctive types of intermediate trophoblast. Hum Pathol 1999;30:687–94.
42. Sienko A, Altshuler G. Meconium induced umbilical vascular necrosis in abortuses and fetuses: a histopathologic study for cytokines. Obstet Gynecol 1999;94:415–20.
43. Stoll C, Alembik Y, Dott B, Roth MP. Risk factors in congenital abdominal wall defects (omphalocele and gastroschisis): a study in a series of 265, 858 consecutive births. Ann Genet 2001;44:201–8.
44. Thureen PJ, Hall DM, Hoffenberg A, Tyson RW. Fatal meconium aspiration in spite of appropriate perinatal airway management: pulmonary and placental evidence of prenatal disease. Am J Obstet Gynecol 1997;176:967–75.
45. Tibboel D, Vermey-Keers C, Kluck P, Gaillard JL, Koppenberg J, Molenaar JC. The natural history of gastroschisis during fetal life: development of the fibrous coating on the bowel loops. Teratology 1986;33:267–72.
46. Usher RH, Boyd ME, McLean FH, Kramer MS. Assessment of fetal risk in postdate pregnancies. Am J Obstet Gynecol 1988;158:259–64.
47. Woods JR Jr. Reactive oxygen species and preterm premature rupture of membranes—a review. Placenta 2001;22(Suppl A):S38–44.
48. Xu P, Alfaidy N, Challis JR. Expression of matrix metalloproteinase (MMP)-2 and MMP-9 in human placenta and fetal membranes in relation to preterm and term labor. J Clin Endocrinol Metab 2002;87:1353–61.
49. Yang SS, Levine AJ, Sanborn JR, Delp RA. Amniotic rupture, extra-amniotic pregnancy, and vernix granulomata. Am J Surg Pathol 1984;8:117–22.

8 EMBRYONIC DEVELOPMENT AND PATHOLOGY OF THE UMBILICAL CORD

EMBRYONIC DEVELOPMENT

Early in gestation, the blastocyst is filled with a loose meshwork of extraembryonic mesoderm which surrounds the embryonic disc. Each of the two layers, the endoderm and ectoderm, expands to form a vesicle, the yolk sac and amnionic cavity, respectively. The extraembryonic mesoderm cavitates centrally to form the exocoelom, or chorionic cavity. The extraembryonic mesoderm lining the inside of the trophoblastic shell (chorionic mesoderm) and the mesoderm covering the embryonic structures are connected by a bridge of extraembryonic mesoderm (the connecting stalk), the forerunner of the umbilical cord. The yolk sac and a smaller caudal outgrowth, the allantois, protrude into the connecting stalk. The embryo rotates during development so that the yolk sac, which originally faced the endometrial cavity, ultimately faces the implantation site. The amnion enlarges, and simultaneously, the embryo prolapses into the amnionic cavity, progressively lengthening the connecting stalk (fig. 8-1).

Both the yolk sac and allantois are vascularized, but the allantoic vessels establish continuity with vessels developing in the villi, resulting in the fetoplacental circulation (thus a chorioallantoic circulation). The two umbilical arteries originate from the internal iliac arteries. The right umbilical vein atrophies within the second month, and the left umbilical vein drains into the hepatic vein. The great majority (96 percent) of umbilical arteries are either fused or connected via an anastomosis (Hyrtl's anastomosis), generally within 1.5 cm of the placental insertion site. This connection is important to equalize flow and distribute blood uniformly to the placenta (7,103,106,108,139).

NORMAL UMBILICAL CORD

The normal umbilical cord contains two arteries and one vein suspended in Wharton's jelly, a loosely structured myxoid tissue covered by a layer of amnion (fig. 8-2). Unlike the amnion of the fetal membranes, which is easily detached from the chorion beneath it, the amnion surfacing the umbilical cord is firmly connected. Wharton's jelly is derived from the extraembryonic mesenchyme, and consists of myofibroblasts and abundant ground substance (97,136). The combination of loose gel and contractile cells helps maintain turgor and protects the vessels against compression. Mast cells are numerous, but macrophages are inconspicuous in Wharton's jelly. The umbilical cord is supplied by the diffusion of oxygen and nutrients from the umbilical vessels.

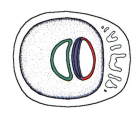
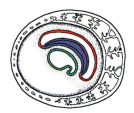
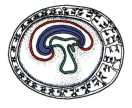
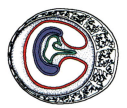

Figure 8-1

FORMATION OF THE UMBILICAL CORD

Extraembryonic mesoderm (dots) surrounds amnionic (red) and yolk sac (green) vesicles (top left).

Extraembryonic mesoderm cavitates to form the exocoelom, leaving the connecting bridge. Allantoic invagination occurs at the caudal end of the embryo (blue) (top right). Yolk sac and allantois protrude into the connecting stalk. Amnion enlarges and nearly surrounds embryo (bottom left). Embryo rotates and prolapses into amnionic cavity. Enlarging amnion largely obliterates exocoelom (bottom right). (Modified from fig. 12.1 from reference 14.)

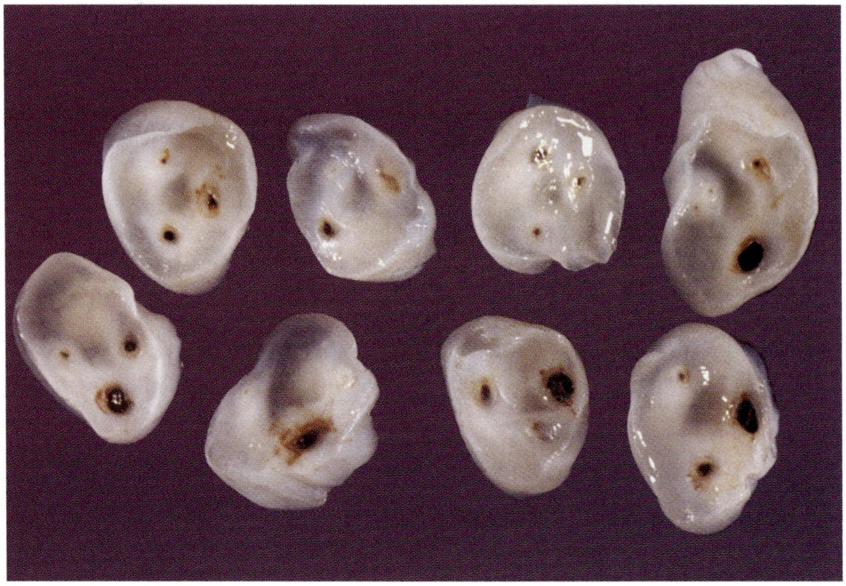

Figure 8-2

NORMAL UMBILICAL CORD

Includes two umbilical arteries and an umbilical vein, surrounded by Wharton's jelly and surfaced by amnion.

The umbilical arteries have no internal elastica, and smooth muscle is concentrated peripherally (98). The umbilical vein has a subintimal elastic layer and the smooth muscle coat is thinner than in the arteries. The endothelial cells of both umbilical arteries and veins are relatively organelle rich, differing from the endothelium of placental vessels (76,100). Umbilical vascular contractility is apparently mediated by local prostaglandin production (52,81), which may be altered in pathologic states such as cigarette smoking, diabetes, and preeclampsia (69,140). No other vessels, specifically vasa vasorum or lymphatics, are found normally in the umbilical cord.

The umbilical cord is normally spiraled, usually counterclockwise (ratio of counterclockwise to clockwise spirals, 7 to 1). The spiral is established early in the first trimester, as demonstrated sonographically (32). It is thought that the fetus establishes the coil by turning when there is ample amnionic fluid and room for movement. The average number of coils is about 0.2 +/- 0.1 coil/cm (82,134). Abnormal coiling is associated with potentially adverse outcomes (28,111,131).

VESTIGIAL REMNANTS

Vestigial remnants that date back to the formation of the connecting stalk and umbilical cord are common microscopic findings. The presence of vestigial remnants has not been correlated with congenital anomalies, maternal age and race, gravidity, or gestational age at delivery.

Allantoic Remnants

Remnants of the allantoic duct, the small rudimentary caudal outgrowth of the yolk sac, are frequent in the proximal portion of the cord, occurring in about 15 percent of umbilical cords (65). They are usually solid, and lined by flat or cuboidal cells often reminiscent of transitional epithelium (fig. 8-3). Allantoic duct remnants are regularly located between the umbilical arteries. Rarely, allantoic remnants are large enough to expand the cord or remain patent, predisposing to urinary leakage from the cord stump.

Omphalomesenteric Remnants

Traces of the omphalomesenteric duct, which connects the fetal ileum and the yolk sac in the early embryo, are infrequent, occurring in 1.5 percent of umbilical cords (65). These remnants are usually discontinuous, located peripherally, and lined by columnar cells resembling intestinal epithelium (fig. 8-4A,B). Omphalomesenteric remnants often have a muscular wall, which occasionally contains ganglion cells (fig. 8-4C). Rarely, omphalomesenteric remnants include mucosa from the liver, pancreas, stomach, or small intestine. Omphalomesenteric remnants are frequently accompanied by vitelline vessels, which are usually paired but

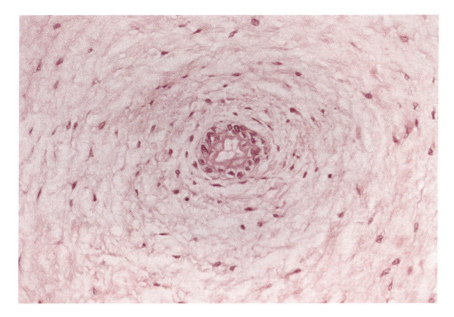

Figure 8-3

ALLANTOIC DUCT REMNANTS

Allantoic duct remnants are typically lined by flat or cuboidal cells.

Figure 8-4

OMPHALOMESENTERIC DUCT REMNANTS

Typical omphalomesenteric duct remnants are lined by columnar epithelium (A), but on occasion, they may contain goblet cells (B) and are often surrounded by smooth muscle (C).

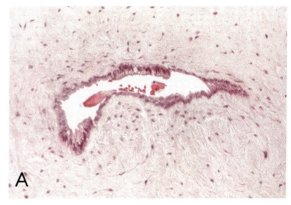

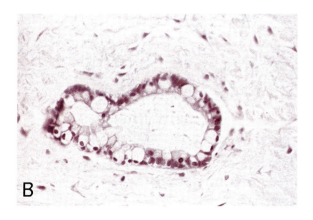

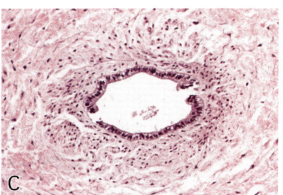

sometimes clustered and lined by endothelium lacking a muscular coat (fig. 8-5).

Omphalomesenteric remnants are of little clinical significance. They are occasionally associated with Meckel's diverticulum, small intestinal atresia, or an intestinal protrusion into the cord that may be inadvertently clamped or cut. Cystic omphalomesenteric remnants are rare, but when they occur, they are more common in males (ratio, 4 to 1). An omphalomesenteric cyst

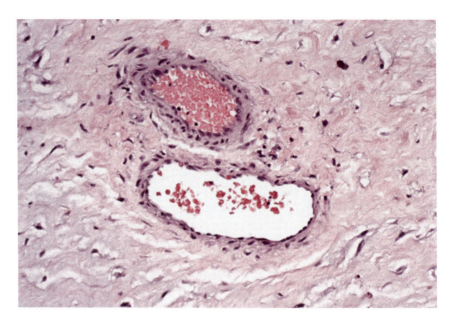

Figure 8-5

VITELLINE VESSEL REMNANTS

Vitelline vessel remnants are typically paired.

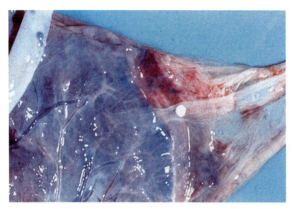
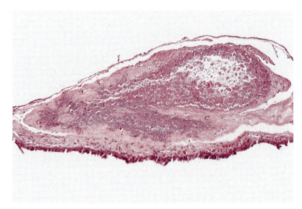

Figure 8-6

YOLK SAC REMNANT

Left: The yolk sac remnant is a tiny white nodule between the amnion and chorion.
Right: It is composed of amorphous basophilic debris.

that contained gastric epithelium and presumably secreted enough acid to erode the umbilical vein, resulting in exsanguination, was the subject of a case report (53,57). The yolk sac remnant, when present, is a small white nodule between the amnion and chorion composed of amorphous basophilic material (fig. 8-6).

INSERTION ANOMALIES

In over 90 percent of placentas, the umbilical cord inserts into the placental disc either centrally or eccentrically.

Velamentous Insertion and Membranous Vessels

Definition. In velamentous insertion, the cord inserts into the fetal membranes rather than onto the placental disc. An associated condition, *vasa previa*, occurs when vessels in the fetal membranes present in advance of a fetal part.

Prevalence. Velamentous insertion is a common anomaly, occurring in about 1 percent of placentas. The incidence is greatly increased in twins, occurring with nine times the frequency than in singletons, and is more frequent as the

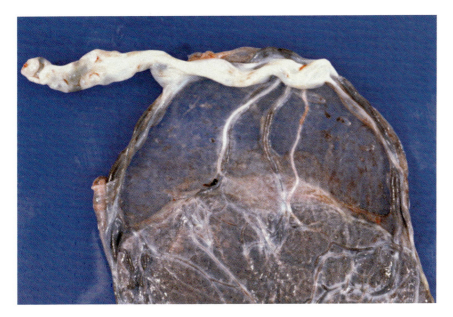

Figure 8-7
VELAMENTOUS INSERTION
This velamentous cord inserted many centimeters from the disc edge.

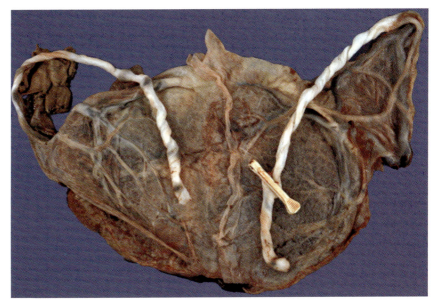

Figure 8-8
VELAMENTOUS INSERTION
Diamnionic monochorionic twin placenta with two velamentously inserted cords. The cord on the left also has a single umbilical artery and is associated with an old laminated blood clot.

proximity of the twins increases. Thus, the frequency is progressively higher in dichorionic separate, dichorionic fused, and monochorionic placentas, and it is increased even further in triplets and higher multiples. Velamentous insertion is also increased in extrachorial placentas, low lying placentas, and cords with a single umbilical artery. Its incidence is reportedly increased in association with cigarette smoking and advanced maternal age (56).

Pathology. After insertion, the umbilical vessels usually branch in the fetal membranes (insertio velamentosa), coursing toward the placenta without the protection of Wharton's jelly and unsupported by villous tissue (figs. 8-7, 8-9). Less commonly, the cord retains its Wharton's jelly, running in the membranes before its vessels branch (interposition) (fig. 8-10). Membranous vessels are vulnerable to traumatic rupture, hemorrhage (figs. 8-8, 8-9), compression, and thrombosis, especially when they traverse the cervical os in advance of the fetus (vasa previa). Most velamentous cords insert relatively close to the placental disc. The distance between cord

Placental Pathology

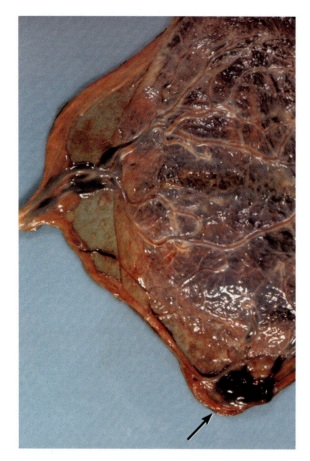

Figure 8-9

VELAMENTOUS INSERTION

This velamentous insertion is associated with rupture and hemorrhage of membranous vessels (arrow).

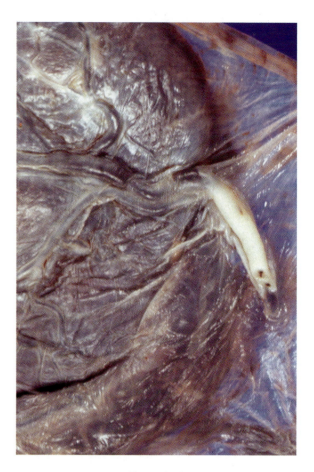

Figure 8-10

INTERPOSITION

This velamentously inserted cord retains its Wharton's jelly and remains intact until it branches when it reaches the placenta.

insertion and the disc margin, the length of the membranous vessels, provides one measure of the degree of their vulnerability. Membranous vessels are not limited to velamentously inserted cords but may arise aberrantly from marginally or even centrally inserted cords (fig. 8-11), and they regularly supply succenturiate lobes. As a site of significant pathologic alterations, membranous vessels should be inspected carefully and included in sections for microscopic examination.

Etiology. According to the abnormal primary implantation (polarity) theory, velamentous cord insertion is the result of malpositioning of the blastocyst at implantation, with consequent aberrant body stalk-placental disc orientation (86). Alternatively, velamentous insertion may result when the placenta "moves" from its initial implantation site, leaving the cord insertion behind (the trophotropism theory). This placental remodeling, probably in response to uterine crowding and/or maternal vascular supply, involves simultaneous atrophy on one aspect and growth/expansion on the other. The increased frequency of velamentous cord insertion in multiples and in uteri with structural defects and foreign bodies (e.g., intrauterine devices) is evidence supporting the trophotropism theory. Sonographic documentation of eccentric placental expansion with conversion of placenta previa to a higher uterine position (but not the opposite) provides support for this mechanism in some cases (72,116,144).

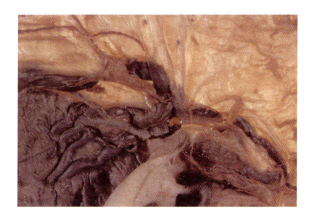 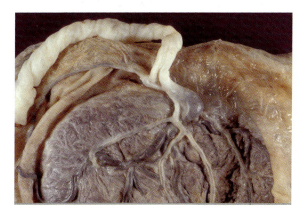

Figure 8-11

MARGINAL INSERTION

Two marginally inserted umbilical cords are associated with membranous vessels.

Clinical Features. Velamentous cord insertion has several important clinical associations. The best documented complications are related to the vulnerability of the membranous vessels, which are subject to compression, trauma, laceration, and thrombosis, especially when they present in advance of fetal parts. Compression with severe fetal distress and a fetal heart rate pattern similar to that in cord compression (6,27), and laceration with blood loss, even exsanguination, may occur suddenly during labor and result in a mortality rate as high as 60 to 70 percent (27,121,137). The diagnosis is rarely made before the onset of bleeding. The Kleihauer-Betke test may identify a fetal blood component, but this is not a routine part of obstetric management (87). Vasa previa may be detected by Doppler imaging (88), but velamentous insertion is almost never detected with routine prenatal ultrasound examination (34). Although bleeding is most common from membranous vessels near the os at the time of labor, bleeding may also occur antepartum and from vessels located higher in the uterus (17). Thrombosis may also occur in membranous arteries and veins, and has been associated with major fetal thromboembolic events, and even fetal death (11,14,112).

Velamentous cord insertion may be used as a marker of poor placentation with decreased chorionic and placental vascularization. This may explain the reported association between velamentous cord insertion and low birth weight, low Apgar scores, and abnormal fetal heart rate patterns (34,58,126). Velamentous cord insertion has also been associated with congenital anomalies (95,118). Structural anomalies occur in as many as 8.5 percent of infants with velamentous cords and in as many as 25 percent of fetuses spontaneously aborted in the first and second trimesters (95). Robinson and colleagues (118) determined that deformations (alteration in the shape of a normally differentiated structure), but not malformations or disruptions, occurred excessively in association with velamentous cord insertion, theorizing that fetal deformations and velamentous insertion both resulted from competition for intrauterine space.

Velamentous cord insertion is significantly more common in monochorionic gestations with the twin-twin transfusion syndrome than in such gestations without it (40). This association has been attributed to the compressibility of the membranous vessels and umbilical cord, resulting in decreased venous flow to the donor, an effect potentiated by discrepant amnionic fluid volumes (80). An additional factor favoring the shunting of blood to the recipient is the decreased placental vascularization and increased resistance (evidenced by increased Doppler S-D ratios) in some placentas with velamentous cord insertion (22).

Marginal Insertion

Marginal (or *Battledore*) cord insertion occurs when the umbilical cord inserts at the edge of the placental disc (figs. 8-11, 8-12). The reported

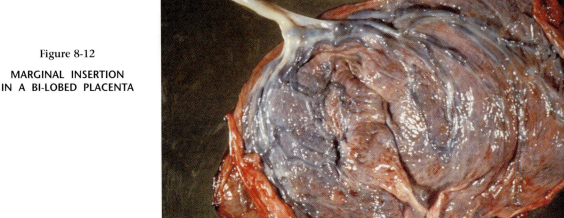

Figure 8-12

MARGINAL INSERTION IN A BI-LOBED PLACENTA

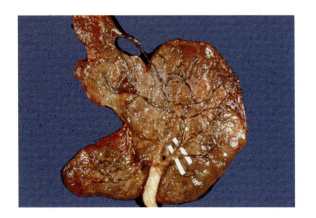
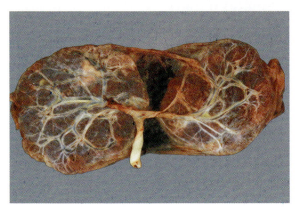

Figure 8-13

FURCATE INSERTION

Left: In furcate cord insertion, umbilical vessels lose Wharton's jelly before reaching the placental disc.
Right: Furcate cord insertion in a bi-lobed placenta.

frequency varies depending on the interpretation of markedly eccentric versus marginal insertion. Overall, marginal insertion occurs in about 7 percent of placentas. Marginal insertion is hypothesized to develop via the same mechanisms as velamentous insertion (abnormal primary implantation versus trophotropism).

The clinical significance of marginal insertion is debated. It has been reported to occur with increased frequency in abortions and malformed infants (94), and in association with neonatal asphyxia and preterm labor, although these associations have not been confirmed by some (39). Peripheral cord insertion (velamentous, marginal, and markedly eccentric) has been associated with discordant growth and small for gestational age in twins (113).

Furcate Insertion

In furcate insertion, the cord loses Wharton's jelly before insertion, leaving the umbilical vessels unsupported (fig. 8-13). Furcate cords may insert velamentously or into the placental disc.

The unsupported vessels are subject to trauma, and examples of fetal hemorrhage have been reported (39,59,64,135).

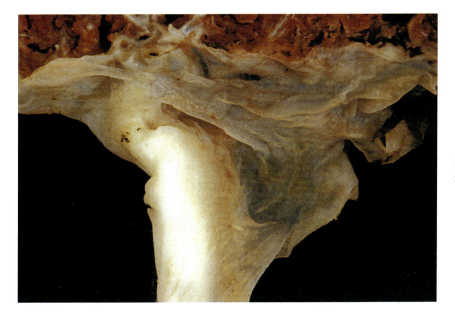

Figure 8-14

TETHERED INSERTION

This amnionic web, or "chorda," binds the cord to the fetal surface of the placenta.

Tethered Insertion ("Amnionic Webs")

Amnionic webs, or chorda, are folds that encase the cord at the insertion site (fig. 8-14). Large tight amnionic webs may limit the mobility of the cord, potentially compromising blood flow (68).

CORD LENGTH

The length of the umbilical cord is an important parameter of potential adverse fetal outcome and is most accurately documented in the delivery room before cord segments are removed for other studies. When the cord is received in several segments, each should be measured and the cord reconstructed as accurately as possible. It is unlikely today that the amount of cord submitted with the placenta is an accurate indicator of its original length.

Cord length reflects factors that influence its growth: mainly tensile forces related to fetal activity and intrauterine conditions affecting fetal movement (90,91,93). Conditions restricting fetal mobility, amnionic bands, oligohydramnios, and crowding (multiple pregnancy), are often associated with relatively short cords. Infants with Down's syndrome reportedly have short cords, and Naeye (94,96) has correlated short cords with subsequent motor and mental impairment. Whether cord length as an indirect indicator of fetal movement correlates ultimately with antenatal neurologic development deserves further study.

Umbilical cord growth slows during the last trimester as room for fetal movement declines, although some cord growth occurs normally until term. Standards for cord length relative to gestational age have been established and should be considered in all cases (92) (see Appendix 7). The mean cord length at term is about 55 to 60 cm. Extremes of cord length have been associated with potentially adverse outcomes, although definitions of an abnormally long or short cord are variable. Some consideration of relative as well as absolute cord length is also appropriate; for example, a long cord with extensive looping may function as a relatively short cord.

Short Cord

Gardiner's (45) calculation that a normal vertex delivery requires a minimum cord length of 32 cm provides the most common definition of an abnormally short cord. Using this definition, between 0.4 and 0.9 percent of umbilical cords are abnormally short. Berg and Rayburn (15) found that 2 percent of cords are less than 35 cm.

Unduly short cords have been linked to fetal distress in some cases (115), although blood pH and base deficit values in short cords are reportedly the same as in cords of normal length (15). Short cords may be associated with rupture or hemorrhage (125). In the absence of fetal anomalies, short cords have been associated with low Apgar scores, neonatal hypotonia, and

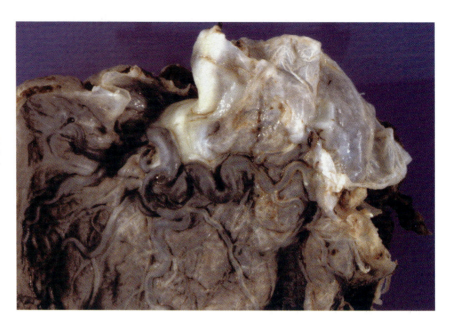

Figure 8-15

SHORT UMBILICAL CORD

This extremely short umbilical cord was associated with a severe abdominal wall defect in a baby who died shortly after birth.

need for resuscitation (120). Reported obstetric conditions associated with short cords include delayed second stage of labor, abruption, and uterine inversion (96). At the extreme, there may be complete or near complete cord absence (acordia), characteristically associated with fetal anterior abdominal wall defects, which may be directly attached to the placenta (fig. 8-15) (117). This is uniformly fatal (46).

Long Cord

Definition and Frequency. Excessive cord length has been variably defined as greater than 80 (15) or 100 (104) cm, with frequencies of 3.7 and 0.5 percent, respectively.

Clinical Features. Abnormally long cords have been associated with excess knotting (fig. 8-16), torsion, encirclement around body parts, prolapse, and vascular occlusion (8,14). Umbilical cord prolapse is an obstetric emergency, defined as presentation of the cord in advance of the presenting fetal part. It occurs in 0.25 to 0.50 percent of deliveries and results in a perinatal mortality rate of 20 percent. Cord prolapse is associated with poor fetal-maternal pelvic fit occurring with abnormal presentation, prematurity, multiparity, and obstetric manipulation (i.e., amniotomy). The diagnosis is established with ultrasound (138), and a cord compression pattern on fetal heart rate monitoring is the associated hemodynamic response (77).

Cord entanglements encircling the fetal neck and extremities are common, occurring in about 23 percent of deliveries (33). The mean umbilical cord length is greater in cases with cord entanglement than in those without entanglement. Ninety percent of very long umbilical cords (more than 115 cm) are associated with at least one nuchal loop. Loose nuchal cords that can be released prior to delivery are usually not clinically significant. Tight nuchal loops are associated with prolonged first stage of labor and, in some instances, increased fetal mortality. Babies with sonographically documented nuchal cords have higher rates of admission to the neonatal intensive care unit and delivery by cesarean section (84). Nuchal cords have been demonstrated as a cause of fetal growth restriction, indicating that the deleterious effect is long term in some cases (130). Cerebral palsy has been linked to nuchal cord entanglement in a recent study (99). Cord entanglement as a cause of early fetal death has also been well documented (14). Excessive cord length and entanglement has been found to be more common in spontaneous abortions than in therapeutic abortion controls (66).

Pathologic Findings. Constriction of the umbilical cord and the encircled fetal part may be dramatic in some cord entanglements. Cord compression may be associated with edema, congestion, hemorrhage or thrombosis of cord

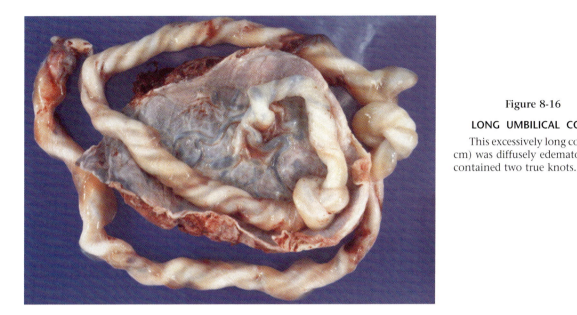

Figure 8-16

LONG UMBILICAL CORD

This excessively long cord (120 cm) was diffusely edematous and contained two true knots.

vessels, thrombosis of large chorionic plate vessels, and hemorrhagic endovasculitis in the placenta.

CORD DIAMETER

Umbilical cord diameter is affected by the number of vessels present and the amount and fluid content of Wharton's jelly. Nomograms generated from uncomplicated pregnancies indicate a progressive increase in sonographic cord diameter and cross sectional area until 32 weeks' gestation, with a decline thereafter presumably due to a reduction in the fluid content of Wharton's jelly (107). Patel and colleagues (101) established the normal cord circumference to be 37.7 ± 7.73 mm. Silver and colleagues (129) determined that cord diameter ranged from 1.25 to 2.00 cm and circumference from 2.4 to 4.4 cm. The factors that determine the amount of Wharton's jelly and its water content are poorly understood. Edema is more common in premature infants, and there is a tendency for Wharton's jelly to decrease late in gestation.

A thin ("lean") cord with decreased or absent Wharton's jelly may be associated with intrauterine growth restriction (29,49,51). At present, a lean cord is defined as one with a cross-sectional area less than the 10th percentile as assessed sonographically (107). The diminished size appears to be due to a reduction in Wharton's jelly and the size of the umbilical vein as the umbilical arteries are usually unaffected. Lean cords tend to have a lower coiling index and reduced umbilical vein flow, normalized for fetal weight (30). Wharton's jelly may be focally deficient, with separation of the vessels (fig. 8-17) (74) or, rarely, it is completely absent, an anomaly that has been associated with fetal death in utero.

Cord edema, focal or diffuse (fig. 8-16), occurs inconsistently in a variety of clinical situations, especially with maternal diabetes, but often the cause is unknown. More cord jelly and vascular spiraling has been associated with better fetal outcome while compression patterns on fetal heart tracings occur more often when cords have decreased fluid content (129,131).

NUMERICAL VARIATION IN UMBILICAL VESSELS

Single Umbilical Artery

Definition and Frequency. The presence of a single umbilical artery rather than the normal two arteries is a common and important cord abnormality that can be diagnosed sonographically (67,102). The reported frequency of a single umbilical artery depends on the population studied. In prospective studies of consecutive deliveries, the frequency of single umbilical artery is consistently less than 1 percent, although the frequency is considerably higher in perinatal autopsy studies (2.7 to 12.0 percent)

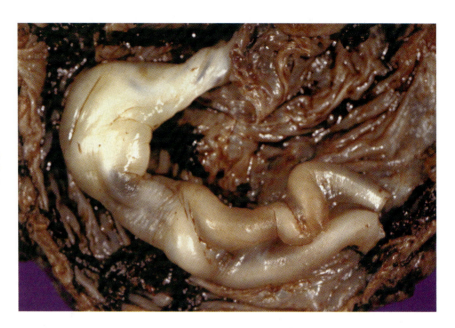

Figure 8-17
DEFICIENT WHARTON'S JELLY
A localized deficiency in Wharton's jelly is associated with separation of umbilical vessels. The baby was alive and well.

and in spontaneous abortions (1.5 to 2.7 percent) (13,23,41).

The method of cord examination influences the frequency with which a single umbilical artery is diagnosed. The likelihood of diagnosing a single umbilical artery is increased when fixed versus fresh cords are examined, and histologic examination provides the most accurate means of establishing the diagnosis (43,73). Cord vascularity should be assessed at least 3 to 5 cm from the placental insertion site because the umbilical arteries frequently fuse close to the placenta. One section taken close to the umbilical cord insertion may lead to an erroneous diagnosis of a single umbilical artery. Rarely, umbilical artery fusion or anastomosis occurs far above the cord insertion site.

The frequency of single umbilical artery also varies with ethnicity, being more common in white women than in blacks or Asians (41,42). Single artery cords are reportedly more common in diabetic mothers and in fetuses with chromosome abnormalities, especially trisomies (42,71,73,123). Many studies have documented an increased frequency of single umbilical artery in twins, although this is disputed by others.

Etiology. Whether a single umbilical artery is due to primary aplasia or secondary atrophy has long been debated. When specifically sought, histologic evidence of vascular remnants are demonstrable in a high percentage of single artery cords, supporting the secondary atrophy theory in many instances (4). Conversely, its absence in such carefully studied cases would support primary aplasia as a mechanism. The higher incidence of single umbilical artery in fetuses as compared to early embryos provides circumstantial evidence that single umbilical artery may be an acquired defect.

Pathology. Histologic sections of the cord confirm the presence of one umbilical artery (fig. 8-18). Muscular or elastic remnants of an atrophied vessel or a small vessel with an obliterated lumen are seen in some cases (fig. 8-19). Single artery cords have a high frequency of velamentous insertion (as high as 12 percent) (83), circumvallation (16), and a magistral pattern of chorionic blood vessels (119). On occasion, two umbilical arteries are present but are of different size. A difference of at least 1 mm in the diameter of the umbilical arteries, as established sonographically, is considered discordance (fig. 8-20) (110). A marked discrepancy in the diameter of the umbilical arteries may be associated with fetal anomalies similar to those encountered with a single umbilical artery (fig. 8-21).

Clinical Features. *Congenital Malformations.* There is a well-documented association between single umbilical artery and fetal malformations, but there is no particular organ or specific abnormality characterizing this association. Any organ system may be affected, and the malformations are frequently multiple (23,24,41,78). Congenital malformations are

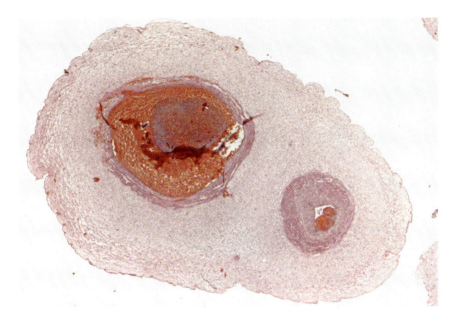

Figure 8-18

SINGLE UMBILICAL ARTERY

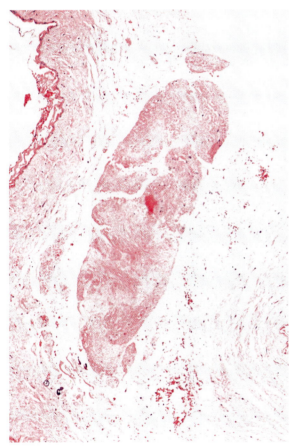

Figure 8-19

SINGLE UMBILICAL ARTERY

Fetal artery remnant in an umbilical cord with a single umbilical artery.

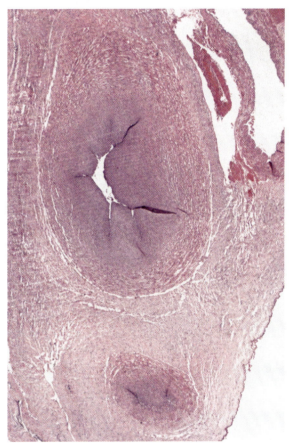

Figure 8-20

DISCORDANT UMBILICAL ARTERIES

Placental Pathology

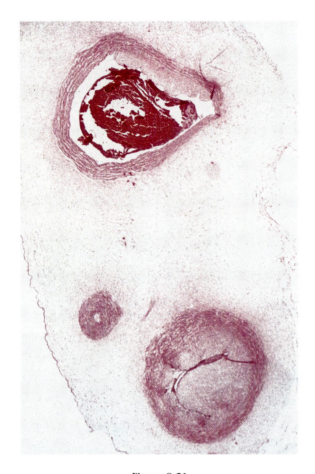

Figure 8-21

DISCORDANT UMBILICAL ARTERIES

Markedly discordant umbilical arteries in a baby with multiple congenital anomalies including an abdominal wall defect.

most numerous and most severe in stillborn infants, aborted fetuses, and infants dying in the neonatal period (24,41,42). Infants with single artery cords but no detectable abnormalities at birth who survive the neonatal period may have clinically silent renal anomalies (19,78), but are unlikely to have other subsequent significant abnormalities (24,41). It has been suggested that complex abnormalities are more often associated with the absence of the left umbilical artery (1). A single umbilical artery is almost invariable in sirenomelic and acardiac fetuses. Whether a single umbilical artery plays a role in the development of congenital malformations or is just another manifestation of them is unclear.

Perinatal Mortality. The perinatal mortality rate of infants with a single umbilical artery is high (11 to 41 percent). This is attributable to associated major malformations in most instances, although otherwise normal infants with single umbilical artery have a high perinatal mortality rate as well (23,42,54,79). The recent sonographic demonstration of decreased Wharton's jelly in single artery cords may contribute to increased cord vulnerability (107).

Low Birth Weight. A single umbilical artery is associated with low birth weight even when infants with malformations are excluded from analysis (23,42,48,60,115,119).

Supernumerary Vessels

The phenomenon of supernumerary cord vessels has not been extensively studied. Meyer (89) reported a fourth vessel in 16 of 310 cords and Gupta (5,50) described more than three vessels in 40 of 644 cords; most are thought to represent a persistent right umbilical vein. Vascular dissection has demonstrated that most extravascular profiles are due to vessel branching. Redundancy and looping of vessels are common in the umbilical cord and should be excluded before a cord is considered to have supernumerary vessels. Supernumerary cord vessels are reported to be associated with fetal anomalies (39).

FOCAL LESIONS

The umbilical cord should be carefully examined along its entire length as clinically significant lesions may be focal. All cord lesions should be carefully assessed for evidence of functionally significant alterations in blood flow. Clinically significant circulatory compromise is often accompanied by pathologic changes, including thrombosis, edema, congestion, or hemorrhage. The availability of increasingly sophisticated imaging techniques provides opportunities for better assessment of the relationship between pathologic aberrations and significant alterations in blood flow.

Knots

Frequency and Etiology. Between 0.35 and 0.50 percent of umbilical cords contain true knots (21,25,85). True knots (fig. 8-22) should be distinguished from false knots, which are focal accentuations of the vascular spiral, a

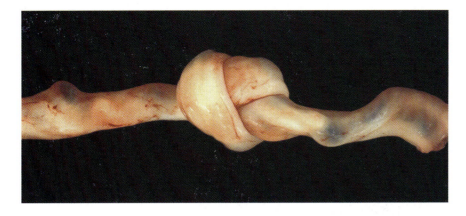

Figure 8-22
TRUE KNOT

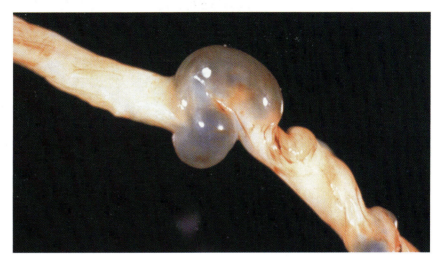

Figure 8-23
FALSE KNOT
False knot due to accentuation of a vascular spiral.

varicosity, or excess Wharton's jelly (figs. 8-23, 8-24). True knots are thought to be related to fetal movement and are increased in multigravidae, long cords (fig. 8-25), male fetuses, monoamnionic twins, and an excess of amniotic fluid. They occur with equal frequency in abortions and term deliveries, indicating that they probably develop early in pregnancy when there is ample opportunity for movement.

Pathology. Umbilical cord knots should be assessed for evidence of chronicity, tightness, and circulatory compromise. In longstanding tight knots, there is grooving and loss of Wharton's jelly with constriction of blood vessels, changes that persist when the knot is untied. Longstanding and acutely tightened knots may be associated with venous distention distal to the knot, edema, and thrombosis, changes that are characteristic of knots with clinical significance (fig. 8-26). There may be thrombosis and calcification of chorionic plate vessels, and hemorrhagic endovasculitis in the placenta. True knots are more common in excessively long umbilical cords.

Clinical Significance. True knots are associated with an overall perinatal mortality rate of 8 to 11 percent, attributable to their potential for fetal circulatory obstruction (39,62). Either an acutely tightened or longstanding knot may be responsible for intrauterine or intrapartum fetal death. False knots are generally of no clinical significance and only rarely cause thrombosis (53,141).

Abnormal Torsion

Definition and Frequency. The normal umbilical cord averages about 0.2 coils/cm (see Appendix 9 and chapter 1) (27,35,75,82,111,134). The degree of cord torsion can be assessed sonographically. Hypercoiled cords are generally considered to be those in which the coiling index is greater than the 90th percentile, and hypocoiled cords are those in which the coiling

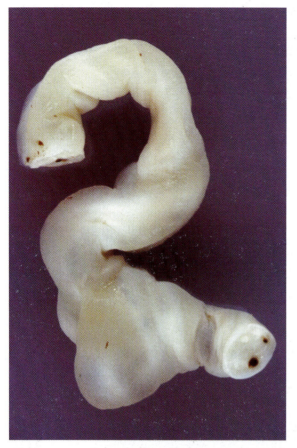

Figure 8-24

FALSE KNOT

False knot due to accentuation of Wharton's jelly.

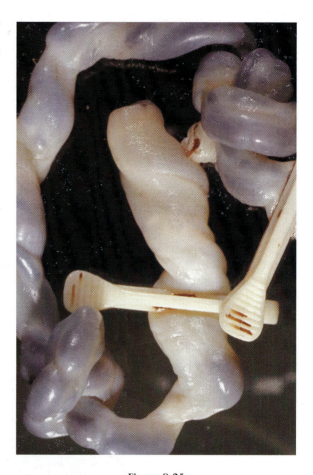

Figure 8-25

TRUE KNOTS

Excessively long umbilical cord with two true knots.

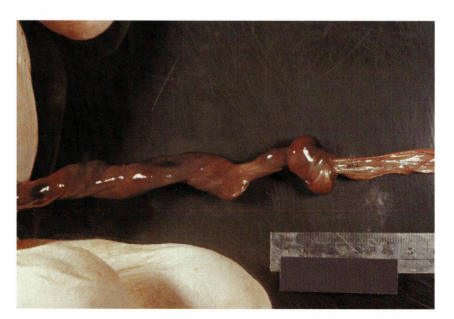

Figure 8-26

TRUE KNOT

This true knot is associated with vascular occlusion and cord congestion, and resulted in fetal death in utero.

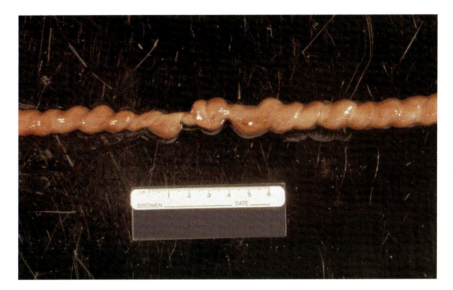

Figure 8-27

HYPERCOILED CORD

This markedly hypercoiled cord was associated with fetal death in utero. (Courtesy of Dr. Phyllis Huettner, St. Louis MO.)

index is less than the 10th percentile. The frequency of noncoiled cords is 4.3 to 4.9 percent (111,134). In one study, 7.5 percent of 120 unselected placentas had hypocoiled cords and 20 percent had hypercoiled cords (82). Umbilical cord coiling is thought to reflect fetal movement; it is decreased in association with uterine constriction or fetal abnormalities that affect movement. Hypercoiled cords are more common in multigravidae, presumably because there is more room for fetal movement; in association with maternal cocaine use; in gestations with long umbilical cords; and in male infants. Hypocoiled cords have been reported to occur more commonly in twins and in babies with chromosomal abnormalities (12,127)

Pathology. Hypercoiling may affect the entire cord (fig. 8-27), but it is commonly localized to the fetal end (18), where it may be associated with stricture (fig. 8-28) and thrombosis of umbilical and chorionic plate vessels. Intimal cushions and calcification in thrombosed vessels suggest a chronic process. Hypocoiled cords are frequently thin, with decreased Wharton's jelly, and may be thrombosed, although umbilical vein thrombosis is said to be less common and more acute in hypocoiled as compared to hypercoiled cords. Stenosis is not seen in hypocoiled cords, but decreased Wharton's jelly and lesser resilience may increase the susceptibility of the cord to kinking, compression, and stasis.

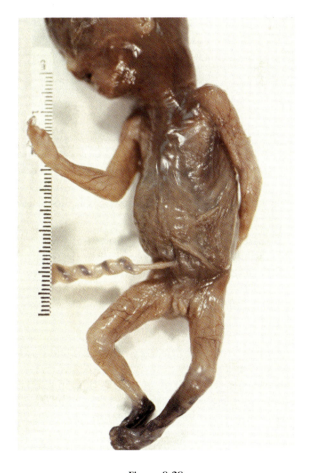

Figure 8-28

HYPERCOILED CORD

Hypercoiled cord with a short stricture at the fetal end caused fetal death in utero. (Courtesy of Dr. Alexander Miller, Downers Grove, IL.)

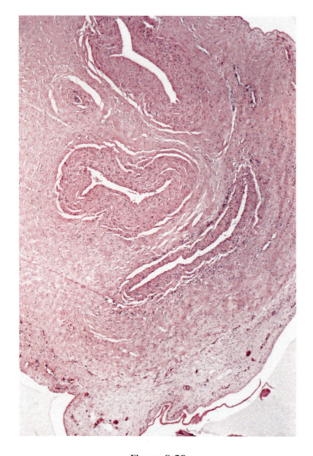

Figure 8-29

UMBILICAL CORD STRICTURE

Umbilical cord stricture with diminished Wharton's jelly.

Clinical Significance. Abnormal coiling, both hypocoiling and hypercoiling, is significantly associated with adverse fetal outcome, principally fetal growth restriction, intolerance of labor, and fetal death (36,47,82).

Stricture

Definition and Etiology. An umbilical cord stricture is a sharply defined, usually short narrowed segment with decreased Wharton's jelly and vascular constriction (fig. 8-28). The etiology is unknown, but it has been hypothesized to be the result of a primary deficiency of Wharton's jelly, perhaps an exaggeration of the gradual loss of Wharton's jelly at the fetal end of the umbilical cord. Umbilical cord stricture rarely occurs outside the setting of hypercoiling.

Frequency. The frequency of cord stricture has not been established.

Gross Findings. Strictures are most common at the fetal end of the cord, although occasionally they occur at the placental end or elsewhere. They are frequently associated with excessively long and hypercoiled cords. Many are seen in association with macerated fetuses, although the abnormality is not confined to abortions.

Microscopic Findings. The strictured segment shows decreased Wharton's jelly and vascular, especially venous, compression (fig. 8-29). Placental surface vessels may be thrombosed with cushions.

Clinical Significance. Umbilical cord strictures are often associated with abortion (142). Strictures have recurred in successive pregnancies (10,61), and have been proposed as a cause of nonimmune hydrops (26).

Hematoma

Definition and Frequency. Umbilical cord hematomas are accumulations of blood in Wharton's jelly. They are uncommon lesions, but their precise frequency is unknown.

Etiology. The etiology of umbilical cord hematoma is unknown in most instances. In the great majority of cases, an obvious source is not apparent (125). Rarely, hemorrhage has a demonstrable origin from an umbilical vein or artery, and an origin from omphalomesenteric vessels has been proposed. Rupture of a varix, traumatic or mechanical damage at the time of amniocentesis or percutaneous umbilical cord sampling, and inflammation or structural anomalies of a vessel wall have been suggested as possible etiologic mechanisms.

Pathology. Most umbilical cord hematomas present as red-purple fusiform swellings, usually at the fetal end (figs. 8-30, 8-31). They are usually single, but may be multiple or even involve the full length of the umbilical cord. They are generally confined to the cord, but on occasion may rupture into the amnionic cavity. Small collections of fresh blood are the frequent result of cord blood sampling and traction at the time of delivery.

Clinical Significance. A perinatal mortality rate of 40 to 50 percent has been reported in association with umbilical cord hematomas (31, 122,124). Fetal death may be due to blood loss or compression of umbilical vessels resulting in circulatory compromise.

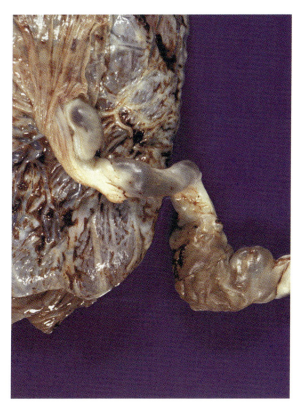 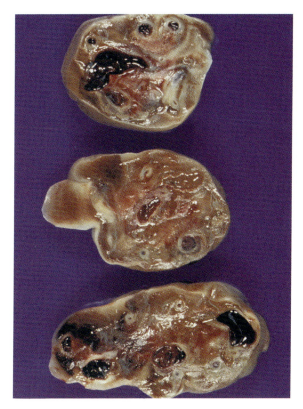

Figure 8-30

UMBILICAL CORD HEMATOMA

Localized umbilical cord hematoma (in cross section [right]) and from a live baby.

Hemangioma

Definition. Hemangiomas are benign lesions composed of vascular channels sometimes associated with marked myxoid degeneration of Wharton's jelly (*angiomyxoma*).

Etiology. Hemangiomas arise from aberrant vessels branching off an umbilical artery and from vessels associated with omphalomesenteric vitelline remnants.

Pathology. Hemangiomas present as a fusiform swelling of the umbilical cord, sometimes associated with a pseudocyst that can attain substantial proportions (900 g in one report [143]) (fig. 8-32). Microscopically, these benign tumors show features seen in benign hemangiomas at other body sites.

Clinical Significance. Hemangiomas with myxoid degeneration (angiomyxoma) can be associated with hemorrhage, increased alpha-fetoprotein levels, and occasionally, fetal hydrops.

ABNORMALITIES IN UMBILICAL CORD VESSELS

Aneurysms

Umbilical cord aneurysms are rare. They may be large enough to compress the adjacent vein resulting in fetal death (12,38,128).

Segmental Thinning

Quereshi and Jacques (105) reported segmental thinning of umbilical vessels, with virtual absence of the media, in 1.5 percent of consecutively examined placentas (fig. 8-33). The umbilical vein was involved in the majority of cases, although on occasion, one or both arteries exhibited identical changes. Both the superficial and medial aspects of the vessels exhibited wall deficiencies. Segmental vascular thinning was accompanied by fetal malformations in a significant number of cases, and there was a high incidence of fetal distress.

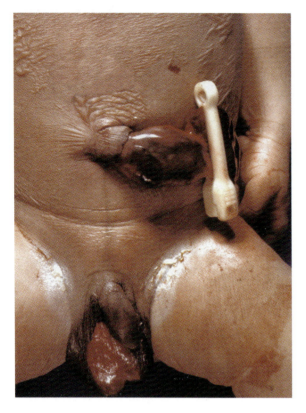

Figure 8-31

UMBILICAL CORD HEMATOMA

The fusiform purple hematoma at the fetal end of the umbilical cord caused fetal death in utero.

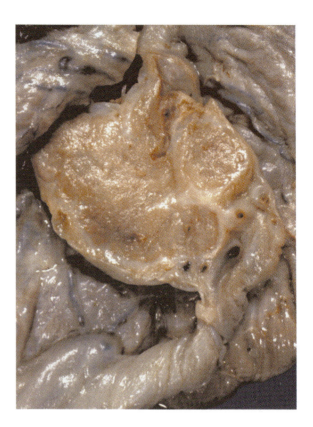

Figure 8-32

UMBILICAL CORD HEMANGIOMA

Umbilical cord hemangioma in an uncomplicated term pregnancy.

Meconium-Induced Necrosis

Segmental muscle necrosis occurs on the superficial aspect (facing the cord surface) in umbilical arteries with longstanding meconium exposure (see chapter 7) (2,3).

Ulceration

Myonecrosis of the umbilical arteries, with linear ulceration of the overlying Wharton's jelly, has been described in association with fetal intestinal atresia (11,70). The resulting arterial necrosis and aneurysmal dilatation may result in intra-amnionic hemorrhage, profound fetal anemia, and fetal death in utero (fig. 8-34).

Thrombosis

Definition. Clotting in umbilical vessels may be occlusive or nonocclusive, and is often associated with similar changes in the chorionic plate or villous vessels.

Frequency. Thrombosis of umbilical cord vessels is uncommon. In one large study, thrombosis occurred in 1 in 1,300 deliveries, 1 in 938 perinatal autopsies, and 1 in 250 high-risk pregnancies (55).

Etiology. Thrombi may be associated with cord compression, abnormal coiling, knots, torsion, stricture, hematoma, funisitis, anomalous insertion, amnionic bands, or entanglements. Other factors such as thrombophilic states could act synergistically to precipitate thrombosis (20). In many instances, the etiology is obscure.

Pathology. Thrombi more commonly involve the umbilical vein alone (71 percent), with a lesser frequency of combined vein and artery thrombosis (18 percent) or arterial thrombosis alone (11 percent). The chorionic plate and villous vessels may be similarly affected. Thrombi are associated with vessel calcification, and on

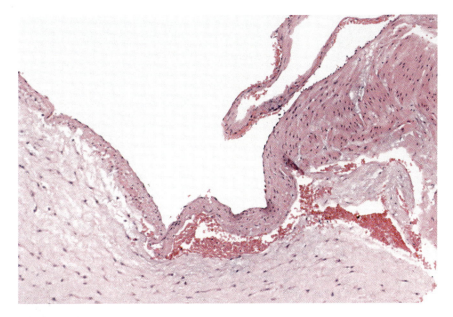

Figure 8-33

SEGMENTAL THINNING

This umbilical cord exhibited multiple foci of venous segmental thining. The full-term baby died during labor and delivery.

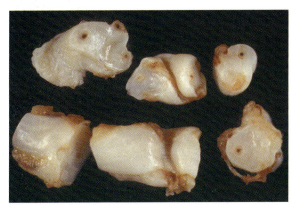 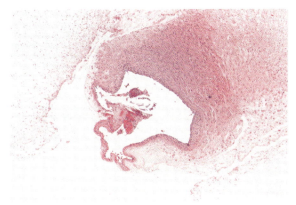

Figure 8-34

ULCERATION

Left: Necrosis and deep depression of Wharton's jelly over the umbilical arteries was associated with bloody amnionic fluid and fetal death. The baby had duodenal atresia.
Right: Loss of superficial Wharton's jelly with thinning of the vessel wall, focal rupture, and thrombosis.

occasion, the thrombosed vessel has a completely necrotic wall (figs. 8-35, 8-36).

Clinical Significance. Fetal morbidity and mortality are very high. Two thirds of affected infants are stillborn and nearly one third experience neonatal distress or die in the newborn period. The mortality rate is particularly high if both umbilical arteries are occluded. Thrombi have been associated with infarcts in fetal organs, cerebral palsy, massive fetomaternal hemorrhage, and fetal growth restriction (63,112).

Rupture

Complete cord rupture is rare (9), but its precise frequency is unknown. Most cord ruptures complicate precipitous delivery, but rarely, rupture occurs in the early stages of labor or before labor begins (37,44,114). Rupture usually occurs at the fetal end of the cord. Torsion, short cord, trauma, or inflammation are some postulated etiologic factors. Partial rupture, with the formation of hemorrhage and hematoma, is more common than complete rupture.

Placental Pathology

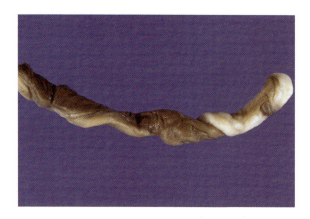
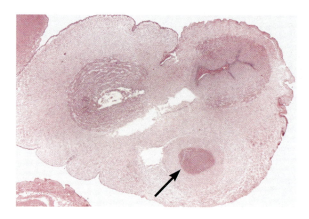

Figure 8-35

THROMBOSED UMBILICAL ARTERY

Left: A thrombosed umbilical artery, cause undetermined, is visible as a dark spiral.
Right: The artery is thrombosed and necrotic (arrow).

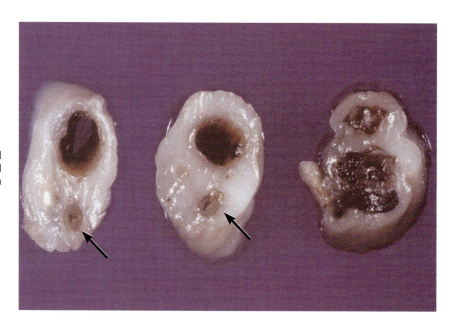

Figure 8-36

THROMBOSED UMBILICAL ARTERY

The thrombosed umbilical artery is visible only as a small yellow dot in cross section (arrows).

REFERENCES

1. Abuhamad AZ, Shaffer W, Mari G, Copel JA, Hobbins JC, Evans AT. Single umbilical artery: does it matter which artery is missing? Am J Obstet Gynecol 1995;173:728–32.
2. Altshuler G, Arizawa M, Molnar-Nadasdy G. Meconium-induced umbilical cord vascular necrosis and ulceration: a potential link between the placenta and poor pregnancy outcome. Obstet Gynecol 1992;79:760–6.
3. Altshuler G, Hyde S. Meconium-induced vasocontraction: a potential cause of cerebral and other fetal hypoperfusion and of poor pregnancy outcome. J Child Neurol 1989;4:137–42.
4. Altshuler G, Tsang RC, Ermocilla R. Single umbilical artery. Correlation of clinical status and umbilical cord histology. Am J Dis Child 1975;129:697–700.
5. Ami MB, Perlitz Y, Matilsky M. Prenatal sonographic diagnosis of persistent right umbilical vein with varix. J Clin Ultrasound 1999;27:273–5.

6. Antoine C, Young BK, Silverman F, Greco MA, Alvarez SP. Sinusoidal fetal heart rate pattern with vasa previa in twin pregnancy. J Reprod Med 1982;27:295–300.
7. Arts NF. Investigations on the vascular system of the placenta. I. General introduction and the fetal vascular system. Am J Obstet Gynecol 1961;82:147–58.
8. Baergen RN, Malicki D, Behling C, Benirschke K. Morbidity, mortality, and placental pathology in excessively long umbilical cords: retrospective study. Pediatr Dev Pathol 2001;4:144–53.
9. Bahary CM, Gabbai M, Eckerling B. Rupture of the umbilical cord: report of a case. Obstet Gynecol 1965;26:130–2.
10. Bakotic BW, Boyd T, Poppiti R, Pflueger S. Recurrent umbilical cord torsion leading to fetal death in 3 subsequent pregnancies: a case report and review of the literature. Arch Pathol Lab Med 2000;124:1352–5.
11. Bendon RW, Tyson RW, Baldwin VJ, Cashner KA, Mimouni F, Miodovnik M. Umbilical cord ulceration and intestinal atresia: a new association? Am J Obstet Gynecol 1991;164:582–6.
12. Benirschke K. Obstetrically important lesions of the umbilical cord. J Reprod Med 1994;39:262–72.
13. Benirschke K, Bourne GL. The incidence and prognostic implication of congenital absence of one umbilical artery. Am J Obstet Gynecol 1960;79:251–4.
14. Benirschke K, Kaufmann P. Pathology of the human placenta. New York: Springer; 2000.
15. Berg TG, Rayburn WF. Umbilical cord length and acid-base balance at delivery. J Reprod Med 1995;40:9–12.
16. Bhargava I, Chakravarty A, Raja PT. Anatomy of foetal blood vessels on the chorial surface of the human placenta. IV. With absence of one umbilical artery. Acta Anat (Basel) 1971;80:620–35.
17. Bilek K, Rothe K, Piskazeck K. Insertio-velamentosa-Blutung vor dem Blasensprung. Zentralbl Gyn kol 1962;84:1536–41.
18. Blickstein I, Varon Y, Varon E. Implications of differences in coiling indices at different segments of the umbilical cord. Gynecol Obstet Invest 2001;52:203–6.
19. Bourke WG, Clarke TA, Mathews TG, O'Halpin D, Donoghue VB. Isolated single umbilical artery—the case for routine renal screening. Arch Dis Child 1993;68:600–1.
20. Brewster JA, Quenby SM, Alfirevic Z. Intra-uterine death due to umbilical cord thrombosis secondary to antiphospholipid syndrome. Lupus 1999;8:558–9.
21. Browne FJ. On the abnormalities of the umbilical cord which may cause antenatal death. Br J Obstet Gynaecol 1925;32:17–48.
22. Bruner JP, Anderson TL, Rosemond RL. Placental pathophysiology of the twin oligohydromnios-polyhydramnios sequence and the twin-twin transfusion syndrome. Placenta 1998;19:81–6.
23. Bryan EM, Kohler HG. The missing umbilical artery. I. Prospective study based on a maternity unit. Arch Dis Child 1974;49:844–52.
24. Bryan EM, Kohler HG. The missing umbilical artery. II. Paediatric follow-up. Arch Dis Child 1975;50:714–8.
25. Chasnoff IJ, Fletcher MA. True knot of the umbilical cord. Am J Obstet Gynecol 1977;117:425–7.
26. Collins JH. Prenatal observation of umbilical cord torsion with subsequent premature labor and delivery of a 31-week infant with mild nonimmune hydrops. Am J Obstet Gynecol 1995;172:1048–9.
27. Cordero DR, Helfgott AW, Landy HJ, Reik RF, Medina C, O'Sullivan MJ. A non-hemorrhagic manifestation of vasa previa: a clinicopathologic case report. Obstet Gynecol 1993;82:698–700.
28. Degani S, Lewinsky RM, Berger H, Spiegel D. Sonographic estimation of umbilical coiling index and correlation with Doppler flow characteristics. Obstet Gynecol 1995;86:990–3.
29. Di Naro E, Ghezzi F, Raio L, Franchi M, D'Addario V. Umbilical cord morphology and pregnancy outcome. Eur J Obstet Gynecol Reprod Biol 2001;96:150–7.
30. Di Naro E, Ghezzi F, Raio L, et al. Umbilical vein blood flow in fetuses with normal and lean umbilical cord. Ultrasound Obstet Gynecol 2001;17:224–8.
31. Dippel AL. Hematomas of the umbilical cord. Surg Gynecol Obstet 1940;70:51–7.
32. Dudiak CM, Salomon CG, Posniak HV, Olson MC, Flisak ME. Sonography of the umbilical cord. Radiographics 1995;15:1035–50.
33. Earn AA. The effect of congenital abnormalities of the umbilical cord and placenta on the newborn and mother: a survey of 5676 consecutive deliveries. J Obstet Gynaecol Br Emp 1951;58:456–9.
34. Eddleman KA, Lockwood CJ, Berkowitz GS, Lapinski RH, Berkowitz RL. Clinical significance and sonographic diagnosis of velamentous umbiical cord insertion. Am J Perinatol 1992;9:123–6.
35. Ercal T, Lacin S, Altunyurt S, Saygili U, Cinar O, Mumcu A. Umbilical coiling index: it is a marker for the foetus at risk? Br J Clin Pract 1996;50:254–6.
36. Ezimokhai M, Rizk DE, Thomas L. Maternal risk factors for abnormal vascular coiling of the umbilical cord. Am J Perinatol 2000;17:441–5.

37. Foldes JJ. Spontaneous intrauterine rupture of the umbilical cord: report of a case. Obstet Gynecol 1957;9:608–9.
38. Fortune DW, Östör AG. Umbilical artery aneurysm. Am J Obstet Gynecol 1978;131:339–40.
39. Fox H. Pathology of the placenta. London: W.B. Saunders; 1997.
40. Fries MH, Goldstein RB, Kilpatrick SJ, Golbus MS, Callen PW, Filly RA. The role of velamentous cord insertion in the etiology of twin-twin transfusion syndrome. Obstet Gynecol 1993;81:569–74.
41. Froehlich LA, Fujikura T. Follow-up of infants with single umbilical artery. Pediatrics 1973;52:6–13.
42. Froelich LA, Fujikura T. Significance of a single umbilical artery. Report from the collaborative study of cerebral palsy. Am J Obstet Gynecol 1966;94:274–9.
43. Fujikura T. Single umbilical artery and congenital malformations. Am J Obstet Gynecol 1964;88:829–30.
44. Gallagher JP, Malone RG. Intra-uterine separation of the umbilical cord. Br J Obstet Gynecol 1956;63:287–9.
45. Gardiner JP. The umbilical cord: normal length; length in cord complications; etiology and frequency of coiling. Surg Gynaecol Obstet 1922;34:252–6.
46. Gilbert-Barness E, Drut RM, Drut R, Grange DK, Opitz JM. Developmental abnormalities resulting in short umbilical cord. Birth Defects Orig Artic Ser 1993;29:113–40.
47. Glanfield PA, Watson R. Intrauterine death due to umbilical cord torsion. Arch Pathol Lab Med 1986;110:357–8.
48. Goldkrand JW, Lentz SU, Turner AD, Clements S, Sefter H, Bryant J. Doppler velocimetry in the fetus with a single umbilical artery. J Reprod Med 1999;44:346–50.
49. Goodlin RC. Fetal dysmaturity, "lean cord," and fetal distress. Am J Obstet Gynecol 1987;156:1357.
50. Gupta I, Hillier VF, Edwards JM. Multiple vascular profiles in the umbilical cord; an indication of maternal smoking habits and intrauterine distress. Placenta 1993;14:117–23.
51. Hall SP. The thin cord syndrome. A review with a report of two cases. Obstet Gynecol 1961;18:507–9.
52. Harold JG, Siegel RJ, Fitzgerald GA, Satoh P, Fishbein MC. Differential prostacyclin production by human umbilical vasculature. Arch Pathol Lab Med 1988;112:43–6.
53. Heifetz SA. Pathology of the umbilical cord. In: Lewis SH, Perrin E, eds. Pathology of the placenta. New York: Churchill Livingstone; 1999.
54. Heifetz SA. Single umbilical artery. A statistical analysis of 237 autopsy cases and review of the literature. Perspect Pediatr Pathol 1984;8:345–78.
55. Heifetz SA. Thrombosis of the umbilical cord: analysis of 52 cases and literature review. Pediatr Pathol 1988;8:37–54.
56. Heifetz SA. The umbilical cord: obstetrically important lesions. Clin Obstet Gynecol 1996;39:571–87.
57. Heifetz SA, Rueda-Pedraza ME. Omphalomesenteric duct cysts of the umbilical cord. Pediatr Pathol 1983;1:325–35.
58. Heinonen S, Ryynänen M, Kirkinen P, Saarikoski S. Perinatal diagnostic evaluation of velamentous umbilical cord insertion: clinical, Doppler, and ultrasonic findings. Obstet Gynecol 1996;87:112–7.
59. Herberz O. Über die Insertio furcata funiculi umbilicalis. Acta Obstet Gynecol Scand 1938;18:336–51.
60. Herrmann UJ Jr, Sidiropoulos D. Single umbilical artery: prenatal findings. Prenatal Diagn 1988;8:275–80.
61. Hersh J, Buchino JJ. Umbilical cord torsion/constriction sequence. In: Saul RA, ed. Proceedings of the Greenwood Genetics Conference, Vol. 7. Clinton, SC: Jacobs Press; 1988:181–2.
62. Hershkovitz R, Silberstein T, Sheiner E, et al. Risk factors associated with true knots of the umbilical cord. Eur J Obstet Gynecol Reprod Biol 2001;98:36–9.
63. Hoag RW. Fetomaternal hemorrhage associated with umbilical vein thrombosis. Case report. Am J Obstet Gynecol 1986;154:1271–4.
64. Hyrtl J. Die Blutgefässe der menschlichen Nachgeburt in normalen und abnormen Verhältnissen. Wien: Braumüller; 1870.
65. Jauniaux E, De Munter C, Vanesse M, Wilkin P, Hustin J. Embryonic remnants of the umbilical cord: morphologic and clinical aspects. Hum Pathol 1989;20:458–62.
66. Javert CT, Barton B. Congenital and acquired lesions of the umbilical cord and spontaneous abortion. Am J Obstet Gynecol 1952;63:1065–77.
67. Jones TB, Sorokin Y, Bhatia R, Zador IE, Bottoms SF. Single umbilical artery: accurate diagnosis? Am J Obstet Gynecol 1993;169:538–40.
68. Kaplan CG. Color atlas of gross placental pathology. New York: Igaku-Shoin; 1994:30.
69. Karbowski B, Bauch HJ, Schneider HP. Functional differentiation of umbilical vein endothelial cells following pregnancy complicated by smoking or diabetes mellitus. Placenta 1991;12:405.

70. Khong TY, Ford WD, Haan EA. Umbilical cord ulceration in association with intestinal atresia in a child with deletion 13q and Hirschsprung's disease. Arch Dis Child 1994;71:F212–3.
71. Khong TY, George K. Chromosomal abnormalities associated with a single umbilical artery. Prenatal Diagn 1992;12:965–8.
72. King DL. Placental migration demonstrated by ultrasonography. A hypothesis of dynamic placentation. Radiology 1973;109:167–70.
73. Kristoffersen K. The significance of absence of one umbilical artery. Acta Obstet Gynecol Scand 1969;48:195–214.
74. Labarrere C, Sebastiani M, Siminovich M, Torassa E, Althabe O. Absence of Wharton's jelly around the umbilical arteries: an unusual cause of perinatal mortality. Placenta 1985;6:555–9.
75. Lacro RV, Jones KL, Benirschke K. The umbilical cord twist: origin, direction and relevance. Am J Obstet Gynecol 1987;157:833–8.
76. Las Heras J, Haust MD. Ultrastructure of fetal stem arteries of human placenta in normal pregnancy. Virchows Arch A Pathol Anat Histol 1981;393:133–44.
77. Lee ST, Hon EH. Fetal hemodynamic response to umbilical cord compression. Obstet Gynecol 1963;22:553–62.
78. Leung AK, Robson WL. Single umbilical artery. A report of 159 cases. Am J Dis Child 1989;143:108–11.
79. Lilja M. Infants with single umbilical artery studied in a national registry. 2. Survival and malformations in infants with single umbilical artery. Paediat Perinat Epidemiol 1992;6:416–22.
80. Lopriore E, Vandenbussche FP, Tiersma ES, de Beaufort AJ, de Leeuw JP. Twin-to-twin transfusion syndrome: new perspectives. J Pediatr 1995;127:675–80.
81. Macara LM, Kingdom JC, Kaufmann P. Control of the fetoplacental circulation. Fetal Maternal Med Rev 1993;5:167–79.
82. Machin GA, Ackerman J, Gilbert-Barness E. Abnormal umbilical cord coiling is associated with adverse perinatal outcomes. Pediatr Dev Pathol 2000;3:462–71.
83. Matheus M, Sala MA. The importance of placental examination in newborns with single umbilical artery. Z Geburtshilfe Perinatol 1980;184:231–2.
84. McCurdy C, Anderson C, Borjon N, Brzechffa P, Miller H, McNamara M, Newman A, Seeds J. Antenatal sonographic diagnosis of nuchal cord (abstract 329). Am J Obstet Gynecol 1994;170:366.
85. McLennan H, Price E, Urbanska M, Craig N, Fraser M. Umbilical cord knots and encirclements. Aust and N Z J Obstet Gynecol 1988;28:116–9.
86. McLennan JE. Implications of the eccentricity of the human umbilical cord. Am J Obstet Gynecol 1968;101:1124–30.
87. Messer RH, Gomez AR, Yambao TJ. Antepartum testing for vasa previa: current standard of care. Am J Obstet Gynecol 1987;156:1459–62.
88. Meyer WJ, Blumenthal L, Cadkin A, Gauthier DW, Rotmensch S. Vasa previa: prenatal diagnosis with transvaginal color Doppler flow imaging. Am J Obstet Gynecol 1993;169:1627–9.
89. Meyer WW, Lind J, Moinian M. An accessory fourth vessel of the umbilical cord. A preliminary study. Am J Obstet Gynecol 1969;105:1063–8.
90. Miller ME, Higginbottom M, Smith DW. Short umbilical cord: its origin and relevance. J Pediatr 1981;67:618–21.
91. Miller ME, Jones MC, Smith DW. Tension: the basis of umbilical cord growth. J Pediatr 1982;101:844.
92. Mills JL, Harley EE, Moessinger AC. Standards for measuring umbilical cord length. Placenta 1983;4:423–6.
93. Moessinger AC, Blanc WA, Marone PA, Polsen DC. Umbilical cord length as an index of fetal activity: experimental study and clinical implications. Pediatr Res 1982;16:109–12.
94. Moessinger AC, Mills JL, Harley EE, Ramakrishnan R, Berendes HW, Blanc WA. Umbilical cord length in Down's syndrome. Am J Dis Child 1986;140:1276–7.
95. Monie IW. Velamentous insertion of the cord in early pregnancy. Am J Obstet Gynecol 1965;93:276–81.
96. Naeye RL. Umbilical cord length: clinical significance. J Pediatr 1985;107:278–81.
97. Nanaev AK, Kohnen G, Milovanov AP, Domogatsky SP, Kaufmann P. Stromal differentiation and architecture of the human umbilical cord. Placenta 1997;18:53–64.
98. Nanaev AK, Shirinsky VP, Birukov KG. Immunofluorescent study of heterogeneity in smooth muscle cells of human fetal vessels using antibodies to myosin, desmin and vimentin. Cell Tissue Res 1991;266:535–40.
99. Nelson KB, Grether JK. Potentially asphyxiating conditions and spastic cerebral palsy in infants of normal birth weight. Am J Obstet Gynecol 1998;179:507–13.
100. Parry EW, Abramovich DR. The ultrastructure of human umbilical vessel endothelium from early pregnancy to full term. J Anat 1972;111:29–42.

101. Patel D, Dawson M, Kalyanam P, Lungus E, Weiss H, Flaherty E, Nora EG Jr. Umbilical cord circumference at birth. Am J Dis Child 1989;143:638–9.
102. Pierce BT, Dance VD, Wagner RK, Apodaca CC, Nielsen PE, Calhoun BC. Perinatal outcome following fetal single umbilical artery diagnosis. J Matern Fetal Med 2001;10:59–63.
103. Priman J. A note on the anastomosis of the umbilical arteries. Anat Rec 1959;134:1–5.
104. Purola E. The length and insertion of the umbilical cord. Ann Chir Gynaecol Fenn 1968;57:621–2.
105. Qureshi F, Jacques SM. Marked segmental thinning of the umbilical cord vessels. Arch Pathol Lab Med 1994;118:826–30.
106. Raio L, Ghezzi F, Di Naro E, et al. In-utero characterization of the blood flow in the Hyrtl anastomosis. Placenta 2001;22:597–601.
107. Raio L, Ghezzi F, Di Naro E, et al. Sonographic measurement of the umbilical cord and fetal anthropometric parameters. Eur J Obstet Gynecol Reprod Biol 1999;83:131–5.
108. Raio L, Ghezzi F, Di Naro E, Franchi M, Bruhwiler H. Prenatal assessment of the Hyrtl anastomosis and evaluation of its function: case report. Hum Reprod 1999;14:1890–3.
109. Raio L, Ghezzi F, Di Naro E, Franchi M, Bruhwiler H, Luscher KP. Prenatal assessment of Wharton's jelly in umbilical cords with single artery. Ultrasound Obstet Gynecol 1999;14:42–6.
110. Raio L, Ghezzi F, Di Naro E, Gomez R, Saile G, Bruhwiler H. The clinical significance of antenatal detection of discordant umbilical arteries. Obstet Gynecol 1998;91:86–91.
111. Rana J, Ebert GA, Kappy KA. Adverse perinatal outcome in patients with an abnormal umbilical coiling index. Obstet Gynecol 1995;85:573–7.
112. Rayne SC, Kraus FT. Placental thrombi and other vascular lesions. Classification, morphology, and clinical correlations. Pathol Res Pract 1993;189:2–17.
113. Redline RW, Shah D, Sakar H, Schluchter M, Salvator A. Placental lesions associated with abnormal growth in twins. Pediatr Dev Pathol 2001;4:473–81.
114. Rehn K, Kinnunen O. Antepartum rupture of the umbilical cord: case report. Acta Obstet Gynecol Scand 1962;41:86–9.
115. Rinehart BK, Terrone DA, Taylor CW, Isler CM, Larmon JE, Roberts WE. Single umbilical artery is associated with an increased incidence of structural and chromosomal anomalies and growth restriction. Am J Perinatol 2000;17:229–32.
116. Rizos N, Doran TA, Miskin M, Benzie RJ, Ford JA. Natural history of placenta previa ascertained by diagnostic ultrasound. Am J Obstet Gynecol 1979;133:287–91.
117. Robinson JN, Abuhamad AZ. Abdominal wall and umbilical cord anomalies. Clin Perinatol 2000;27:947–78.
118. Robinson LK, Jones KL, Benirschke K. The nature of structural defects associated with velamentous and marginal insertion of the umbilical cord. Am J Obstet Gynecol 1983;146:191–3.
119. Rolschau J. The relationship between some disorders of the umbilical cord and intrauterine growth retardation. Acta Obstet Gynecol Scand Suppl 1978;72:15–21.
120. Rosen RH. The short umbilical cord. Am J Obstet Gynecol 1955;66:1253–9.
121. Rucker MP, Tureman GR. Vasa previa. Va Med Mon 1945;72:202–7.
122. Ruvinsky ED, Wiley TL, Morrison JC, Blake PG. In utero diagnosis of umbilical cord hematoma by ultrasonography. Am J Obstet Gynecol 1981;140:833–4.
123. Saller DN Jr, Neiger R. Cytogenetic abnormalities among perinatal deaths demonstrating a single umbilical artery. Prenat Diagn 1994;14:13–6.
124. Schreier R, Brown S. Hematoma of the umbilical cord. Report of a case. Obstet Gynecol 1962;20:798–800.
125. Seoud M, Aboul-Hosn L, Nassar A, Khalil A, Usta I. Spontaneous umbilical cord hematoma: a rare cause of acute fetal distress. Am J Perinatol 2001;18:99–102.
126. Shanklin DR. The influence of placental lesions on the newborn infant. Pediatr Clin North Am 1970;17:25–42.
127. Shen-Schwarz S, Ananth CV, Smulian JC, Vintzleos AM. Umbilical cord twist patterns in twin gestations [abstract 538]. Am J Obstet Gynecol 1997;176:S154.
128. Siddiqi TA, Bendon R, Schultz DM, Miodovnik M. Umbilical artery aneurysm: prenatal diagnosis and management. Obstet Gynecol 1992;80:530–3.
129. Silver RK, Dooley SL, Tamura RK, Depp R. Umbilical cord size and amniotic fluid volume in prolonged pregnancy. Am J Obstet Gynecol 1987;157:716–20.
130. Somes T. Umbilical cord encirclements and fetal growth restriction. Obstet Gynecol 1995;86:725–8.
131. Strong TH Jr. Factors that provide optimal umbilical protection during gestation. Contemp Obstet Gynecol 1997;42:82–105.
132. Strong TH Jr, Elliott JP, Radin TR. Non-coiled umbilical blood vessels: a new marker for the fetus at risk. Obstet Gynecol 1993;81:409–11.

133. Strong TH Jr, Finberg HJ, Mattox JH. Antepartum diagnosis of noncoiled umbilical cords. Am J Obstet Gynecol 1994;170:1729–33.
134. Strong TH Jr, Jarles DL, Vega JS, Feldman DB. The umbilical coiling index. Am J Obstet Gynecol 1994;170:29–32.
135. Swanberg H, Wiqvist N. Rupture of the umbilical cord during pregnancy. Acta Obstet Gynecol Scand 1951;30:323–37.
136. Takechi K, Kuwabara Y, Mizuno M. Ultrastructural and immunohistochemical studies of Wharton's jelly umbilical cord cells. Placenta 1993;14:235–45.
137. Torrey WE. Vasa previa. Am J Obstet Gynecol 1952;63:146–52.
138. Uchide K, Ueno H, Inuyama R, Murakami K, Terada S. Cord presentation with posterior placenta previa. Lancet 1997;350:1448.
139. Ullberg U, Sandstedt B, Lingman G. Hyrtl's anastomosis, the only connection between the two umbilical arteries. A study in full term placentas from AGA infants with normal umbilical artery blood flow. Acta Obstet Gynecol Scand 2001;80:1–6.
140. Ulm MR, Plockinger B, Pirich C, Gryglewski RJ, Sinzinger HF. Umbilical arteries of babies born to cigarette smokers generate less prostacyclin and contain less arginine and citrulline compared with those of babies born to control subjects. Am J Obstet Gynecol 1995;172:1485–87.
141. Viora E, Sciarrone A, Bastonero S, Errante G, Campogrande M. Thrombosis of umbilical vein varix. Ultrasound Obstet Gynecol 2002;19:212–3.
142. Weber J. Constriction of the umbilical cord as a cause of foetal death. Acta Obstet Gynecol Scand. 1963;42:259–68.
143. Yavner DL, Redline RW. Angiomyxoma of the umbilical cord with massive cystic degeneration of Wharton's jelly. Arch Pathol Lab Med 1898;113:935–7.
144. Young GB. The peripatetic placenta. Radiology 1978;128:183–8.

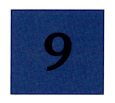

ABORTION, STILLBIRTH, AND INTRAUTERINE FETAL DEATH

INTRODUCTION

Depending upon the sensitivity and sophistication of the diagnostic methods used to confirm the diagnosis of pregnancy, well over half of all conceptions fail (13). Of gestations confirmed in this way, about half actually implant and persist long enough to be recognized clinically. The most common causes of gestational failure are genotypic abnormalities, infections, blood clotting or bleeding in and around the placenta, and autoimmunity or possibly an abnormal alloimmune response to fetal antigens. The relative frequency of these etiologies varies with gestational age. Very early abortions, prior to 6 weeks developmental stage, usually have abnormal karyotypes, while inflammatory causes predominate after 11.5 weeks (57).

The products of conception and decidual tissue are commonly submitted for pathologic examination after spontaneous passage or dilatation and curettage. The pathologic examination serves two purposes: to confirm that the aborted tissue includes chorionic villi and to explain, if possible, why the pregnancy failed. Identification of the cause of pregnancy failure may require specialized studies. For example, microbiologic cultures, karyotyping, and biochemical analyses or molecular biologic studies may identify specific infections, chromosomal trisomies, genetically determined enzyme deficiencies, coagulopathies, or forms of abnormal maternal immune response.

Terminology. The following terms have been commonly used for centuries in clinical settings, but most are imprecise and ambiguous, with shades of meaning that vary depending on the context. The timing of the developmental stages of embryonic or fetal death is also inexact when estimated for specimens in a clinical context.

Abortion denotes the premature spontaneous expulsion of a nonviable human conceptus. While the term applies in all cases of spontaneous fetal loss, abortion is generally reserved for gestations spontaneously expelled early, before the 20th gestational week, prior to the time of legal viability. Most clinically recognized abortions occur between the 8th and 12th weeks, but many more from 2 to 6 weeks pass unnoticed. The legal definition of viability varies in different legal jurisdictions. In some states within the United States abortions are defined in terms of weight, for example, below a weight of 350 g.

The expression *products of conception* is synonymous with all of the spontaneously passed fetal tissues, embryonic, villous, and membranous, including the intermediate trophoblast infiltrating the decidua from the implantation site. *Intrauterine fetal death* (IUFD) generally applies to the loss of older gestations, from the 12th to the 28th week, or even at term. A *miscarriage* is an intrauterine fetal death that occurs after fetal movement has been detected by the mother. A *stillbirth* means that the fetus has been delivered dead, without respirations or heartbeat, and incapable of resuscitation at the time it is delivered. *Premature delivery* refers to a live birth after 20 weeks' gestation, or above a specific weight such as 350 g, in some legal jurisdictions.

The intentional evacuation of a conceptus that is normal or believed to be capable of surviving if the pregnancy continues is not, strictly speaking, an abortion, which is a spontaneous event. This type of procedure may be called an *elective abortion* or, in some cases, a *therapeutic abortion*. Examination of the tissues produced in this way is necessary when performed for specific indications such as intrauterine infections including toxoplasmosis and parvovirus, or for various anomalies.

EARLY SPONTANEOUS ABORTION, PRODUCTS OF CONCEPTION, AND EMBRYONIC DEATH

Definition. The embryonic stage includes the embryo, immature villi, and chorioamnionic membranes through the 8th gestational week. Early abortions include pregnancy losses up to the 12th week. These tissues may be passed

Table 9-1

RELATIVE FREQUENCIES OF CHROMOSOMAL ABERRATIONS ACCORDING TO PHENOTYPE IN SPONTANEOUS ABORTIONS AT GESTATIONAL AGE LESS THAN 28 WEEKS[a]

Specimen Studied	Percent Chromosomally Abnormal (Range)
Intact Empty Sac	57-64%
Ruptured Sac	41-63%
Morphologically Abnormal Embryo	55-71%
Morphologically Normal Embryo	45-60%
Abnormal Fetus	16-25%
Normal Fetus	2-14%

[a]Modified from reference 3.

Table 9-2

RELATIVE FREQUENCIES OF ABNORMAL KARYOTYPES IN CULTURED SPONTANEOUS ABORTIONS[a]

Karyotype	Total Number	Gestational Age <11.5 Weeks	Gestational Age >11.5 Weeks
Normal	318	291	53
Abnormal	350	328	22
Trisomy	225	216	9
Triploidy	43	37	6
Monosomy X	34	28	6
Tetraploid	15	15	0
Others	33	31	2

[a]Modified from reference 57.

spontaneously or may require removal by curettage after intrauterine death has occurred.

Incidence or Prevalence. In a study of early pregnancies whose presence was diagnosed solely on the basis of rising urinary beta-human chorionic gonadotropin (β-HCG) levels, Edmonds et al. (13) concluded that 69.1 percent of conceptuses in a normal population of women attempting to conceive are lost prior to 12 weeks. However, 91 percent of these pregnancy losses are not clinically recognized by any other criteria. In general, about 15 percent of clinically evident pregnancies abort (13).

Clinical Features and Etiology. The death or absence of an embryo (also called a "blighted ovum") is accompanied in the mother by pelvic (uterine) cramping and bleeding (threatened abortion). The conceptus is then often expelled as a mass of soft hemorrhagic tissue (complete abortion). This event is commonly followed or assisted by removing the remaining uterine contents by curettage (incomplete abortion). In some cases, absence of a viable embryo is detected by an early pregnancy ultrasound (missed abortion) for which an elective curettage is usually performed to avoid the excessive bleeding associated with spontaneous passage. Cases without an embryo should be documented, even when recurrent, because these are more likely to represent chance events or chromosomal abnormalities with a low risk of recurrence.

Over half of aborted embryos and fetuses have abnormal karyotypes. Karyotyping the chromosomes of the conceptus involves the use of cultured, dividing fetal or placental trophoblastic cells. The chromosomes are examined morphologically, and counted to identify deletions of all or part of a specific chromosome, the presence of extra chromosomes, or polyploidy. Large studies using karyotyping indicate that these abnormalities are a common cause of early pregnancy loss, especially when the aborted tissue is grossly abnormal, as when the embryo is deformed or absent (Table 9-1). Abnormal karyotypes are a relatively uncommon cause of third trimester fetal loss or stillbirth (73). In a series of 668 spontaneous abortions, 350 (51 percent) had an abnormal karyotype, most of which were trisomies, with smaller numbers of triploid, monosomy X, and tetraploid karyotypes (Table 9-2) (58). The 318 (49 percent) abortions with normal karyotype in this series included more with an older gestational stage, and had a variety of inflammatory lesions as described below (see figs. 9-13–9-15). The abortions with normal karyotype occurred in younger women, many of whom had autoimmune markers identified serologically. Some trisomic chromosomes, such as trisomy 16 or 21, are relatively common while trisomy 1 occurs rarely, if at all (Table 9-3). The occurrence of two or more sets of cells with different karyotypes in the same individual is called a mosaic. Mosaics, most in the form of a trisomy mixed with a line of cells with normal karyotype, represent about 8 to 10 percent of abortions with abnormal karyotypes.

In selected cases when a karyotype has not been obtained, trisomies can be identified in formalin-fixed archival tissues by fluorescence in situ hybridization (FISH) using commercially prepared probes specific for the centromeric regions of individual chromosomes. With the addition of multiple specific molecular probes (spectral karyotyping) (62), more subtle abnormalities can be demonstrated. The technique of comparative genomic hybridization, when combined with flow cytometry, promises to provide even better results, with a lower failure rate (41). This would be especially useful if it can be applied to formalin-fixed archival tissues.

Maternal coagulopathies (thrombophilias), both inherited and acquired (antiphospholipid antibodies), are another major etiologic factor for abortion as well as for later fetal loss (8,10, 21, 40,49,52,58,59,69). All of the known thrombophilic abnormalities have been implicated: the C677T mutated methylenetetrahydrofolate reductase *(MTHFR)* gene, activated protein C resistance, factor V Leiden, and the prothrombin gene mutation are the most common. As with other placental lesions related to clotting, homozygosity, multiple coagulopathies, and the chance association of more than one lesion or condition enhance the potential for harm.

The notion that immune rejection of the fetoplacental allograft is a cause of abortion, especially repeated abortion, remains attractive, if for no other reason than it has been difficult to explain why the placental attachment is ever immunologically permitted. Studies of women with multiple consecutive abortions have lead to the recognition of variations in the immune response. Local and systemic immunoregulation of T-cell responses, variations in subsets of immunocompetent cells (23,55), certain human leukocyte antigen (HLA) haplotypes (7), and possible relationships with intervillous macrophage accumulation (11) have all been studied, with inconclusive results. The potential role for maternal immunization by paternal leukocytes (4) remains controversial, with recommendations that this theory be abandoned (15).

The observation that T-cell–mediated rejection of all implantations in mice occur rapidly when an inhibitor of the tryptophan-catabolizing enzyme produced by trophoblast and macrophages at the implantation site is introduced is an intriguing discovery. This suggests that the normally occurring breakdown of tryptophan at the implantation site suppresses T-cell activity, defending the fetus from rejection (48). The same processes occur in human placental tissue (34).

The Purpose of Examining Aborted Tissue. The main goal, and very often the only goal, of aborted tissue examination is to confirm that

Table 9-3

RELATIVE FREQUENCIES OF CHROMOSOMAL TRISOMY IN 563 SPONTANEOUS ABORTIONS[a]

Chromosome	Trisomies Reported	Percent
1	0	0.0
2	20	3.6
3	6	1.1
4	17	3.0
5	1	0.2
6	4	0.7
7	23	4.1
8	22	3.9
9	15	2.7
10	10	1.8
11	2	0.3
12	7	1.2
13	22	3.9
14	31	5.5
15	44	7.8
16	167	29.7
17	3	0.5
18	26	4.6
19	1	0.2
20	11	1.9
21	59	10.5
22	69	12.3
X	3	0.5
Total	563	100.0

[a]Modified from reference 3.

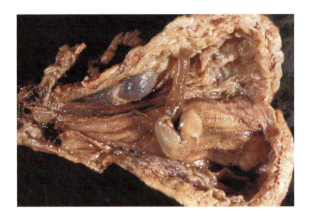

Figure 9-1

SPONTANEOUSLY PASSED "UTERINE CAST"

Much of the soft pale tan tissue is decidua. The primitive umbilical cord is edematous, and the embryo is deformed. The karyotype is likely to be abnormal in this case. Specimen is partially fixed in formalin.

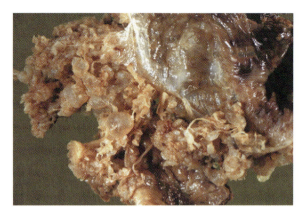

Figure 9-2

SPONTANEOUS ABORTION (HYDROPIC ABORTION, POSSIBLE CHROMOSOMAL TRISOMY)

The amnionic sac was ruptured and empty. Some of the villi are hydropic. A diploid true mole is unlikely in the presence of the well-formed amnionic sac.

an early intrauterine pregnancy has aborted. This is usually achieved by identifying immature chorionic villi. In some cases, all of the villous component may have been expelled, but the curetted uterine decidua usually contains enough placental site trophoblast tissue to confirm an intrauterine pregnancy. Immunostaining for keratin, human placental lactogen (HPL), or HCG may assist in doubtful cases (29, 30). If pregnancy testing is positive, the absence of any trophoblastic tissue after all tissue has been examined histologically suggests the possibility of an ectopic pregnancy, and therefore must be reported. Conversely, the demonstration of villi in curettings does not exclude the presence of an ectopic pregnancy (22), especially in the context of assisted (ovulation induction) pregnancy (39). Significant histologic findings are the presence of embryonic or fetal tissue, the absence of unsuspected uterine pathology such as intrauterine infection and endometrial neoplasms, and the relevant pathology of abortions described below.

Gross Findings. Spontaneously passed tissue may include an intact gestational sac with or without an embryo in the sac. The tissue is a soft, dark red, often hemorrhagic mass, which includes decidua that may conform to the shape of the uterine cavity and variable amounts of blood clot (fig. 9-1). Both the immature placental tissues and the embryo, if present, require evaluation.

Curetted tissues often include a pale spongy mass (the villi) attached to a glistening translucent membrane (the chorionic plate with amnion). The decidual component is folded sheets or strips of soft pink tissue with a smooth surface and a shaggy underside. Careful inspection of the gross fragments ensures adequate villous sampling, high quality specimens for karyotyping, and prompt identification of the villi in ectopic pregnancy specimens.

Gross evidence of villous hydropic change (figs. 9-2–9-5) suggests a partial or complete hydatidiform mole and requires more complete sampling. Vesicular villi are more readily appreciated when floating in water (figs. 9-3, 9-5). The presence of a large hematoma (fig. 9-6) should be documented, noting whether it is intraplacental or extraplacental, deforming the placental mass, or just an extraneous clot.

The embryo or fetus should be inspected for anomalies that might suggest a chromosomal defect. Certain abnormalities are distinctive, though not specific. Marked hydropic changes with cystic hygroma are typical of monosomy X (fig. 9-7). A triploid fetus often has facial clefts, syndactyly of digits 3 and 4, and a large head (figs. 9-3, 9-8); both the placenta and the fetus are small for the gestational age. The fetus with trisomy 13 has features of cyclopia, polydactyly, and cleft lip and palate (figs. 9-9, 9-10). The prenatal ultrasound may identify cardiac

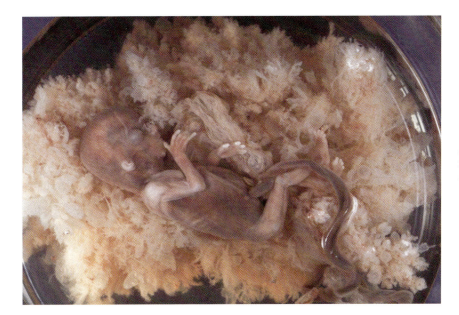

Figure 9-3

SPONTANEOUS ABORTION OF A TRIPLOID FETUS AT 11 WEEKS' GESTATION

There is syndactyly of digits 3 and 4, and scattered hydropic villi intermixed with more normal-appearing smaller villi.

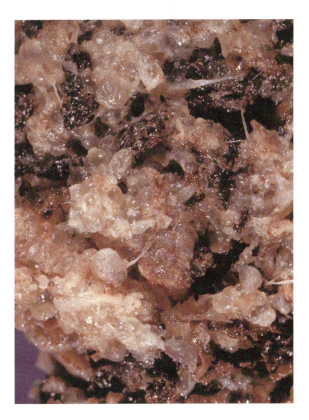

Figure 9-4

EARLY COMPLETE HYDATIDIFORM MOLE

Early complete hydatidiform mole, postcurettage, at 11 weeks, with abnormal vesicular villi intermixed with blood clot. It is difficult to be sure whether there might be a component of more normal nonhydropic villi. Compare with figure 9-5.

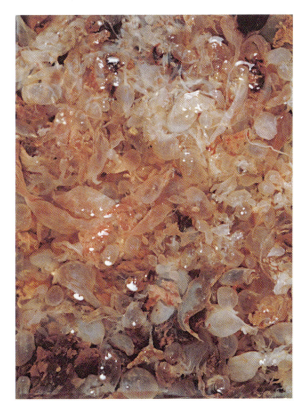

Figure 9-5

COMPLETE HYDATIDIFORM MOLE

Complete hydatidiform mole, floating in water. All villi are clearly abnormal and vesicular. Compare with figure 9-4.

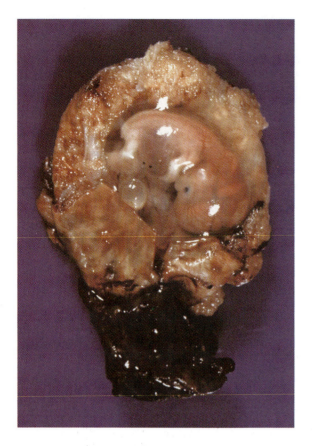

Figure 9-6

SPONTANEOUS ABORTION OF AN INTACT SAC WITH NORMAL-APPEARING EMBRYO

The hematoma at the bottom involved the immature placental component. An abnormal karyotype is less likely; the clot may be the significant factor.

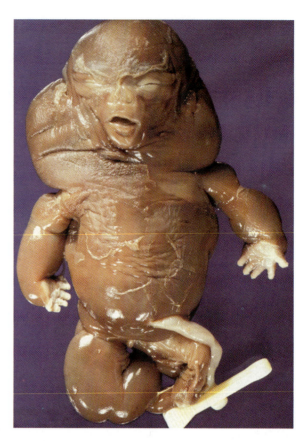

Figure 9-7

MACERATED HYDROPIC FETUS

Macerated hydropic fetus with large cystic hygroma and 45X0 karyotype.

and renal abnormalities; cerebral anomalies such as holoprosencephaly, with a large single ventricle; and other anomalies (fig. 9-11). The presence of an intact but empty sac or a grossly disorganized nodular embryonic structure (fig. 9-12) suggests that an abnormal karyotype is likely, while a grossly normal embryo in both size and morphologic detail is much more likely to be karyotypically normal. The extensively illustrated reviews of karyotype-correlated embryonic and fetal anomalies by Baldwin (3), Keeling (30), and Dimmick and Kalousek (9) provide a useful atlas-format resource for classifying the possible genotype of a malformed fetus.

Microscopic Findings. Dysmorphic villi are especially common in very early abortions (less than 6 weeks) with abnormal karyotypes. Villi that appear histologically normal for gestational age, especially in a miscarriage at or after a gestational age of 11 weeks, strongly suggest a normal karyotype (56,60). Abnormalities suggesting some other type of clinical problem (decidual vasculitis, villous infarcts, chronic intervillositis, abundant perivillous fibrin, decidual plasma cells) are also more frequent in chromosomally normal gestations (figs. 9-13–9-15). The near absence of implantation site trophoblast (intermediate trophoblast) is an unexplained feature in occasional spontaneous abortions; the pathogenesis and significance of this feature are unknown (fig. 9-16). Large clots in the intervillous space may in some cases be related to maternal coagulopathies (fig. 9-17).

Dysmorphic features suggesting abnormal karyotypes include enlarged vesicular villi with hydropic stroma, often with irregular villous

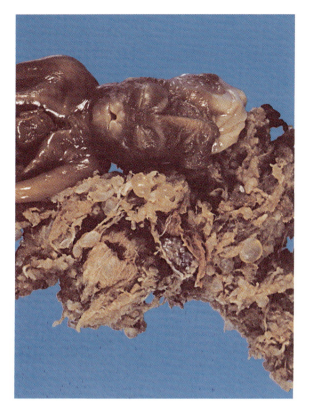

Figure 9-8

MACERATED TRIPLOID FETUS

Macerated triploid fetus with bilateral facial cleft fusion defect and a component of vesicular villi.

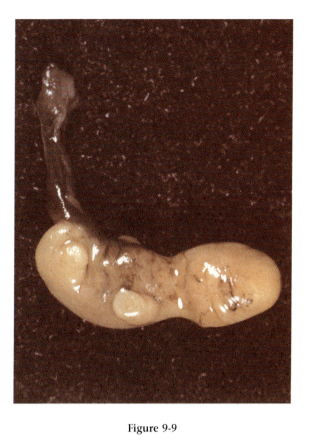

Figure 9-9

TRISOMY 13

Embryo with ocular fusion and stunted deformed limb buds, consistent with trisomy 13.

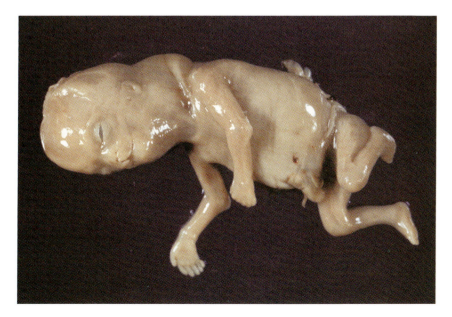

Figure 9-10

TRISOMY 13

Trisomy 13 fetus with a facial cleft deformity, supernumerary digits, malformed low-set ears, and small cervical hygroma.

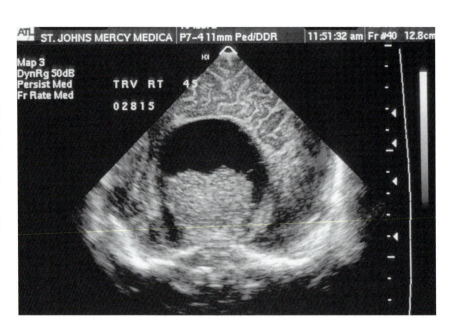

Figure 9-11

ALOBAR HOLOPROSENCEPHALY

The ultrasound image shows a single large ventricle, fused thalami (center), and absent corpus callosum, falx, septum, and interhemispheric fissure. Various abnormal karyotypes occur, involving chromosomes 13 and 18 especially. The karyotype in this case was not analyzed. Placental lesions (not necessarily related) included fetal thrombotic vasculopathy, one infarct, and chorangiosis.

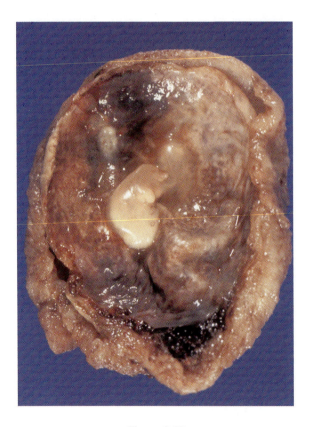

Figure 9-12

SPONTANEOUS ABORTION WITH ABNORMAL EMBRYO

The umbilical stalk is edematous, protruding from a hypoplastic caudal pole. The chorionic sac is abnormally dilated. The gross appearance is not specific, but suggestive of an abnormal karyotype.

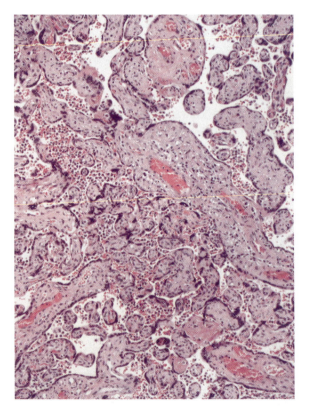

Figure 9-13

CHRONIC INTERVILLOSITIS

Clusters of mononuclear cells form small masses in the intervillous space. There are a few small clumps of fibrin attached to the villi. Fetal vessels remain open.

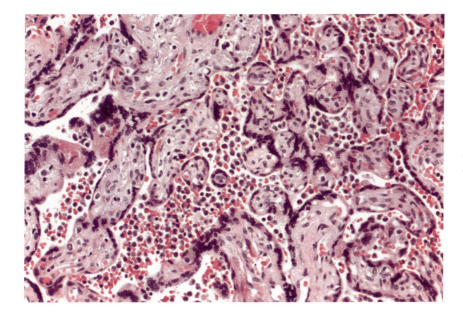

Figure 9-14

CHRONIC INTERVILLOSITIS
Higher magnification of figure 9-13 shows mononuclear cells in the intervillous space.

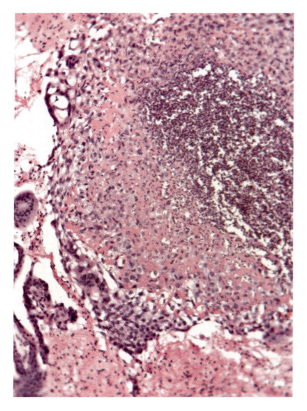

Figure 9-15

SEPTIC ABORTION CAUSED BY SEVERE INTRAUTERINE BACTERIAL INFECTION
Masses of degenerating neutrophils form small abscesses, with focal necrosis of villi.

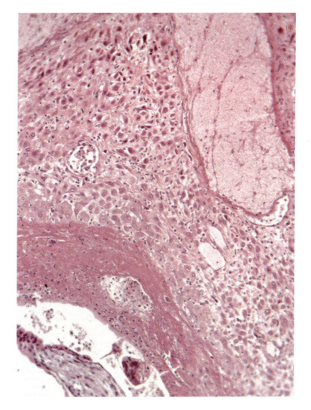

Figure 9-16

SPONTANEOUS ABORTION
Spontaneous abortion associated with marked reduction of placental site (intermediate) trophoblast. The few trophoblast cells appear small and poorly developed. Immune mechanisms have been suggested, but not proven, as an etiology.

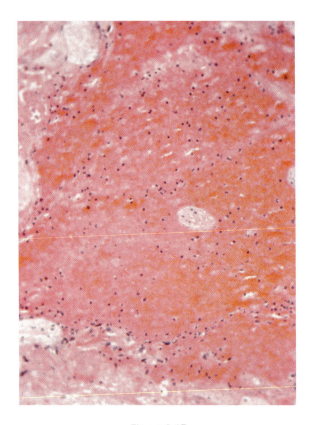

Figure 9-17

SPONTANEOUS ABORTION

A large hematoma expands the intervillous space, separating the villi, which have begun to degenerate. This was the third consecutive spontaneous abortion in a woman with a coagulopathy caused by the *MTHFR* gene mutation.

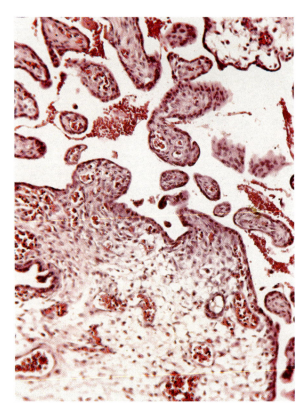

Figure 9-18

TRIPLOID ABORTION (69XXY KARYOTYPE)

The large vesicular villus at the bottom contains two small, rounded, trophoblastic "inclusions," which are actually in-vaginations. There is a distinct separate component of smaller, more normal-sized villi at the top.

contours; large irregular stromal vascular spaces; and trophoblastic invaginations intermixed with groups of smaller more normal-sized villi (figs. 9-18–9-25). This pattern is typical of chromosomal triploidy, including triploid partial moles, which have two sets of paternally derived chromosomes (digynic triploid villi are essentially of normal size and shape) (45,75). Avascular villi, with lesser degrees of swelling and myxoid stroma invaded by occasional large mononuclear trophoblast cells, are common in fetuses with trisomy karyotype (figs. 9-21–9-25). Trophoblastic hyperplasia is especially prevalent in complete and partial moles, as well as in triploid and tetraploid abortions, but it also occurs to a lesser extent in some trisomies (54). These histologic abnormalities do not have a useful predictive value for identifying specific karyotypes (70,74).

The gross and microscopic features of classic, fully developed, complete hydatidiform moles are very different from the above (figs. 9-26, 9-27). This subject is presented in detail in Fascicle 3, third series, by Silverberg and Kurman (64).

Differential Diagnosis. The most important clinical role for the histopathologic evaluation of abortions is in the identification of early complete and partial hydatidiform moles, at which time the distinction between the two is often difficult. The increasing use of diagnostic ultrasound in early pregnancy results in early identification and evacuation of abnormal gestations with no identifiable embryo or fetus. In this context, the clinically important distinction between partial moles, complete moles, and hydropic abortions has become much more difficult than it was previously, when abnormal gestations were allowed to progress until

Abortion, Stillbirth, and Intrauterine Fetal Death

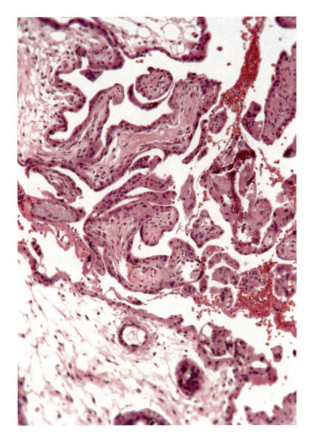

Figure 9-19

TRIPLOID PARTIAL MOLE

There are irregular scalloped villous outlines, trophoblastic invaginations in the large villus, and a separate component of smaller villi at center, right.

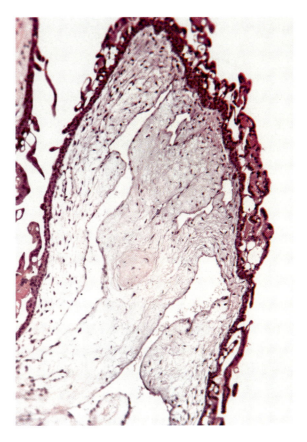

Figure 9-20

TRIPLOID PARTIAL MOLE

This hydropic villus contains large prominent endothelial-lined vascular spaces which, typically, are empty.

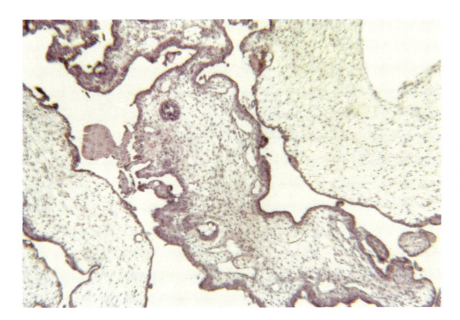

Figure 9-21

TRIPLOID PARTIAL MOLE

The large vesicular villi have irregular scalloped margins, with a "cistern" at the upper right and trophoblastic invaginations in the villus at center.

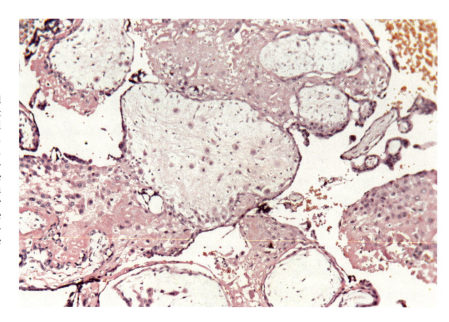

Figure 9-22

HYDROPIC ABORTION

The villous stroma is myxoid and slightly edematous, but villous enlargement is minimal and there are no cisterns, vessels, or trophoblastic invaginations. The trophoblast layer is discontinuous. Clumps of fibrin are prominent. The mother was a XX/XXX mosaic with three prior abortions, and the aborted tissue is trisomic (47XX, +22). (Figs. 9-22 and 9-23 are from the same patient.)

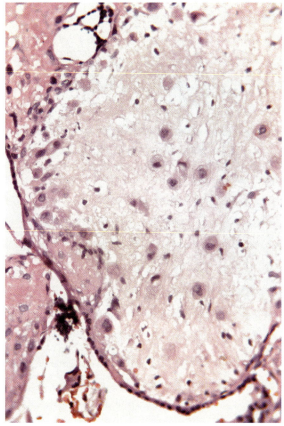

Figure 9-23

HYDROPIC ABORTION

Mononuclear trophoblast cells are present in the villous stroma.

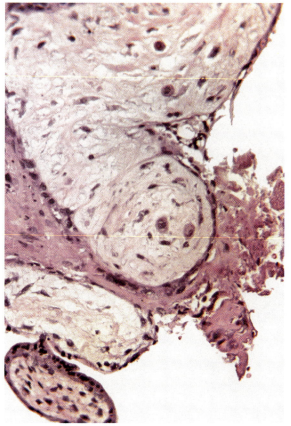

Figure 9-24

HYDROPIC ABORTION

Hydropic abortion, with chromosomal trisomy (47XY, + 2). The stroma is fibrotic and avascular, with mononuclear trophoblast cells. (Figs. 9-24 and 9-25 are from the same patient.)

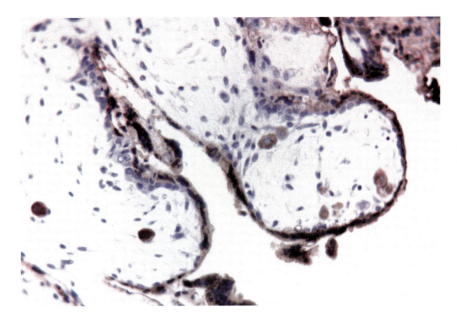

Figure 9-25

HYDROPIC ABORTION

Antihuman placental lactogen immunostain confirms the trophoblastic origin of the large mononuclear cells in the stroma.

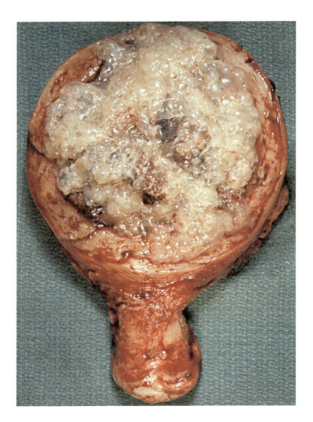

Figure 9-26

CLASSIC COMPLETE HYDATIDIFORM MOLE

Hysterectomy specimen contains a classic complete hydatidiform mole. About half of the burgeoning molar tissue has been removed in order not to hide the uterus. The mole had begun to abort at 5 months' gestation. There is no problem with diagnosis in these circumstances.

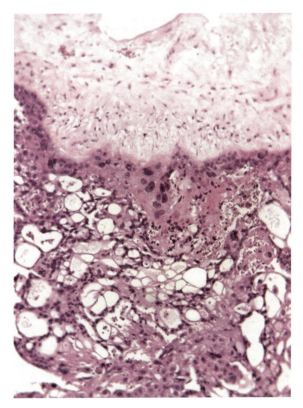

Figure 9-27

CLASSIC HYDATIDIFORM MOLE

Villus from a classic hydatiform mole shows massive vesicular change in the villous stroma, with part of a cistern at the top margin. There is marked trophoblastic hyperplasia and nuclear atypia. The karyotype was 46XX.

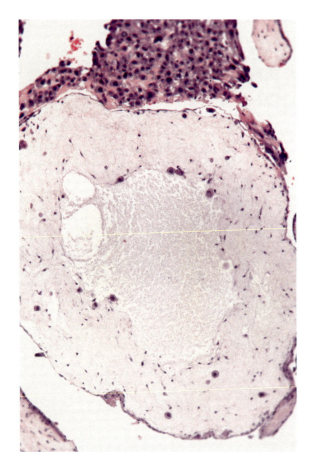

Figure 9-28

EARLY COMPLETE HYDATIDIFORM MOLE

Only a few small vesicular villi were evident grossly and the amount of tissue was relatively scant. Even though this villus is small, it has a cistern and an asymmetric clump of hyper-plastic trophoblast at top. (Courtesy of Drs. B. M. Ronnett and R. J. Kurman, Baltimore, MD.) (Figs. 9-28–9-31 are from the same patient.)

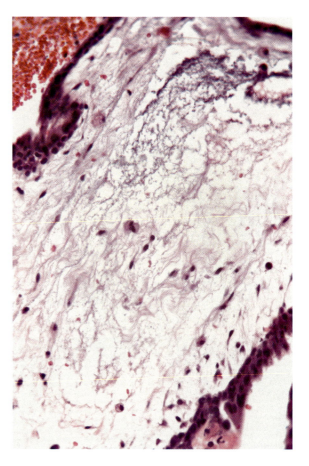

Figure 9-29

EARLY COMPLETE HYDATIDIFORM MOLE

Stromal cells are degenerating (apoptotic). (Courtesy of Drs. B. M. Ronnett and R. J. Kurman, Baltimore, MD.)

clinical and morphologic differences became more apparent. All three of these lesions have in common the presence of swollen, hydropic villi and some degree of trophoblastic hyperplasia. Early lesions are grossly indistinguishable.

At early stages, complete moles may have a uniform population of enlarged hydropic villi. However, at very early stages, the stroma may be hypercellular, with a light blue background matrix. Subsequently, the matrix breaks down and both the villous stromal cells and residual capillary endothelial cells show nuclear karyorrhexis. Even the earliest specimens have at least focal hyperplasia and nuclear atypia of both the villous and implantation site trophoblast (figs. 9-28–9-31) (47,63). A distinctive but inconstant feature is branching and clubbing of villous outlines separated by linear seams of trophoblast (fig. 9-32) (31). Embryonic or fetal tissues are characteristically absent, although a normal twin may occur with a complete mole. These differences are summarized in Table 9-4 and figures 9-17–9-32.

Early partial moles, in contrast, characteristically have two distinct populations of villi by size (figs. 9-17–9-19) and circumferential mild trophoblastic hyperplasia; scalloped villous outlines, trophoblastic invaginations, and stromal cisterns are also present (figs. 9-20, 9-21) (5). Dilated vascular spaces with irregular outlines are distinctive but infrequent. Embryonic or fetal tissue may be present (fig. 9-20).

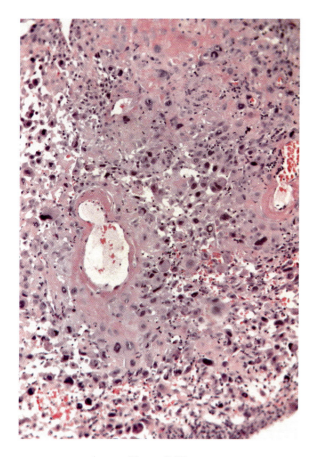

Figure 9-30

EARLY COMPLETE HYDATIDIFORM MOLE

There is marked atypia of the implantation site (intermediate) trophoblast. (Courtesy of Drs. B. M. Ronnett and R. J. Kurman, Baltimore, MD.)

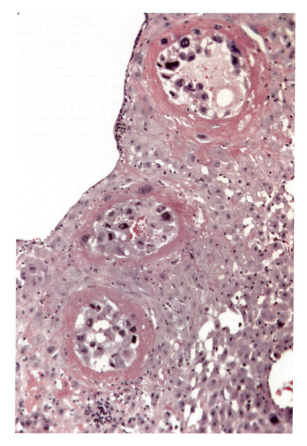

Figure 9-31

EARLY COMPLETE HYDATIDIFORM MOLE

There is marked atypia of the intermediate trophoblast within spiral arterioles. (Courtesy of Drs. B. M. Ronnett and R. J. Kurman, Baltimore, MD.)

The villi of hydropic abortions are only slightly enlarged and never identifiable grossly as vesicular. Trophoblastic hyperplasia, if any, is focal. The villous stroma may be myxoid or fibrotic, and sparsely cellular (figs. 9-22–9-25). Most hydropic abortions are the result of abnormal karyotypes.

Special Techniques. Conventional karyotyping of fresh tissue provides the most specific means of distinguishing between diploid (diandric) complete moles, triploid (diandric) partial moles, and hydropic abortions with other karyotypes. The technique of comparative genomic hybridization, in combination with flow cytometry, can detect essentially the same chromosomal abnormalities without the need for tissue culture, and may be especially helpful in evaluating macerated fetuses (6,38) and even archival tissues (42).

Flow cytometry examination of tissue from paraffin blocks is an effective means of distinguishing between diploid and triploid or tetraploid cell lines (35,36). The distinction between diploid and triploid karyotypes is also easily made on microscopic sections by image analysis, which in our experience also eliminates potential contamination by maternal cells and can identify mosaics (26,28). FISH may be used to identify trisomies on formalin-fixed paraffin-embedded tissue (25,32). Centromeric probes sufficient to specifically identify all chromosomes are available (50). Multicolor FISH analysis probing for only five chromosomes can identify 95 percent of clinically relevant chromosomal abnormalities (68). A potential source of fetal DNA not to be forgotten is the maternal blood. Fetal cells circulate in all pregnant

Placental Pathology

Table 9-4

COMPARISON OF HISTOLOGIC FEATURES OF COMPLETE MOLE, PARTIAL MOLE, AND HYDROPIC ABORTION

	Complete Mole	Partial Mole	Hydropic Abortion
Trophoblastic Hyperplasia	+++	++ Circumferential	+ Focal
Trophoblastic Atypia	+ to +++	0	0
Villous Size	Uniformly large	Large and small	Mostly small
Villous Outlines	Round or oval	Irregular	Round or oval
Karyorrhexis of Stromal and Endothelial Cells	++	0	0

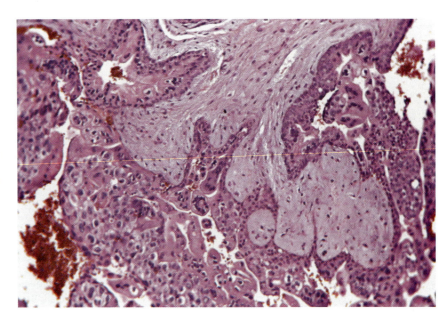

Figure 9-32

EARLY KARYOTYPED (46XX) COMPLETE MOLE

Tissue was scant, with no grossly evident vesicular change. Hydropic change is minimal, but the villous clubbing characterized by plump lobulations is a distinctive feature when present.

women. Techniques to concentrate these fetal cells for immunohistochemical and genetic analysis hold promise for detailed prenatal diagnosis (71). Various applications for the evaluation of fetal DNA are under study (51).

Prenatal ultrasound studies have become increasingly common; pathologists should be aware of the utility of ultrasound in evaluating fragmented or macerated fetuses (67). A pathologist embarking upon an autopsy and placental examination of a stillborn fetus would be well advised to check on the possible existence of predelivery ultrasound findings such as cerebral calcifications, cardiac malformations, bladder dilatation, and large retroplacental hematomas, which can be overlooked on gross examination unless they are looked for specifically.

LATE SPONTANEOUS ABORTION (MISCARRIAGE, STILLBIRTH, AND INTRAUTERINE FETAL DEATH)

Definition. An intrauterine fetal death is commonly recognized by the absence of fetal activity and fetal heartbeat or other evidence of life after quickening has been recognized by the mother. After the stage of legal viability (at 20 weeks in most jurisdictions) the delivered dead fetus is commonly classified as a stillbirth. Usage varies considerably. A widely recognized definition of livebirth includes all instances, irrespective of gestational age, in which the newborn breathes or shows intrapartum evidence of heartbeat, movement of muscles, or cord pulsations (19). A liveborn infant who dies within 4 weeks of birth is classified as a neonatal death.

Perinatal deaths are the sum of late fetal deaths and neonatal deaths within the first week of life. Precise definitions are often not followed, even by those who know them; as a result, worldwide perinatal mortality statistics are inexact and vary widely (19).

Incidence or Prevalence. Quoted rates for stillbirth in different countries vary from 4 to 40 in 1,000 live births (65). In the United States, quoted figures vary from 5 to 10 in 1,000 (24,53). The stillbirth rate over a 10-year period at a university hospital in Ireland subjected to thorough analysis was 12 in 1,000 (43). Neonatal mortality rates in most developed countries have been approximately the same as stillbirth rates during the last half of the 20th century (65).

Clinical Features and Etiology. The most common causes of or associations with late spontaneous abortion include intrauterine infections, thromboses, abruptions and other forms of clot, vascular lesions, and maternal hypertension, isoimmunization, and diabetes. Many et al. (44) found a significant association between unexplained third trimester intrauterine fetal death and maternal thrombophilias. Malformations, intrauterine growth restriction, fetomaternal hemorrhage, genetically determined metabolic disorders, cord accidents, and maternal drug abuse are less frequent causes (1). Chromosomal abnormalities still occur in the third trimester (trisomy 18 is most common), and even at term, but are much less common after the 20th week, accounting for less than 5 percent of stillbirths.

Gross and Microscopic Findings. Placental lesions associated with the various specific disease conditions listed above are described under the appropriate headings elsewhere in this volume. Pathologic changes in the placenta related to fetal death vary depending on gestational age and the time elapsed between death and delivery. Fetal death, regardless of cause, leads to involution of the fetal vessels progressively and diffusely throughout the placenta. This alteration begins with karyorrhexis (irregular clumps of fragmented nuclear debris) in villous capillaries, followed by septation in larger vessels, ultimately ending in fibrous obliteration of vascular walls and lumens (figs. 9-33–9-35). The sequence of histologic changes is identical to that which occurs in a localized manner in

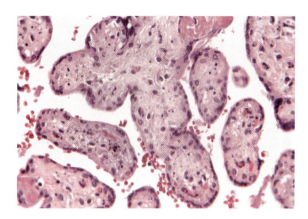

Figure 9-33

PLACENTAL VILLI AFTER RECENT INTRAUTERINE FETAL DEATH

Most capillary endothelial cells have disappeared. Karyorrhexis, characterized by numerous scattered fragments of nuclear debris in and adjacent to vascular spaces, indicates that fetal death occurred at least 6 hours prior to delivery, when this pattern is present diffusely in all areas of the placenta (16).

downstream vessels and villi following thrombotic occlusion of a single large stem vessel or surface vessel (see chapter 6).

Genest et al. (16–18) have detailed the evolution of gross and microscopic changes over time in both the placenta and fetus following instances of intrauterine fetal death in cases with a known death to delivery interval. Significant placental histologic markers included intravascular karyorrhexis (presumably from degenerating nuclei of intravascular leukocytes and endothelial cells) at 6 hours (fig. 9-33) and septation of stem vessel lumens after 48 hours (fig. 9-34). Extensive fibrosis of the villous stroma (fig. 9-35) indicated a prolonged interval, more than 2 weeks. Our experience with instances of stillbirths with a known death to delivery interval supports these findings. These observations are approximate, but sufficiently predictive to be useful for many purposes. For instance, the finding of clustered fibrotic villi, stem vessels, and septation in a placenta when the death to delivery interval is less than 48 hours is sufficient to confirm that a prenatal vascular lesion occurred (33).

Extensive illustrations of the characteristic fetal malformations and deformities associated with a wide array of cytogenetic abnormalities

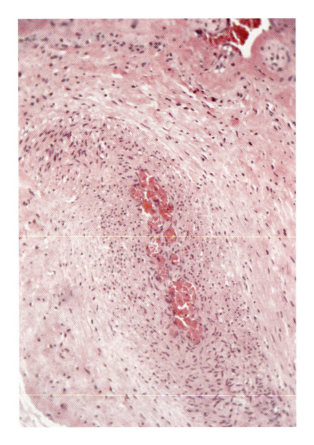 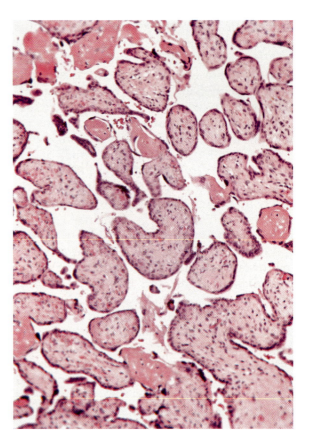

Figure 9-34

PLACENTAL STEM VILLUS AFTER INTRAUTERINE FETAL DEATH

The pattern of septation produced by ingrowth of spindle-shaped endothelial or fibroblastic cells forms multiple channels or loculations. This correlates with death occurring more than 48 hours prior to delivery, when multiple vessels with this pattern are evident in most or all areas of the placenta.

Figure 9-35

PLACENTAL VILLI AFTER INTRAUTERINE FETAL DEATH

Extensive areas of avascular villi with villous stromal fibrosis indicate that the intrauterine fetal death occurred more than 2 weeks prior to delivery. A few red blood cell fragments persist in the stroma, but the capillaries have disappeared and the stroma is nearly acellular.

are presented in the monograph originally prepared by D. W. Smith, now compiled by Jones (66). Smith's monograph on deformations of nongenetic origin is now revised by Graham (20).

Differential Diagnosis: The Causes of Perinatal Death. It is often difficult, and sometimes impossible, to determine the cause of a stillbirth, but it is always important (61). The impact on the parents is devastating. An explanation, when possible, is reassuring, and assists with closure for the family. The perinatal autopsy and placental pathologic findings are indispensable components in this process (24,53,61).

The most common causes of stillbirth are infections, malformations incompatible with life, the effects of hemorrhage or thrombosis, and less frequent lesions that cause extensive destruction of a functional placenta, such as massive perivillous fibrin deposition and massive chronic villitis. Both of these lesions may result in repeated late abortion, in which case attentive perinatal care may be lifesaving (fig. 9-36). The frequency with which an acceptable cause is found varies with the intensity and completeness of the search. With adequate clinical data, an autopsy, and placental pathology, Rayburn et al. (53) found an explanation for 88 of 89 stillbirths delivered by induction shortly after the fetal death, reducing the effects of maceration. In less selective studies, inconclusive results were more common, from

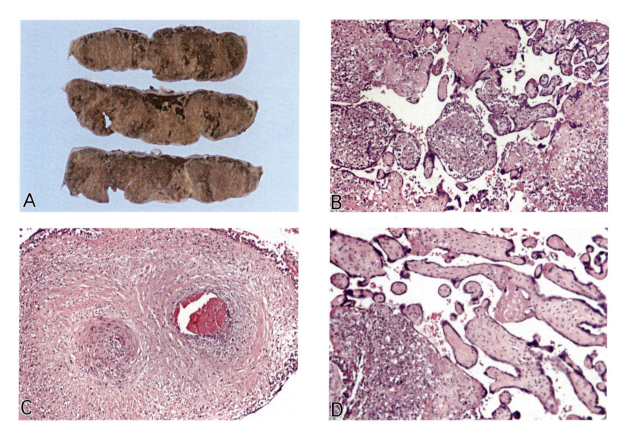

Figure 9-36

MASSIVE CHRONIC VILLITIS

A: Massive chronic villitis as a cause of repeated sudden late miscarriage. Two otherwise asymptomatic prior pregnancies both ended in sudden intrauterine fetal death at term. Massive chronic villitis was present in both. The third pregnancy was normal until the mid 34th week when an abnormal nonstress test was followed by immediate cesarean section. All cut sections of this placenta were extensively solidified by firm gray tissue. The immediate cesarean section was probably life-saving.

B: The villi and intervillous space are obliterated by an extensive necrotizing lymphohistiocytic inflammatory infiltrate.

C: Inflammation in stem vessels resulted in thrombosis.

D: Some villi not involved by the inflammatory process are avascular and fibrotic, presumably because they are downstream from occluded stem vessels.

24 to 36 percent (24,61). A recent review of the costs and benefits of the model comprehensive stillbirth assessment program in Wisconsin indicates substantial benefits (46). Any computation of the cost of no program should include the cost of litigation incurred when parents feel that their need to know and understand as much as possible has been ignored.

The need for other laboratory data depends upon the clinical features together with a review of autopsy and placental abnormalities. In the appropriate context, we have found the assistance of detailed coagulation studies (2,44), assessment of autoimmune antibodies, carefully obtained cultures of placenta and other fetal organs, cytogenetics, and a review of predelivery ultrasound or Doppler examinations to be very useful. In contrast, immunologic screening for congenital TORCH (toxoplasmosis, other infections, rubella, cytomegalovirus, herpes simplex) infections has little value in the absence of suggestive clinical or pathologic data (24). A Kleihauer-Betke test for fetomaternal hemorrhage should probably be performed on all stillbirths (1), but is especially useful when an otherwise normal-appearing stillborn infant is very pale, or when there is a history of maternal trauma.

Kalousek (27,37) has described a specific form of genetic abnormality affecting only the placenta, called *confined placental mosaicism*, which is associated with stillbirth, intrauterine growth restriction, and premature labor. Placental cells trisomic for chromosomes 7, 16, and 18 are most prevalent, while the somatic cells of the fetus have a normal karyotype. In a series of 2,612 cases studied by chorionic villus sampling, there were 51 (1.9 percent) instances of confined placental mosaicism (72). No specific pathologic abnormalities have as yet been described in the affected placentas. If the placenta has not been karyotyped, the identification of placental trisomies can be accomplished by comparative genomic hybridization (38) and FISH analysis using commercially prepared probes specific for the centromeric regions of individual chromosomes (12).

Screening for the more common trisomies involved can also be accomplished efficiently by comparative genomic hybridization (38). The technique is applicable even to macerated fetuses (6). More frequent use of the FISH technique on archival paraffin-embedded tissues, perhaps screening for the most frequently involved chromosomal trisomies, may identify a reason for the demise of some of these "normal"-appearing stillbirths (14).

REFERENCES

1. Ahlenius I, Floberg J, Thomassen P. Sixty-six cases of intrauterine fetal death. A prospective study with an extensive test protocol. Acta Obstet Gynecol Scand 1995;74:109–17.
2. Arias F, Romero R, Joist H, Kraus FT. Thrombophilia: a mechanism of disease in women with adverse pregnancy outcome and thrombotic lesions in the placenta. J Matern Fetal Med 1998;7:277–86.
3. Baldwin VJ, Kalousek DK, Dimmick JE, Applegarth DA, Hardwick DF. Diagnostic pathologic investigation of the malformed conceptus. Perspect Pediatr Pathol 1982;7:65–108.
4. Beer AE. Immunologic aspects of normal pregnancy and recurrent spontaneous abortion. Semin Reprod Endocrinol 1988;6:163–80.
5. Chew SH, Perlman EJ, Williams R, Kurman RJ, Ronnett BM. Morphology and DNA content analysis in the evaluation of first trimester placentas for partial hydatidiform mole (PHM). Hum Pathol 2000;31:914–24.
6. Christiaens GC, Vissers J, Poddighe PJ, de Pater JM. Comparative genomic hybridization for cytogenetic evaluation of stillbirth. Obstet Gynecol 2000;96:281–6.
7. Christiansen OB. The possible role of classical human leukocyte antigens in recurrent miscarriage. Am J Reprod Immunol 1999;42:110–15.
8. deVries JI, Dekker GA, Huijgens PC, Jakobs C, Blomberg BM, van Geijn HP. Hyperhomocysteinaemia and protein S deficiency in complicated pregnancies. Br J Obstet Gynaecol 1997;104:1248–54.
9. Dimmick JE, Kalousek DK, eds. Developmental pathology of the embryo and fetus. Philadelphia: JB Lippincott Co; 1992.
10. Dizon-Townson DS, Meline L, Nelson LM, Varner M, Ward K. Fetal carriers of the factor V Leiden mutation are prone to miscarriage and placental infarction. Am J Obstet Gynecol 1997;177:402–5.
11. Doss BJ, Greene MF, Hill J, Heffner LJ, Bieber FR, Genest DR. Massive chronic intervillositis associated with recurrent abortions. Hum Pathol 1995;26:1245–51.
12. Drut RM, Harris CP, Drut R, Meisner L. Use of fluorescent in situ hybridization to detect trisomy 13 in archival tissues for cytogenetic analysis. Pediatr Pathol 1992;12:799–805.
13. Edmonds DK, Lindsay KS, Miller JF, Williamson R, Wood PJ. Early embryonic mortality in women. Fertil Steril 1982;38:447–53.
14. Fejgin MD, Kidron D, Kedar I, et al. Genetic diagnosis from formalin-fixed fetal tissue using FISH; a new tool for genetic counseling in subsequent pregnancies. Eur J Obstet Gynecol Reprod Biol 1996;64:221–4.
15. Fraser EJ, Grimes DA, Schulz KF. Immunization as therapy for spontaneous abortion: a review and meta-analysis. Obstet Gynecol 1993;82:854–9.
16. Genest DR. Estimating the time of death in stillborn fetuses: II. Histologic evaluation of the placenta; a study of 71 stillborns. Obstet Gynecol 1992;80:585–92.
17. Genest DR, Singer DB. Estimating the time of death in stillborn fetuses: III. External fetal examination; a study of 86 stillborns. Obstet Gynecol 1992;80:593–600.
18. Genest DR, Williams MA, Greene MF. Estimating the time of death in stillborn fetuses: I. Histologic evaluation of fetal organs; an autopsy study of 150 stillborns. Obstet Gynecol 1992;80:575–84.

19. Golding J. Epidemiology of fetal and neonatal death. In: Keeling JW, ed. Fetal and neonatal pathology, 2nd ed. New York: Springer-Verlag; 1993:165–82.
20. Graham JM Jr, ed. Smith's recognizable patterns of human deformation, 2nd ed. Philadelphia: Saunders; 1988.
21. Gris JC, Quere I, Monpeyroux F, et al. Case-control study of the frequency of thrombophilic disorders in couples with late foetal loss and no thrombotic antecedent—the Nimes Obstetricians and Haematologists Study 5 (NOHA5). Thromb Haemost 1999;81:891–9.
22. Gruber K, Gelven PL, Austin RM. Chorionic villi or trophoblastic tissue in uterine samples of four women with ectopic pregnancies. Int J Gynecol Obstet 1997;16:28–32.
23. Hill JA, Polgar K, Anderson DJ. T-helper 1-type immunity to trophoblast in women with recurrent spontaneous abortion. JAMA 1995;273:1933–6.
24. Incerpi MH, Miller DA, Samadi R, Settlage RH, Goodwin TM. Stillbirth evaluation: what tests are needed? Am J Obstet Gynecol 1998;178:1121–5.
25. Jalal SM, Law ME. Utility of multicolor fluorescent in situ hybridization in clinical cytogenetics. Gen Med 1999;1:181–6.
26. Jeffers MD, Michie BA, Oakes SJ, Gillan JE. Comparison of ploidy analysis by flow cytometry and image analysis in hydatidiform mole and nonmolar abortion. Histopathology 1995;27:415–21.
27. Kalousek DK, Barrett I. Confined placental mosaicism and stillbirth. Pediatr Pathol 1994;14:151–9.
28. Kaspar HG, Kraemer BB, Kraus FT. DNA ploidy by image cytometry and karyotype in spontaneous abortion. Hum Pathol 1998;29:1013–6.
29. Kaspar HG, To T, Dinh TV. Clinical use of immunoperoxidase markers in excluding ectopic gestation. Obstet Gynecol 1991;78:433–7.
30. Keeling JW. Fetal pathology. Edinburgh: Churchill Livingstone; 1994.
31. Keep D, Zaragoza MV, Hassold T, Redline RW. Very early complete hydatidiform mole. Hum Pathol 1996;27:708–13.
32. Kopf I, Hanson C, Delle U, Verbiene I, Weimarck A. A rapid and simplified technique for analysis of archival formalin-fixed, paraffin-embedded tissue by fluorescence in situ hybridization (FISH). Anticancer Res 1996;16:2533–6.
33. Kraus FT, Acheen VI. Fetal thrombotic vasculopathy in the placenta: cerebral thrombi and infarcts, coagulopathies, and cerebral palsy. Hum Pathol 1999;30:759–69.
34. Kudo Y, Boyd CA, Sargent IL, Redman CW. Tryptophan degradation by human placental indoleamine 2,3-dioxygenase regulates lymphocyte proliferation. J Physiol 2001;535:207–15.
35. Lage JM, Driscoll SG, Yavner DL, Olivier AP, Marks D, Weinberg DS. Hydatidiform moles. Application of flow cytometry in diagnosis. Am J Clin Pathol 1988;89:596–600.
36. Lage JM, Popek EJ. The role of DNA flow cytometry in evaluation of partial and complete hydatidiform moles and hydropic abortions. Semin Diag Pathol 1993;10:267–74.
37. Lestou VS, Kalousek DK. Confined placental mosaicism and intrauterine fetal growth. Arch Dis Child Fetal Neonatal Ed 1998;79:F223–6.
38. Lestou VS, Lomax BL, Barrett IJ, Kalousek DK. Screening of human placentas for chromosomal mosaicism using comparative genomic hybridization. Teratology 1999;59:325–30.
39. Levy G, Muller G, Pigaglio O. [Simultaneous intrauterine and extrauterine pregnancies.] Rev Fr Gynecol Obstet 1987;82:729–32. (French.)
40. Lissak A, Sharon A, Fruchter O, Kassel A, Sanderovitz J, Abramovici H. Polymorphism for mutation of cytosine to thymine at location 677 in the methylenetetrahydrofolate reductase gene is associated with recurrent early fetal loss. Am J Obstet Gynecol 1999;181:126–30.
41. Lomax B, Tang S, Separovic E, et al. Comparative genomic hybridization in combination with flow cytometry improves results of cytogenetic analysis of spontaneous abortions. Am J Hum Genet 2000;66:1516–21.
42. Loukianova A, Tang SS, Kuchinka B, Kalousek DK, Ma S. Comparative genomic hybridization universal DOP-PCR genome amplification and specific SRY-PCR sex confirmation [Abstract]. Placenta 2001;22:A73.
43. Magani IM, Rafla NM, Mortimer G, Meehan FP. Stillbirths: a clinicopathological survey (1972-1982). Pediatr Pathol 1990;10:363–74.
44. Many A, Elad R, Yaron Y, Eldor A, Lessing JB, Kupferminc MJ. Third-trimester unexplained intrauterine fetal death is associated with inherited thrombophilia. Obstet Gynecol 2002;99:684–7.
45. McFadden DE, Pantzar JT. Placental pathology of triploidy. Hum Pathol 1996;27:1018–20.
46. Michalski ST, Porter J, Pauli RM. Costs and consequences of comprehensive stillbirth assessment. Am J Obstet Gynecol 2002;186:1027–34.
47. Montes M, Roberts D, Berkowitz RS, Genest DR. Prevalence and significance of implantation site trophoblastic atypia in hydatidiform moles and spontaneous abortions. Am J Clin Pathol 1996;105:411–6.
48. Munn DH, Zhou M, Attwood JT, et al. Prevention of fetal rejection by tryptophan catabolism. Science 1998;281:1191–3.

49. Nayar R, Lage JM. Placental changes in a first trimester missed abortion in maternal systemic lupus erythematosus with antiphospholipid syndrome; a case report and review of the literature. Hum Pathol 1996;27:201–6.
50. Nietzel A, Rocci M, Starke H, et al. A new multicolor-FISH approach for the characterization of marker chromosomes: centromere specific multicolor-FISH (cen M-FISH). Hum Genet 2001;108:199–204.
51. Pertl B, Bianchi DW. Fetal DNA in maternal plasm: emerging clinical applications. Obstet Gynecol 2001;98:483–90.
52. Rand JH, Wu XX, Andree HA, et al. Pregnancy loss in the antiphospholipid-antibody syndrome—a possible thrombogenic mechanism. N Eng J Med 1997;337:154–60.
53. Rayburn W, Sander C, Barr M Jr, Rygiel R. The stillborn fetus: placental histologic examination in determining a cause. Obstet Gynecol 1985;65:637–41.
54. Redline RW, Hassold T, Zaragoza M. Determinants of villous trophoblastic hyperplasia in spontaneous abortions. Mod Pathol 1998;11:762–8.
55. Redline RW, Lu CY. Localization of fetal major histocompatibility complex enzymes and maternal leukocytes in murine placenta. Implications for maternal-fetal immunological relationship. Lab Invest 1989;61:27–36.
56. Redline RW, Wilson-Costello D, Borawski E, Fanaroff AA, Hack M. Placental lesions associated with neurologic impairment and cerebral palsy in very low-birth-weight infants. Arch Pathol Lab Med 1998;122:1091–8.
57. Redline RW, Zaragoza M, Hassold T. Prevalence of developmental and inflammatory lesions in nonmolar first-trimester spontaneous abortions. Hum Pathol 1999;30:93–100.
58. Ridker PM, Miletich JP, Buring JE, et al. Factor V Leiden mutation as a risk factor for recurrent pregnancy loss. Ann Intern Med 1998;128: 1000–3.
59. Rotmensch S, Liberati M, Mittelmann M, Ben-Rafael Z. Activated protein C resistance and adverse pregnancy outcome. Am J Obstet Gynecol 1997;177:170–3.
60. Salafia C, Maier D, Vogel C, Pezzullo J, Burns J, Silberman L. Placental and decidual histology in spontaneous abortion: detailed description and correlations with chromosome number. Obstet Gynecol 1993;82:295–303.
61. Saller DN Jr, Lesser KB, Harrel U, Rogers BB, Oyer CE. The clinical utility of the perinatal autopsy. JAMA 1995;273:663–5.
62. Schrock E, Veldman T, Padilla-Nash H, et al. Spectral karyotyping refines cytogenetic diagnostics of constitutional chromosomal abnormalities. Hum Genet 1997;101:255–62.
63. Sheikh SS, Lage JM. Diagnosis of early complete hydatidiform mole. A study of 35 cases. Mod Pathol 1998;11:114A.
64. Silverberg SG, Kurman RJ. Tumors of the uterine corpus and gestational trophoblastic disease. 3rd Series, Fascicle 3. Washington DC. Armed Forces Institute of Pathology; 1992.
65. Singer DB, MacPherson T. Fetal death and the macerated stillborn fetus. In: Wigglesworth JS, Singer DB, eds. Textbook of fetal and perinatal pathology, 2nd ed. Malden, Mass: Blackwell Science; 1998:233–50.
66. Smith DW, Graham JM. Smith's recognizable patterns of human deformation. 2nd ed. Philadelphia: Saunders; 1988.
67. Sun CC, Grumbach K, DeCosta DT, Meyers CM, Dungan JS. Correlation of ultrasound diagnosis and pathologic findings in fetal anomalies. Pediatr Dev Pathol 1999;2:131–42.
68. Thilaganathan B, Sairam S, Ballard T, Peterson C, Meredith R. Effectiveness of prenatal chromosomal analysis using multicolor fluorescent in situ hybridization. BJOG 2000;107:262–6.
69. Unfried G, Griesmacher A, Weismuller W, Nagele F, Huber JC, Tempfer CB. The C677T polymorphism of the methylenetetrahydrofolate reductase gene and idiopathic recurrent miscarriage. Obstet Gynecol 2002;99:614–9.
70. van Lijnschoten G, Arends JW, Leffers P, De La Fuente AA, Van Der Looij HJ, Geraedts JP. The value of histomorphological features of chorionic villi in early spontaneous abortion for the prediction of karyotype. Histopathology 1993;22:557–63.
71. Vona G, Beroud C, Benachi A, et al. Enrichment, immunomorphological, and genetic characterization of fetal cells circulating in maternal blood. Am J Pathol 2002;160:51–8.
72. Wang BB, Rubin CH, Williams J 3rd. Mosaicism in chorionic villus sampling: an analysis of incidence and chromosomes involved in 2612 consecutive cases. Prenat Diagn 1993;13:179–90.
73. Warburton D. Chromosomal causes of fetal death. Clin Obstet Gynaecol 1987;30:268–77.
74. Warren CJ, Kraus FT, Taysi K, et al. Histologic-karyotypic correlations in spontaneous abortions. Mod Pathol 1990;3:105A.
75. Zaragoza MV, Surti U, Redline RW, Millie E, Chakravarti A, Hassold TJ. Parental origin and phenotype of triploidy in spontaneous abortions: predominance of diandry and association with the partial hydatidiform mole. Am J Hum Genet 2000;66:1807–20.

10 FETAL AND PLACENTAL HYDROPS

INTRODUCTION

Fetal hydrops, also known as *hydrops fetalis*, is a state of profound generalized fetal edema, with a marked accumulation of fluid in subcutaneous tissue and all body cavities. It represents the end stage of a variety of fetal disease states including fetal cytogenetic anomalies, anemias, hypoproteinemia, and cardiac failure. A clear distinction between fetal hydrops and cystic hygroma as well as more localized body cavity effusions is not always possible. The placenta and umbilical cord become edematous, an appearance called *placental hydrops*. The placenta does not always have the gross features of hydrops, even when the fetus is severely hydropic, as in many instances of monosomy X, but villous edema is usually evident histologically.

The gross appearance of a hydropic placenta is the same, regardless of cause. Microscopic differences may be subtle but provide clues to the etiology and potentially assist in the management of some cases.

Many cases are now diagnosed by prenatal ultrasound. Prenatal investigation to assign a specific cause is urgent, because a large proportion of cases are potentially treatable. Assignment of a cause in fatal cases, assisted by a detailed autopsy, is important for parental counseling and management of future pregnancies. For these reasons, an understanding of the different causes of hydrops is necessary for a pathologist confronted with a hydropic placenta. Even though there may be no specific placental histopathology, the pathologist has a primary role in the coordination of other forms of laboratory testing, including cytogenetics, fluorescence in situ hybridization, immunohistochemistry, and microbiologic studies (10).

Incidence figures for *nonimmune hydrops* vary from 1 in 1,400 (7) to 1 in 3,748 births (6). Maternal isoimmunization (*immune hydrops*) still occurs, but most cases now go unreported.

A hydropic placenta is often massively enlarged, soft, and friable, weighing in excess of 1,000 g. The cut surface is typically pale and bloodless. The degree of hydropic change varies considerably, in most cases in step with the severity of the underlying cause (fig. 10-1A). Intervillous thrombi are common. In some instances, the gross appearance associated with all of the basic lesions described below may be nearly normal.

Microscopically, villous diameters are enlarged, focal syncytiotrophoblast cell necrosis is present, cytotrophoblast cells are increased with occasional mitoses, villous capillaries are reduced, and Hofbauer cells are numerous. Villous capillaries contain numerous immature erythroid cells, which may focally form small clusters that distend capillary lumens (fig. 10-1). The villous stroma is edematous. Histologic variations associated with various subtypes follow.

IMMUNE HYDROPS (ERYTHROBLASTOSIS FETALIS, HEMOLYTIC DISEASE OF THE NEWBORN)

Immune hydrops was formerly the most common variation of fetal hydrops. The introduction of maternal prophylaxis with anti-D gammaglobulin (Rhogam) has successfully reduced the prevalence of this disease. The cause of the hydrops in this context is a severe hemolytic anemia in an Rh-positive fetus with an Rh-negative mother, who has become sensitized to the Rh (mainly D) antigen expressed by the fetal red blood cells. Transplacental passage of maternal anti-Rh (D) antibodies back into the fetal circulation causes the hemolysis. Much less commonly, an incompatibility of ABO and other red blood cell antigens can have a similar, usually less severe, effect. There are no specific histologic features in the placenta (fig. 10-1). Prenatal diagnosis is based on the indirect Coombs test (antibody screen) of the mother's serum, with evaluation of ABO, Rh (D), and other blood group antigen determinations as needed.

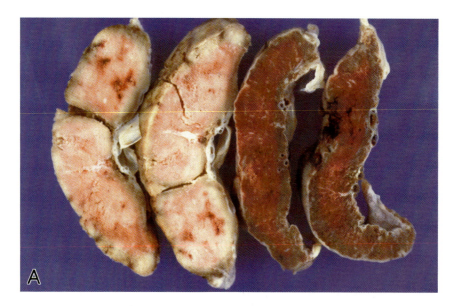
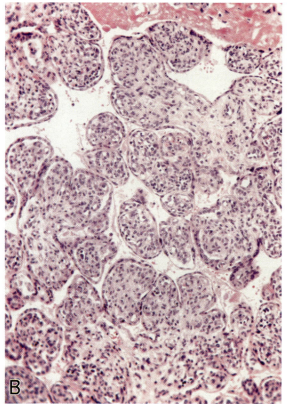
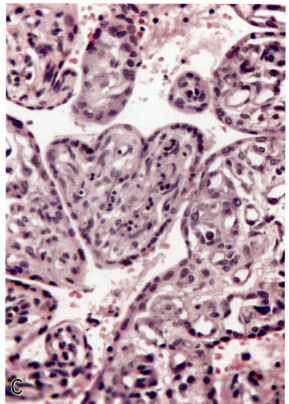

Figure 10-1

PLACENTAL HYDROPS IN DICHORIONIC TWINS, CAUSED BY RH (ANTI-D) ISOIMMUNIZATION

A: The gestational age was 34 weeks. Hydrops and anemia were severe in placenta A, at left, which weighed 733 g, but only mild in placenta B, at right (285 g). The discordance illustrates the result of differences in the immune responses of these dizygotic twin fetuses, which coincidentally were different sexes.

B: The chorionic villi of placenta A have increased diameters, and appear very cellular due to numerous erythroblasts and stromal cells. Note the near absence of red blood cells.

C: At higher magnification, the intravascular location and immaturity of the erythroblasts is evident in placenta A.

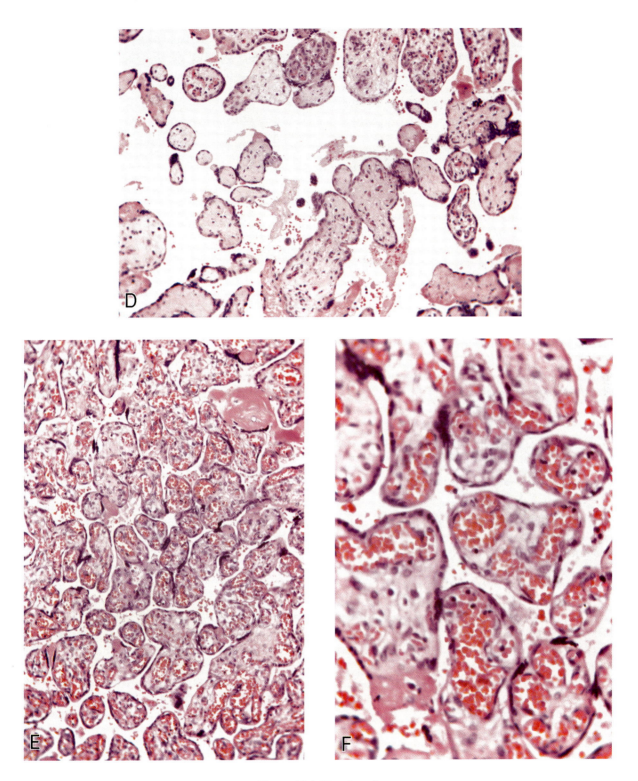

Figure 10-1 (Continued)

D: Small foci of fetal thrombotic vasculopathy were also present in placenta A.

E: The chorionic villi of placenta B are smaller, with more numerous red blood cells and little evidence of edema.

F: Higher magnification of villi of placenta B. There are relatively few normoblasts and only rare immature erythroblasts in the fetal capillaries.

NONIMMUNE HYDROPS

This very heterogeneous group of uncommon nonimmune causes of fetal and placental hydrops now makes up the majority of cases. Machin (12) presents a detailed listing of over 100 specific entities based upon a comprehensive literature review of case reports and series published in the 1980s. These are grouped into three categories (Table 10-1), based on pathophysiologic mechanisms: cardiac failure, anemia, and hypoproteinemia. The prevalence of some types of nonimmune hydrops varies with geographic location. For example, alpha-thalassemia is more prevalent in Southeast Asia. There is necessarily some overlap (parvovirus causes both infection and anemia; cardiac failure also occurs with severe anemia).

An autopsy study of fetuses with fatal nonimmune hydrops found pathologic evidence of intrauterine brain injury in 60 percent of 38 cases (11). The typical features of leukomalacia were the most common findings, with microcalcifications and small vessel thrombi in some cases. Clinical features in common with anemia, hypoproteinemia, and cardiac failure with hypotension suggested that brain hypoperfusion and hypoxia were the likely basis for neurologic injury.

Cardiovascular

The full range of congenital cardiac anomalies may lead to congestive heart failure, resulting in fetal and placental hydrops. The 1,204-g placenta in figure 10-2 belonged to a stillborn infant with large interatrial and interventricular septal defects. Fetal cardiac arrhythmias, especially tachycardias, also cause hydrops. The specific anatomic diagnoses are often made prenatally by ultrasound evaluation. High-output cardiac failure results from large hemangiomas and other large tumors, such as sacrococcygeal teratomas. Rare instances of cardiomyopathy and cardiac rhabdomyoma in tuberous sclerosis can impair cardiac function prenatally (13).

Fetal Anemias

Hemoglobinopathies. The anemia caused by homozygous alpha-thalassemia (fig. 10-3) is a common cause of hydrops and should be considered first among ethnic Southeast Asian parents. The fetus with homozygous sickle cell disease or beta-thalassemia (Cooley's anemia)

Table 10-1

POTENTIAL CAUSES OF NONIMMUNE HYDROPS[a]

	Number of Cases	%
Cardiovascular Lesions	331	22.5
Anemias	185	12.6
Fetal Infections	58	3.9
Pulmonary, Thoracic Lesions	236	16.0
Chromosomal Anomalies	155	10.5
Urinary Tract Malformations	39	2.6
Other (Tumors, Storage Diseases, Metabolic)	89	11.8
Not Determined	293	19.9

[a]Adapted from reference 12.

is protected from hemolysis prior to birth by the presence of fetal hemoglobin.

Parvovirus Anemia. Parvovirus B-19 is responsible for 14 to 18 percent of cases of nonimmune placental and fetal hydrops (9,17). The hydrops occurs in the second trimester and is usually fatal to the fetus. In addition to typical hydropic villi, an important histologic characteristic of parvovirus infection is the presence of viral inclusions in the numerous fetal nucleated red blood cells (figs. 10-4, 10-5) that cluster prominently in villous capillaries. The presence of viral DNA is confirmed by polymerase chain reaction studies of placental or other fetal tissues soon after onset of illness (3), or the viral antigens may be demonstrated in tissue sections by immunostaining (fig. 10-6). Viral DNA and antigens are usually not detectable in third trimester placentas. Even if maternal infection is proven and fetal hydrops is present (3), the virus does not appear to persist to term.

Maternal infection does not always lead to fetal hydrops. Anemia occurs only in those fetuses whose red blood cells express an antigen of the blood group P system, the P antigen. The P antigen functions as a receptor for the virus (1), and is expressed on the surface membrane of megakaryocytes, endothelial cells, fetal liver and heart, and placenta. This may explain an instance in which only one of a set of dichorionic twins became infected (16).

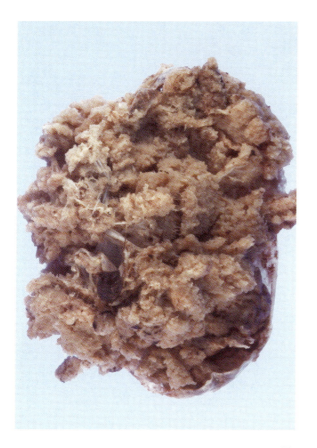
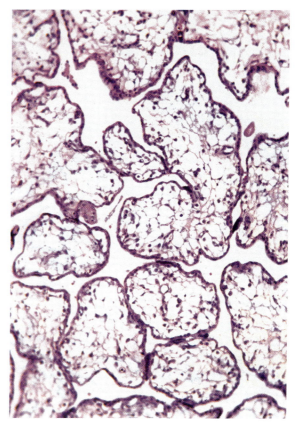

Figure 10-2

CARDIOVASCULAR-ASSOCIATED HYDROPS

Left: The massively hydropic, 1,204-g placenta at 24 weeks was associated with large atrial and ventricular septal defects, resulting in intrauterine fetal death from cardiac failure. The fragmentation is related to difficulty in removing the placenta, which is very common in cases of placental hydrops, regardless of cause.

Right: The villi of the placenta are immature as well as markedly edematous.

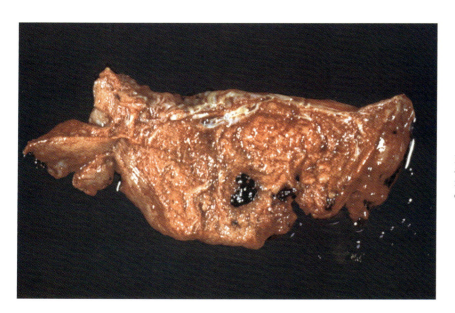

Figure 10-3

ALPHA-THALASSEMIA–ASSOCIATED HYDROPS

The villi of this hydropic placenta of a newborn with alpha-thalassemia are uniformly swollen. There is a recent hematoma near the center.

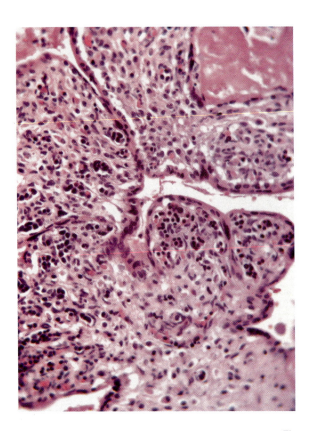
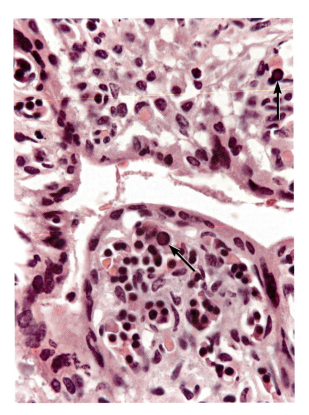

Figure 10-4

PARVOVIRUS-ASSOCIATED HYDROPS

Left: Parvovirus infection caused intrauterine fetal death at 24 weeks. The villous capillaries are stuffed with immature erythroblasts and fetal erythroblasts are almost absent.

Right: At higher magnification, many normoblasts are seen and an immature erythroblast in the dilated vessel at center contains a pale eosinophilic intranuclear inclusion. Miscarriage in the second trimester is typical, and inclusions at this time are usually easily demonstrated. (Figs. 10-4 and 10-5 are from the same patient.)

Figure 10-5

PARVOVIRUS-ASSOCIATED HYDROPS

The central capillary contains several erythroblasts, most of which contain typically ill-defined inclusions. Trophoblast nuclei are fragmented, indicating focal necrosis.

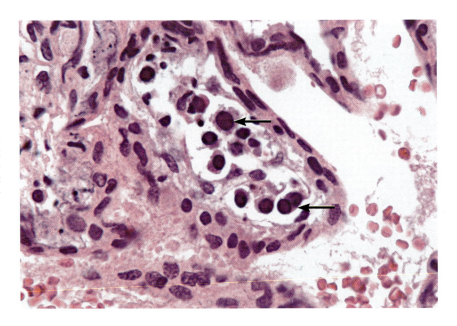

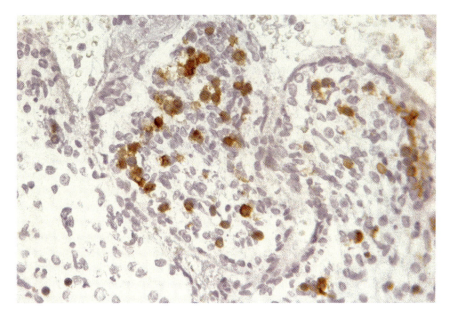

Figure 10-6

PARVOVIRUS-ASSOCIATED HYDROPS

Immunohistochemical staining confirms the presence of parvovirus.

Although the disease caused by parvovirus B-19 is an infection, the lesion is presented here because the result is fetal hydrops, and the mechanism of the hydrops is the severe hemolytic anemia. Involvement of cardiac muscle (14,15), resulting in myocardial dysfunction, may also contribute to the hydropic state. Maternal infection is detected by demonstration of serum IgM antibodies.

Fetomaternal Hemorrhage. A massive, acute, transplacental hemorrhage from the fetal into the maternal circulation is commonly fatal and represents one of the causes of otherwise unexplained stillbirth. Intraplacental hematomas associated with this are described in chapter 6. When a massive hemorrhage occurs more slowly, the profound anemia causes cardiac failure, resulting in placental and fetal hydrops. A Kleihauer-Betke test to quantitate the amount of fetal blood in the maternal circulation is confirmatory; the newer flow cytometric assay (2) appears to be more precise. The diagnosis of hydrops can be confirmed by ultrasound. Intrauterine transfusion has been successful in treating the anemia, and can reverse the placental hydrops as well (5). There are no specific histopathologic variations in placental hydrops.

Twin-Twin Transfusion. Monozygotic twins with monochorionic placentas have shared circulations, as described in detail in chapter 12. If an adequate balance between the two circulations is not maintained, the recipient twin becomes plethoric at the expense of the donor twin. Cardiac dysfunction caused by circulatory overload in the recipient frequently results in cardiac dysfunction (18). The results of this circulatory overload include cardiac failure, polyhydramnios, edema, pleural and peritoneal effusions, and placental hydrops.

The placental examination in this case must be detailed and correlate with the specific twin. The cords must be carefully labeled in the delivery room, with all tissue blocks keyed individually and specifically. The analysis in the report must relate the findings to the specific twin, and be correlated with the clinical status of each twin, as detailed in chapter 13. The hydropic histopathology of the placenta has no unique features.

Other Anemias. Fetal and placental hydrops has been reported as a result of the anemias associated with glucose-6-phosphate isomerase deficiency, fetal erythroleukemia, osteopetrosis, and hemorrhage into a fetal neoplasm (12, 13). In addition to hydrops and anemia, infantile sialic acid storage disease causes extensive cytoplasmic vacuolation of essentially all types of fetal cells, including trophoblast and stromal cells of the placental villi (4).

Fetal Infections

Intrauterine infections caused by cytomegalovirus, *Toxoplasma*, herpes simplex virus, *Treponema pallidum* (syphilis), and rubella virus are occasional causes of hydrops. Specific histopathologic features, if any, are described in chapter 5.

Pulmonary Lesions and Other Intrathoracic Causes

Congenital cystic adenomatoid malformation and pulmonary sequestration were the most common pulmonary lesions to cause hydrops in the large collected review by Machin (13). A variety of intrathoracic tumors or space-occupying lesions capable of compressing the heart or great vessels, including chylothorax, chondrodysplasia, and diaphragmatic hernia, together make up a major cause of hydrops. The placental histopathology is nonspecific.

Major Chromosomal Disorders

A significant proportion of fetuses with Down's syndrome (trisomy 21) and Turner's syndrome have hydropic placentas (8). Those with trisomy 18, triploidy, and trisomy 13, though less common, characteristically have villous edema with some other variations, as described in chapter 9. Numerous rare chromosomal anomalies occasionally cause hydrops (8).

Other Congenital Anomalies and Genetic Metabolic Diseases

Rarely, urinary tract anomalies, certain dystrophic muscle syndromes, and lysosomal storage disorders such as Gaucher's disease (19) lead to fetal hydrops (12). Thyrotoxicosis in pregnancy represents a treatable form of nonimmune hydrops (20).

Fetal Tumors

Large neoplasms that occur prenatally cause hydrops, mainly through the mechanism of high-output cardiac failure (13). Sacrococcygeal teratomas and angiomas are the most common, but instances of neuroblastoma and even glioblastoma multiforme have been reported (13).

REFERENCES

1. Brown KE, Hibbs JR, Gallinella G, et al. Resistance to parvovirus B19 infection due to lack of virus receptor (erythrocyte P antigen). N Engl J Med 1994;330:1192–6.
2. Davis BH, Olsen S, Bigelow NC, Chen JC. Detection of fetal red cells in fetomaternal hemorrhage using a fetal hemoglobin monoclonal antibody by flow cytometry. Transfusion 1998;38:749–56.
3. Essary LR, Vnencak-Jones CL, Manning SS, Olson SJ, Johnson JE. Frequency of parvovirus B19 infection in nonimmune hydrops fetalis and utility of three diagnostic methods. Hum Pathol 1998;29:696–701.
4. Hale LP, van de Ven CJ, Wenger CJ, Bradford WD, Kahler SG. Infantile sialic acid storage disease: a rare cause of cytoplasmic vacuolation in pediatric patients. Pediatr Pathol Lab Med 1995;15:443–53.
5. Hartung J, Chaoui R, Bollmann R. Nonimmune hydrops from fetomaternal hemorrhage treated with serial fetal intravascular transfusion. Obstet Gynecol 2000;96:844.
6. Hutchison AA, Drew JH, Yu VY, Williams ML, Fortune DW, Beischer NA. Nonimmunologic hydrops fetalis: a review of 61 cases. Obstet Gynecol 1982;59:347–52.
7. Iliff P, Nicholls JM, Keeling JW, Gough JD. Nonimmunologic hydrops fetalis: a review of 27 cases. Arch Dis Child 1983;58:979–82.
8. Jauniaux E, Van Maldergem L, De Munter C, Moscoso G, Gillerot Y. Nonimmune hydrops fetalis associated with genetic abnormalities. Obstet Gynecol 1990;75:568–72.
9. Jordan JA. Identification of human parvovirus B-19 infection in idiopathic nonimmune hydrops fetalis. Am J Obstet Gynecol 1996;174:37–42.
10. Lallemand AV, Doco-Fenzy M, Gallard DA. Investigation of nonimmune hydrops fetalis; multidisciplinary studies are necessary for diagnosis—review of 94 cases. Pediatr Dev Pathol 1999;2:432–9.
11. Larroche JC, Aubry MC, Narcy F. Intrauterine brain damage in nonimmune hydrops fetalis. Biol Neonate 1992;61:273–80.
12. Machin GA. Hydrops, cystic hygroma, hydrothorax, pericardial effusions, and fetal ascites. In: Gilbert-Barness E, ed. Potter's pathology of the fetus and infant. St. Louis: Mosby; 1997:163–81.
13. Machin GA. Hydrops revisited: literature review of 1,414 cases published in the 1980s. Am J Med Genet 1989;34:366–90.
14. Morey AL, Porter HJ, Keeling JW, Fleming KA. Non-isotopic in situ hybridisation and immunophenotyping of infected cells in the investigation of human fetal parvovirus infection. J Clin Pathol 1992;45:673–8.
15. Murry CE, Jerome KR, Reichenbach DD. Fatal parvovirus myocarditis in a 5-year-old girl. Hum Pathol 2001;32:342–5.
16. Pustilnik TB, Cohen AW. Parvovirus B19 infection in a twin pregnancy. Obstet Gynecol 1994;83:834–6.
17. Rogers BB, Mark Y, Over CE. Diagnosis and incidence of fetal parvovirus infection in an autopsy series: I. Histology. Pediatr Pathol 1993;13:371–9.
18. Simpson LL, Marx GR, Elkadry EA, D'Alton ME. Cardiac dysfunction in twin-twin transfusion syndrome: a prospective, longitudinal study. Obstet Gynecol 1998;92:557–62.
19. Soma H, Yamada K, Osawa H, Hata T, Oguro T, Kudo M. Identification of Gaucher cells in the chorionic villi associated with recurrent hydrops fetalis. Placenta 2000;21:412–6.
20. Stulberg RA, Davies GA. Maternal thyrotoxicosis and fetal nonimmune hydrops. Obstet Gynecol 2000;95:1036.

11 TUMOR-LIKE LESIONS AND METASTATIC NEOPLASMS

Primary nontrophoblastic tumors of the placenta are rare, and the neoplastic status of all of the candidate lesions, including hemangiomas, has been questioned. The pathologic features of primary neoplasms of trophoblastic origin, including choriocarcinoma, placental site trophoblastic tumor, hydatidiform mole, and related lesions are presented in the Atlas of Tumor Pathology Fascicle, *Tumors of the Uterine Corpus and Gestational Trophoblastic Disease* (23).

PUTATIVE PRIMARY PLACENTAL NEOPLASMS

Hemangioma (Chorangioma)

Placental hemangiomas, which have perhaps the best credentials as neoplasms, have never been subjected to clonality studies to prove their neoplastic status. By custom, the common, small, isolated, intraplacental, circumscribed nodular mass of vessels has been widely regarded as a neoplasm. The distinction, if any, between this and similar lesions that seem to expand villi more diffusely (hemangiomatosis, chorangiomatosis) may be difficult and sometimes arbitrary. For these reasons, the discussion of hemangiomas is presented in chapter 4 in order to facilitate comparison with the other similar, but clearly non-neoplastic, vascular lesions that must be considered in the differential diagnosis.

Intraplacental Leiomyoma

Four placental lesions with the morphologically typical histologic features of leiomyoma have been reported, one in the membranes external to decidua (19), and three within the placental mass (7,10,26). The possibility that these actually were detached primary uterine leiomyomas was considered in all cases, but rejected in three of the reports because they separated so easily from the uterus. They also appeared to be unencapsulated, with infiltrative finger-like extensions into the adjacent placenta, and were covered by decidua at the maternal surface of the placenta (figs. 11-1, 11-2). However, molecular studies confirmed the maternal origin of the lesion reported by Ernst et al. (7), casting doubt upon a placental origin in any of the cases. The Y chromosome of the male fetus was not expressed by the tumor (fig. 11-2D).

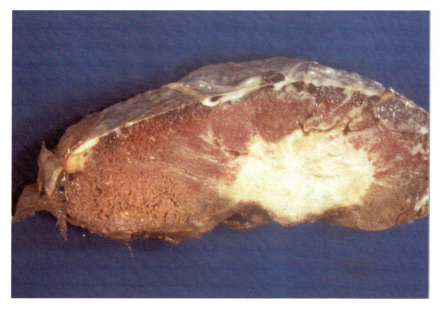

Figure 11-1

INTRAPLACENTAL LEIOMYOMA

This firm solid tumor is enveloped by the placental tissue of a male fetus. The irregular margins and the intraplacental location suggest origin from the placenta. However, absence of Y chromosome DNA in the tumor, although present throughout the placenta, confirms a maternal origin from myometrium. (Fig. 1 from Ernst LM, Hui P, Parkash V. Intraplacental smooth muscle tumor. Int J Gynecol Pathol 2001;20:284–8.) (Figs. 11-1 and 11-2 are from the same patient.)

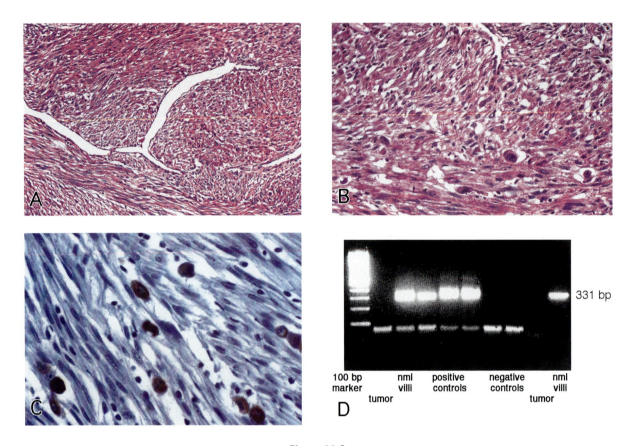

Figure 11-2

INTRAPLACENTAL LEIOMYOMA

A: The microscopic features are consistent with a uterine smooth muscle origin, with immunoreactivity for smooth muscle actin and desmin.

B: Epithelioid cells are intermixed with the smooth muscle component.

C: Reactivity for cell adhesion molecule (CAM) 5.2 (shown here) as well as human placental lactogen (HPL) supports an intermediate trophoblast phenotype for the epithelioid cells.

D: Gel showing polymerase chain reaction (PCR) results. The Y chromosome is a band with about 331 base pairs in the normal villi, at far right. The tumor (second band from left) has no comparable DNA component, consistent with a maternal origin. (A–D courtesy of Dr. Vinita Parkash, New Haven, CT.)

TERATOMAS (OR ACARDIAC TWINS?)

Nodular masses of variably disorganized tissue elements, with prominent components of ectodermal, mesodermal, and endodermal tissue, occur on the fetal aspect of the placenta, between the amnion and the chorionic plate, as well as attached to the umbilical cord. It is generally conceded that those that have both an identifiable umbilical cord attachment and contain axially oriented skeletal structures are correctly regarded as acardiac twins (described in chapter 12). Several accounts of such a mass lacking any axial orientation or evidence of an umbilical cord-like structure have been reported; these are classified as teratomas of the placenta or cord (8,14,28).

This classification, however, is widely disputed because pedunculated structures with what appear to be obvious umbilical cords may lack axial organization, and reviews of large numbers of reports indicate "an anatomical continuum" between acardiac twins and placental teratomas (3,25). Karyotypes of acardiacs and their co-twins, as reviewed by Benirschke (3), present complex results which so far fail to settle the subject. One case report is of note in that it describes an immature teratoma, Norris grade 3, in typical subamnionic continuity with

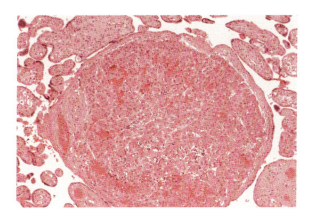 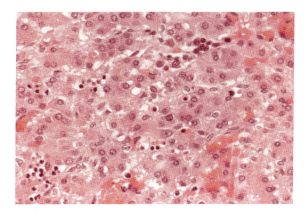

Figure 11-3

LIVER ADENOMA

Left: Cytologic features and hepatocellular cord architecture are suggestive of fetal liver. Hepatic identification was further confirmed by immunostaining for alpha-fetoprotein, alpha-1-antitrypsin, and carcinoembryonic antigen, as well as cytokeratins. There were no portal or central areas. (Adapted from case 1 from Khalifa MA, Gersell DJ, Hansen CH, Lage JM. Hepatic (hepatocellular) adenoma of the placenta: a study of four cases. Int J Gynecol Pathol 1998;17:241–4.)

Right: At higher magnification, foci of extramedullary hematopoiesis are evident at top center and lower left.

the placenta and with a definite blood supply from a fetal artery on the surface of the placenta (29). The authors concluded that the immature malignant histology confirmed a neoplastic origin. Unfortunately, no photomicrographs were included.

At this time, it appears that acardiac fetuses are not rare, and are well understood and widely accepted, while the existence of teratomas of the placenta and cord is questionable, and so far not proven. Regardless of how these lesions are classified, their clinical significance depends on the size and extent to which the circulation of the parasitic mass interferes with the growth and development of the "pump" twin.

ADENOMA (CHORISTOMA?)

Hepatocellular Adenoma (Heterotopic Liver)

Rarely, single, well-circumscribed, encapsulated nodules composed of liver cells have occurred in the placenta. Most are small, up to 1 cm in diameter (13); the eighth case, however, reported in 2000, measured 7 cm in greatest diameter (4). Hepatocellular adenomas do not include portal areas, bile ducts, or central veins, but may contain foci of hematopoiesis (fig. 11-3). Immunostaining for cytokeratin, alpha-fetoprotein, alpha-1-antitrypsin, and carcinoembryonic antigen, typical of fetal liver, is present. A comparable lesion, more compatible with heterotopic liver, with portal and central areas, occurred in an umbilical cord (fig. 11-4). A nodular mass of liver has also been reported in the umbilicus (22). Heterotopic liver nodules may occur in the chest as well as in other less common locations in the fetus. The pathogenesis of these interesting curiosities is unexplained.

Heterotopic Adrenal Cortex

Tiny nodules of heterotopic adrenal cortex are a common autopsy finding in fetuses and newborns. They are conspicuous in the retroperitoneum because of their golden color. They are most common near the adrenal glands and gonads, but in rare cases are found almost anywhere, including the placenta (fig. 11-5) (21). Embolic spread of adrenal precursor cells via fetal vascular connections has been proposed as the most likely mechanism (9); monodermal teratoma and aberrant differentiation of extraembryonic mesoderm have also been suggested.

METASTATIC NEOPLASMS

About 1 in 1,000 women of childbearing age develop a cancer (2). Congenital cancers in the newborn are much less common. Metastases from either rarely occur in the placenta.

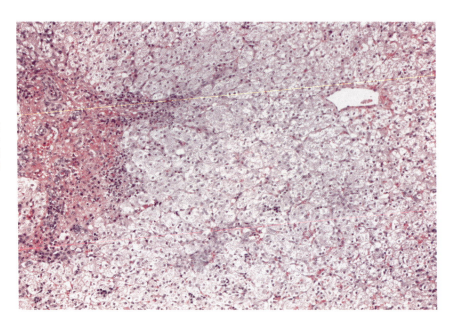

Figure 11-4

HETEROTOPIC LIVER

Heterotopic liver, located near the fetal end of the umbilical cord. In contrast to cases of liver adenoma, both portal and central areas are present.

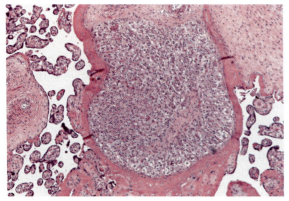 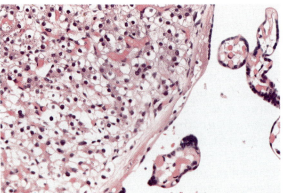

Figure 11-5

HETEROTOPIC ADRENAL CORTEX

Left: An adrenal cortical origin was presumed on the basis of cytology and architecture, in the absence of positive immunostaining for other possible tissue types. (Adapted from case 1 from Qureshi F, Jacques SM. Adrenocortical heterotopia in the placenta. Pediatr Pathol Lab Med 1995;15:51–6.)

Right: Higher magnification shows clear cytoplasm; contrast with the liver cells in figures 11-3, 11-4.

Fetal Primary Tumors Involving the Placenta

The most common congenital cancers are, in order of incidence, neuroblastoma, lymphoma/leukemia, various soft tissue sarcomas, brain tumors, and, in some series, teratomas (11). Placental metastases are extremely rare. Congenital neuroblastoma has been reported most frequently, with 11 cases listed in a review in 1997 (18). Instances of congenital hepatoblastoma (6), sacrococcygeal teratoma (17), and leukemia (15,16) have also been reported.

Nonimmune hydrops is consistently associated with metastatic malignant neoplasms from the fetus, regardless of the nature of the neoplasm. The metastatic cancer typically distends, but remains confined to, fetal vessels of the placenta (figs. 11-6, 11-7). Only rarely does invasion of the villous stroma occur from neuroblastomas (18).

Giant congenital "bathing trunk" nevi of the fetus are associated with benign intraplacental deposits of pigmented nevi that expand the villous stroma (fig. 11-8). These deposits do not involve vessels, and are probably not metastases

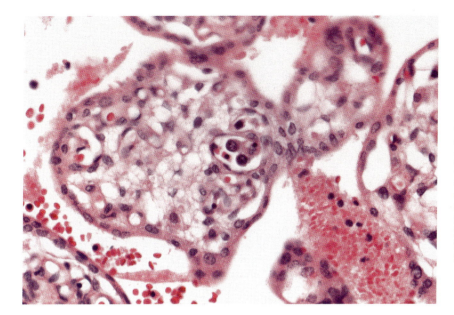

Figure 11-6

METASTATIC HEPATOBLASTOMA

This primary tumor in the fetus, otherwise limited to the liver, had been identified by ultrasound prior to delivery. Both the 33-week fetus and the placenta (1,190 g) were grossly hydropic. The villi are immature and hydropic. Clustered tumor cells are confined within vessels. (Adapted from case 1 from Doss BJ, Vicari J, Jacques SM, Qureshi F. Placental involvement in congenital hepatoblastoma. Pediatr Dev Pathol 1998;1:538–42.)

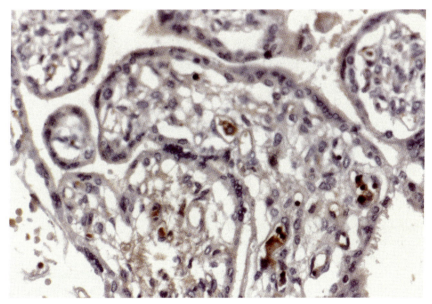

Figure 11-7

METASTATIC HEPATOBLASTOMA

Alpha-fetoprotein immunostain is positive.

(24). Although some giant congenital nevi are malignant, extended follow-up of the cases with placental involvement indicates that these particular giant nevi are benign (24).

Other sources of melanin should be considered in the differential diagnosis of melanocytic cells in the placenta. A study of placental melanin pigment that perhaps deserves to be repeated found surprising amounts of melanin, as identified by Fontana-Masson stain, in Hofbauer cells, basement membrane of villi, trophoblastic knots, and intervillous fibrin deposits, a condition the authors called *dermatopathic melanosis of the placenta* (12). In this series, 25 (88 percent) of 29 women with a history of dermatologic disease, had placentas containing histologic evidence of melanin, while only 4 (3 percent) of 125 women with no dermatopathic history had placentas with melanin.

Maternal Primary Tumors Involving the Placenta

In a collected review of case reports from 1866 to 1989 Dildy et al. (5) found 52 cases of

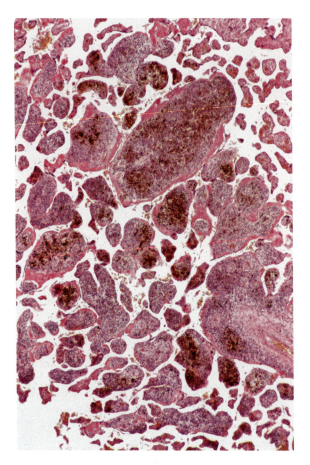 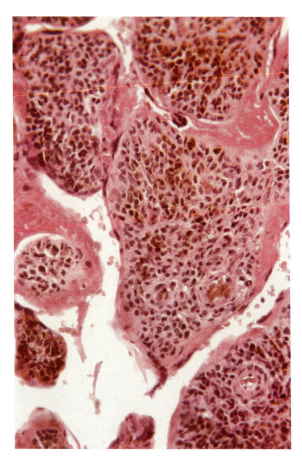

Figure 11-8

INTRAPLACENTAL NEVUS ASSOCIATED WITH A GIANT CONGENITAL NEVUS OF THE FETUS

Left: The pigmented nevus cells occupy the villous stroma. Compare with the metastatic malignant melanoma of maternal origin seen in figure 11-11.

Right: Higher magnification shows benign cytologic features and well-defined vessels. The consistent lack of vessel involvement supports migration of neural crest elements early in gestation, as opposed to metastasis from the giant nevus. Compare with fetal malignant melanoma in figure 11-13.

malignancy metastatic to the placenta. In 2002, the total reported increased to 68 (27). The most common primary neoplasm was malignant melanoma (23 percent), while leukemias and lymphomas, breast carcinoma, and lung carcinoma were each represented about half as frequently. This is surprising because primary cancer of the breast, cervix, and lymphoma-leukemia together account for about 25 percent of cancers in pregnant women in contrast to malignant melanoma, which is only 8 percent. There have been 14 case reports of transplacental metastases to the fetus (27). These are disproportionately represented by malignant melanoma (1). Lymphomas and leukemias have also spread transplacentally to the fetus (5).

Metastatic malignant melanoma may form large pigmented deposits (fig. 11-9). Other metastases, most often from breast or lung, may form small scattered nodules (fig. 11-10), but in most cases the tumor is not evident grossly. Tumor masses were present in 8 of 20 placentas with metastatic melanoma reviewed by Baergen et al (1), of which 5 were pigmented. Lymphomas may produce white nodular masses (20). There is no association with hydrops, in contrast to metastatic neoplasms from the fetus.

Microscopically, metastatic tumor deposits from the mother are distributed within the maternal intervillous space (figs. 11-11, 11-12). Invasion of villous tissue may occur, but it does not correlate well with spread to the fetus (1).

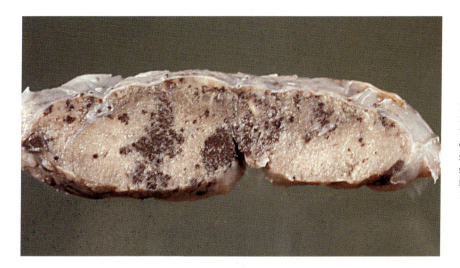

Figure 11-9

METASTATIC MATERNAL MALIGNANT MELANOMA

Gross appearance of metastatic malignant melanoma, forming relatively large, deeply pigmented nodules. The mother had disseminated metastases, and died soon after delivery. The newborn survived and was well several months later. (Figs. 11-9 and 11-11 are from the same patient.)

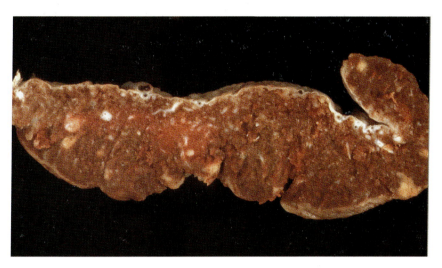

Figure 11-10

METASTATIC BREAST CARCINOMA

Gross appearance of metastatic breast carcinoma in this placenta, which produced numerous, very small, firm gray nodules (center, far left, and far right). The newborn was not affected. (Figs. 11-10 and 11-12 are from the same patient.)

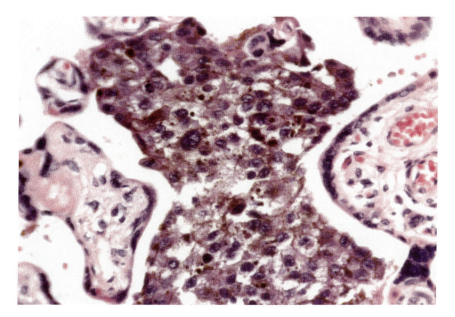

Figure 11-11

METASTATIC MATERNAL MALIGNANT MELANOMA

Masses of pigmented malignant cells are distributed in clumps within the maternal intervillous space.

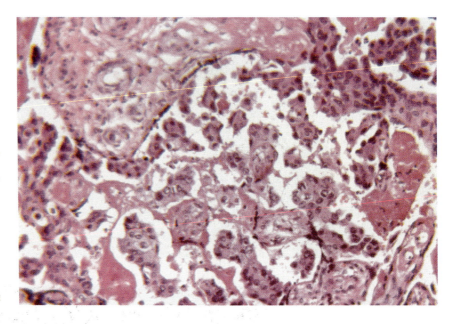

Figure 11-12

METASTATIC BREAST CARCINOMA

Poorly differentiated adenocarcinoma cells form small masses, intermixed with fibrin, and confined to the intervillous space.

The massive melanocytic lesion of the fetal scalp in figure 11-13A is different from the usual giant melanocytic nevus described above in that diffuse involvement of the villous stroma led to obliteration of vascular spaces (fig. 11-13B), and the cytologic features appeared malignant (fig. 11-13C). Foci of fetal thrombotic vasculopathy (FTV) (fig. 11-13D) suggest that tumor thrombi may have been responsible for the FTV by causing occlusive tumor thrombi.

REFERENCES

1. Baergen RN, Johnson D, Moore T, Benirschke K. Maternal melanoma metastatic to the placenta: a case report and review of the literature. Arch Pathol Lab Med 1997;121:508–11.
2. Barber HR. Malignant disease in pregnancy. J Perinat Med 2001;29:97–111.
3. Benirschke K, Kaufmann P. Pathology of the human placenta. New York: Springer; 2000:853–8.
4. Dargent JL, Verdebout JM, Barlow P, Thomas D, Hoorens A, Goossens A. Hepatocellular adenoma of the placenta: report of a case associated with maternal bicornuate uterus and fetal renal dysplasia. Histopathology 2000;37:287–9.
5. Dildy GA 3rd, Moise KJ Jr, Carpenter RJ Jr, Klima T. Maternal malignancy metastatic to the products of conception: a review. Obstet Gynecol Surv 1989;44:535–40.
6. Doss BJ, Vicari J, Jacques SM, Qureshi F. Placental involvement in congenital hepatoblastoma. Pediatr Dev Pathol 1998;1:538–42.
7. Ernst LM, Hui P, Parkash V. Intraplacental smooth muscle tumor: a case report. Int J Gynecol Pathol 2001;29:284–8.
8. Fox H, Butler-Manuel R. A teratoma of the placenta. J Pathol Bacteriol 1964;88:137–40.
9. Guschmann M, Vogel M, Urban M. Adrenal tissue in the placenta: a heterotopia caused by migration and embolism? Placenta 2000;21:427–31.
10. Harirah HM, Jones DC, Donia SE, Bahado-Singh R. Intraplacental smooth muscle tumor: a case report. J Reprod Med 2001;46:937–40.
11. Isaacs H Jr. Tumors. In: Gilbert-Barness E, ed. Potter's pathology of the fetus and infant. St Louis: Mosby; 1997:1242–339.
12. Ishizaki Y, Belter LF. Melanin deposition in the placenta as a result of skin lesions (dermatopathic melanosis of the placenta). Am J Obstet Gynecol 1960;79:1074–7.
13. Khalifa MA, Gersell DJ, Hansen CH, Lage JM. Hepatic (hepatocellular) adenoma of the placenta: a study of four cases. Int J Gynecol Pathol 1998;17:241–4.
14. Kreczy A, Alge A, Menardi G, Gassner I, Gschwendtner A, Mikuz G. Teratoma of the umbilical cord. Case report with review of the literature. Arch Pathol Lab Med 1994;118:934–7.

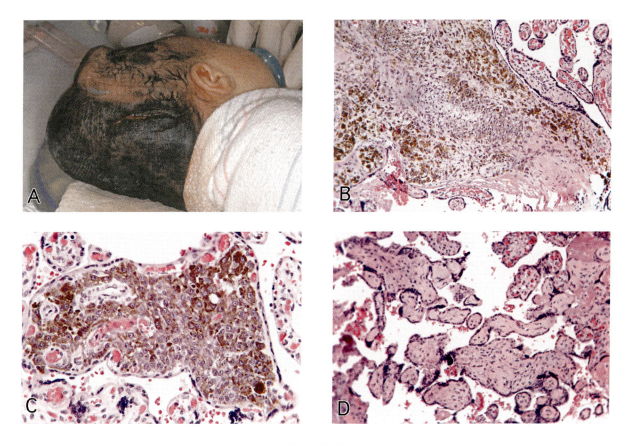

Figure 11-13

METASTATIC MALIGNANT MELANOMA OF FETAL SCALP

A: Congenital malignant melanoma forms a hugh scalp mass. (Courtesy of Dr. M. J. Bell, St. Louis, MO.)

B: Histologic pattern of placental metastasis from the tumor in figure A. The wall of a fetal vessel is invaded and its lumen is obliterated.

C: The melanocytic cells of this tumor have large nuclei, prominent nucleoli, and thick nuclear membranes, representing malignant cytologic features.

D: The presence of foci of fetal thrombotic vasculopathy further denote fetal vascular involvement, resulting in the diagnosis of malignant melanoma primary in the fetus.

15. Las Heras J, Leal G, Haust MD. Congenital leukemia with placental involvement. Report of a case with ultrastructural study. Cancer 1986;58:2278–81.
16. Lentz SE, Coulson CC, Gocke CD, Fantaskey AP. Placental pathology in maternal and neonatal myeloproliferative disorders. Obstet Gynecol 1998;91:863.
17. Leung JC, Mann S, Salafia CM, Brion LP. Sacrococcygeal teratoma with vascular placental dissemination. Obstet Gynecol 1999;93:856.
18. Lynn AA, Parry SI, Morgan MA, Mennuti MT. Disseminated congenital neuroblastoma involving the placenta. Arch Pathol Lab Med 1997;121:741–4.
19. Misselevich I, Abramovici D, Reiter A, Boss JH. Leiomyoma of the fetal membranes: report of a case. Gynecol Oncol 1989;33:108–11.
20. Nishi Y, Suzuki S, Otsubo Y, et al. B-cell-type malignant lymphoma with placental involvement. J Obstet Gynaecol Res 2000;26:39–43.
21. Qureshi F, Jacques SM. Adrenocortical heterotopia in the placenta. Pediatr Pathol Lab Med 1995;15:51–6.
22. Shaw A, Pierog S. "Ectopic" liver in the umbilicus: an unusual focus of infection in a newborn infant. Pediatrics 1969;44:448–50.
23. Silverberg SG, Kurman RJ. Tumors of the uterine corpus and gestational trophoblastic disease. 3rd Series, Fascicle 3. Washington DC: Armed Forces Institute of Pathology; 1992.

24. Sotelo-Avila C, Graham M, Hanby DE, Rudolph AJ. Nevus cell aggregates in the placenta. A histochemical and electron microscopic study. Am J Clin Pathol 1988;89:395–400.
25. Stephens TD, Spall R, Urfer AG, Martin R. Fetus amorphus or placental teratoma? Teratology 1989;40:1–10.
26. Tapia RH, White VA, Ruffolo EH. Leiomyoma of the placenta. South Med J 1985;78:863–4.
27. Walker JW, Reinisch JF, Monforte HL. Maternal pulmonary adenocarcinoma metastatic to the fetus: first recorded case report and literature review. Pediatr Pathol Molec Med 2002;21:57–69.
28. Wang L, Du X, Li M. Placental teratoma. A case report and review of the literature. Path Res Pract 1995;191:1267–70.
29. Williams VL, Williams RA. Placental teratoma: prenatal ultrasonographic diagnosis. J Ultrasound Med 1994;13:587–9.

12 MULTIPLE PREGNANCY

Multiple gestations are common and becoming more so with assisted reproductive techniques (ART). In the United States, in 2000, ART accounted for 14 percent of all twin births, and 45 percent of ART births were twins (101). Multiples are associated with a disproportionate share of complications including higher rates of morbidity, mortality, low birth weight, anomalous development, and malformation than singletons (16,33,58,90,97,124). Careful pathologic examination of the placenta(s) can provide important insight into problems peculiar to multiples, and pathologists must be aware of the special considerations required in the examination of such placentas.

TWIN GESTATION

Zygosity

Twins arise from the fertilization of two separate ova (dizygous, or fraternal twins) or from the division of a single fertilized ovum (monozygous, or identical twins). Monozygous twins are genetically and usually phenotypically identical, but dizygous twins are genetically dissimilar, like singleton siblings.

Rare variants of dizygous twinning result when ova are fertilized by sperm from different sources (superfecundation) or when ova are ovulated and fertilized at different times, resulting in twins of disparate developmental ages (superfetation). Monozygous heterokaryotic twins, a rare variant of monozygous twins, have different karyotypes and sometimes even different sex (25,71). These twins are thought to result from chromosome nondisjunction, most commonly involving the sex chromosomes, but on occasion the autosomes as well. There are several recorded instances of 45X/46XY monozygous female/male twins, presumably resulting from Y chromosome loss through nondisjunction in early development (45), and there are many instances of mosaic twins (23).

A third type of twinning, polar body, or dispermic monovular twinning, presumably results from fertilization of an oocyte and a polar body. Bieber (15) described a triploid acardiac/diploid twin gestation resulting from the fertilization of an oocyte and its first polar body. Theoretically, fertilization of the oocyte and second polar body could also occur; the resulting diploid fetuses would be genetically intermediate between monozygous and dizygous twins. The frequency of this phenomenon is unknown. It has been hypothesized that dispermic monovular twins are monochorionic due to the proximity of the oocyte and the polar body, and because cytoplasmic imbalance equips only the oocyte with its more abundant cytoplasm to implant.

Frequency and Etiology

The frequency of monozygous twinning is relatively constant worldwide (about 3.5 in 1,000 pregnancies) (19). However, there are marked geographic differences in the total twinning rate, reflecting excess dizygous twinning in certain populations and families who have a genetic predisposition for high follicle-stimulating hormone (FSH) levels and polyovulation (61,80,91,113). Dizygous twinning is also age related, increasing with maternal age until 35 years, again probably reflecting a role for increasing FSH levels with age. The cause of monozygous twinning is unknown. Monozygous twinning is increased in pregnancies following ART (79). Twins occur in about 1 in 80 Caucasian pregnancies in the United States, and approximately 30 percent of these are monozygotic (83,84).

Placentation

The object of the placental exam in multiple gestation is the same as in singleton gestation: to identify pathologic processes interfering with placental function. The gross and microscopic manifestations of these processes are identical

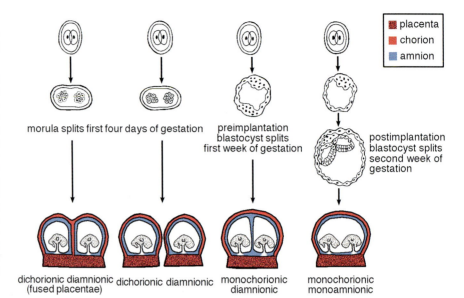

Figure 12-1

PLACENTATION TYPES AND MEMBRANE RELATIONSHIPS IN MONOZYGOUS TWINS

Placentation in monozygous twins depends on when division occurs. If division occurs early, two placentas form that may be separate or fused (left). When division occurs later, there is one placenta (monochorionic) and two amnions (diamnionic). Division occurring after the amnion is formed results in monoamnionic monochorionic placentation, and even later division in conjoined twins. (Modified from fig. 4-2 from Fox H. Pathology of the placenta. Philadelphia: WB Saunders; 1997:80.)

in the placentas of singletons and multiples, although some lesions are particularly pertinent to the problems experienced by multiples. Comparison of the relative distribution of lesions in the two placental territories and correlation with the size and condition of the fetuses are important aspects of placental assessment in multiple gestation. Features unique to multiples include the relationship of the placental discs and fetal membranes, and the pattern and degree of anastomosis of the chorionic vessels.

Chorionicity. Placentas in twin gestation are either monochorionic or dichorionic. All dizygous twins have dichorionic placentas (diamnionic dichorionic [DiDi]). In double ovulation, each blastocyst generates a placenta. If these implant in close proximity, varying degrees of fusion may result (DiDi fused); otherwise they are entirely separate. Monozygous twins may show any type of placentation depending on when division occurs (fig. 12-1). If the single fertilized ovum divides very early before differentiation of the chorion (first 2 or 3 days), the situation is analogous to dizygous twinning: two placentas develop that may be separate or fused. If splitting occurs in the blastocyst stage, after formation of the chorion but before formation of the amnion (3rd to 8th day after fertilization), there will be a single placenta with two amnionic sacs (diamnionic monochorionic [DiMo]). A split after formation of the amnion (between the 8th and 13th day), will result in one placenta with one amnionic cavity (monoamnionic monochorionic [MoMo]), and still later splitting, in conjoined twins.

Virtually all twins with monochorionic placentas, therefore, are monozygous (22) with the exception of monovular dispermic twins. Twins with dichorionic placentas, whether separate or fused, may be either dizygous or monozygous (20). Obviously, different fetal sex establishes a dizygous relation, but further investigation (blood group analysis, human leukocyte antigen [HLA] typing, DNA analysis) is required to determine zygosity in like-sex dichorionic twins (10,35). Studies of the frequencies of different placentation types indicate that about 75 percent of monozygous twins have monochorionic placentas (20). Overall, about 20 percent of twins with dichorionic placentas are monozygous.

Establishment of placentation type is important, not only as an initial step in determining zygosity, but primarily because it has an important relationship to the increased morbidity and mortality that occur in multiple gestations. Many factors contribute to the increased morbidity/mortality in multiples, most importantly the premature onset of labor and delivery, but type of placentation is also a significant risk factor. Twins with monochorionic placentas have much higher mortality rates than those with dichorionic placentas, and monoamnionic placentation is associated with a fetal mortality rate as high as 50 percent (20,40,69,70).

Multiple Pregnancy

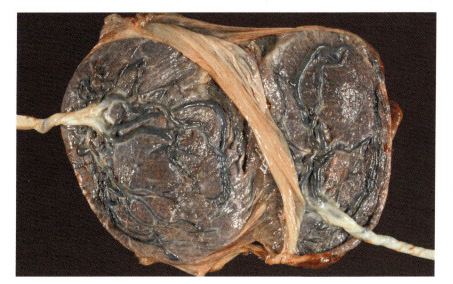

Figure 12-2

DIAMNIONIC DICHORIONIC FUSED TWIN PLACENTAS WITH IRREGULAR CHORIONIC FUSION

Fused membranes extend onto the placenta on the right, presumably due to differential expansion (left greater than right) of membranous sacs.

Figure 12-3

DIAMNIONIC DICHORIONIC TWIN PLACENTAS WITH IRREGULAR CHORIONIC FUSION

Fused membranes overlap placenta on right.

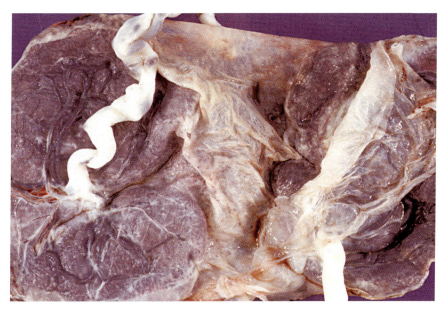

Placentation type can usually be reliably established on gross examination. Two entirely separate placentas are obviously dichorionic, each requiring routine examination (DiDi separate). Frequently, the discs are separate but the placentas have implanted close enough for the membranes to fuse or for the membranes of one twin to overlap the adjacent disc of the co-twin (figs. 12-2, 12-3). The latter phenomenon, termed irregular chorionic fusion, has been attributed to differential amniotic fluid pressure and expansion of the membranous sacs. When the blastocysts implant close to one another, the two placental discs fuse to form an apparently single disc with a dividing septum (DiDi fused). The principal task for the pathologist is to distinguish between the two types of single-disc twin placentas: diamnionic monochorionic and diamnionic dichorionic fused placentas.

The nature of the membranous septum and the pattern of chorionic vascularization are critical in this distinction. The septum in dichorionic fused placentas is relatively thick and variably opaque due to the presence of chorionic tissue between the two amnionic layers (fig. 12-4). Because each of the embryos is developing within its own chorion, any fusion between them will contain chorionic tissue. The chorionic tissue in

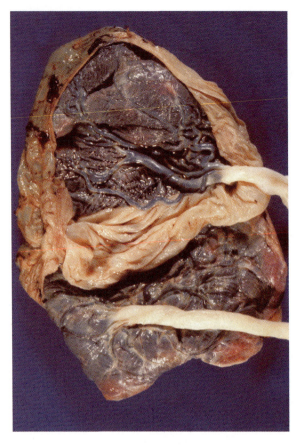

Figure 12-4

DIAMNIONIC DICHORIONIC TWIN PLACENTAS

Thick opaque membranous septum characteristic of diamnionic dichorionic (DiDi) fused twin placentas.

the septum is continuous with the underlying placenta, and therefore, remains firmly attached to the fetal surface. If the amnions are separated, chorionic tissue will remain as a ridge along the base of septal attachment. In contrast, the septum in a DiMo placenta is thin and translucent, composed of only two directly apposed layers of amnion (fig. 12-5). This septum, devoid of chorion, is easily detached from the placental surface. Some pathologists advocate peeling the dividing membrane at gross examination in order to identify placentas that require injection studies (see chapter 13).

The thickness of the membranous septum, and therefore the type of chorionicity, can be established by ultrasound prior to birth (38,110, 125). Histologic examination of the membranous septum confirms the gross impression. This is most easily accomplished in a section of rolled septal membranes (figs. 12-6–12-8), although identical information may be obtained from a section of the T zone where the septum meets the fetal surface (fig. 12-9). The latter method is particularly useful when the septal membrane has been torn or otherwise distorted and cannot be rolled, but this approach is technically more difficult, especially in monochorionic placentas. Fused chorion intervening between the amnions in the septum of dichorionic fused placentas is usually obvious (fig. 12-6), but on occasion, it may be scant or incomplete (fig. 12-7).

Figure 12-5

DIAMNIONIC MONOCHORIONIC TWIN PLACENTA

Velamentous cord inserts into a thin, transparent septum.

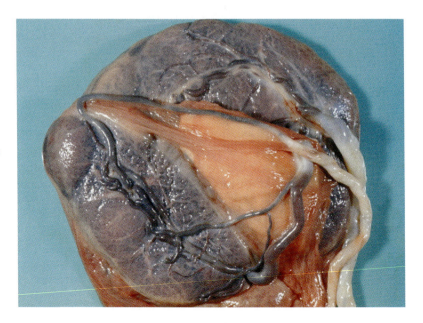

Multiple Pregnancy

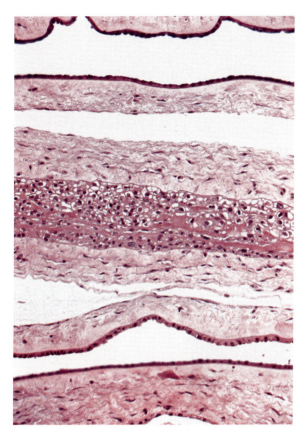

Figure 12-6

DIAMNIONIC DICHORIONIC TWIN PLACENTAS

Fused membranes with central fused chorion between amnions.

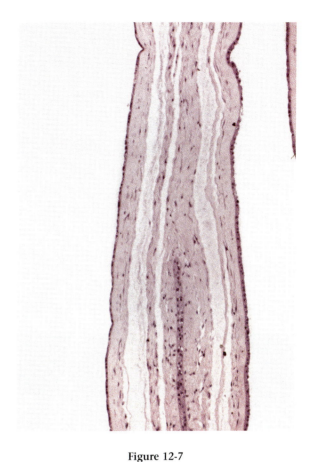

Figure 12-7

DIAMNIONIC DICHORIONIC TWIN PLACENTAS

The intervening chorion is usually abundant in DiDi septal membranes, but on occasion, it may be subtle or incomplete, as in this example.

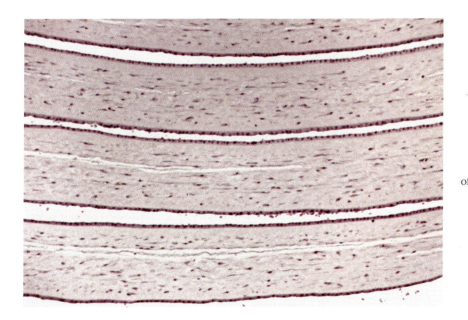

Figure 12-8

DIAMNIONIC MONOCHORIONIC TWIN PLACENTA

The septum has two layers of directly apposed amnions.

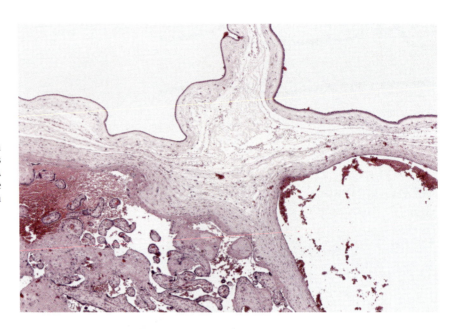

Figure 12-9

T ZONE IN DIAMNIONIC MONOCHORIONIC PLACENTA

The T zone is the region where the septal membranes intersect the chorionic plate. A section through the T zone provides the same information as a roll of septal membranes.

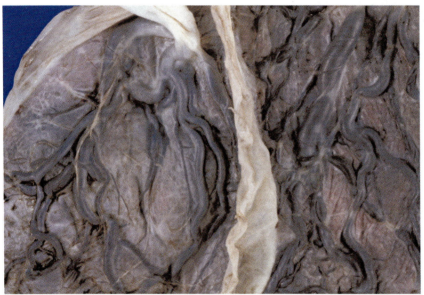

Figure 12-10

DIAMNIONIC DICHORIONIC FUSED PLACENTA

The vascular territories are discrete; they approach but do not cross the area of fusion.

The distribution of the fetal vessels on the chorionic plate is equally helpful in distinguishing DiDi fused from DiMo placentas. In dichorionic placentas, the septum represents the intimately apposed borders of the two fused placentas and, as such, defines the vascular equator of the two placentas. Therefore, in DiDi fused placentas, fetal chorionic vessels approach, but do not cross, the area of fusion (figs. 12-10, 12-11). In DiMo placentas, portions of the placenta are shared by both fetuses, and the two vascular districts are intimately intermingled (fig. 12-12). The position of the membranous septum in the DiMo placenta is independent of, and does not necessarily conform to, the vascular equator.

Vascular Anastomoses. An important feature of monochorionic placentas is the presence of vascular communications between the two fetal circulations. The fetal circulation is established when small vessels developing independently within the villous mesenchyme connect with larger vessels in the chorionic plate and body stalk. When twins share the same placenta (monochorionic), the potential exists for the

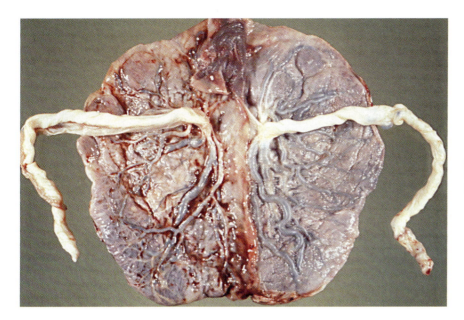

Figure 12-11
DIAMNIONIC DICHORIONIC FUSED TWIN PLACENTAS
The chorionic vascular pattern is better appreciated when the amnion is stripped, as on the left.

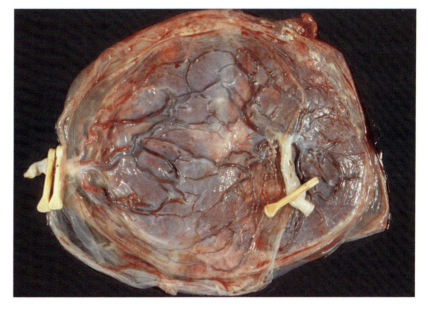

Figure 12-12
DIAMNIONIC MONOCHORIONIC TWIN PLACENTA
There is often intimate intermingling of the vascular districts to such a degree that it may be difficult to define a vascular equator.

two developing circulations to merge in a number of different ways. For example, the capillary bed supplied by an artery from one twin might establish continuity with a vein returning to its co-twin, resulting in a parenchymal arteriovenous anastomosis. Whether these connections are established purely by chance or are related to other factors, such as blood pressure or regional factors, is unknown. In contrast, the two circulations in dichorionic twins are established independently, explaining why vascular communications in DiDi fused placentas are absent, with rare exception.

It is generally agreed that some degree of vascular communication occurs in all monochorionic placentas, although the number, size, and type of anastomoses are highly variable. Anastomoses between large chorionic plate vessels are common. The majority of superficial large vessel anastomoses are between arteries; vein-to-vein anastomoses are much less common (fig. 12-13). Of greater physiologic significance are the arteriovenous anastomoses that occur within capillaries deep within the shared villous parenchyma (fig. 12-13). Vascular anastomoses may

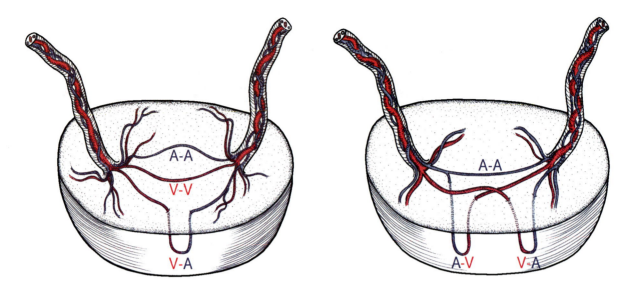

Figure 12-13

TYPES OF VASCULAR ANASTOMOSES IN MONOCHORIONIC PLACENTAS

Left: Large vessel anastomoses (artery-to-artery and vein-to-vein) are easily identified on gross exam. Arteriovenous anastomoses occur between capillaries deep in shared placental lobules. These cannot be seen on gross exam, but the presence of an unpaired artery penetrating the chorionic plate in the vicinity of an unpaired vein from its co-twin suggests the possibility of an underlying anastomosis.

Right: Superficial large vessel and deep capillary anastomoses may involve the same vessels (left).

be compound, with surface (large vessel) and parenchymal (villous capillary) connections involving the same vessels (fig. 12-13). Estimates of the frequencies of the types of inter-twin blood vessel anastomoses vary, but artery to artery anastomoses alone (20 to 28 percent of anastomoses) and artery to artery with arteriovenous anastomoses (25 to 40 percent) are the most common. Arteriovenous anastomoses alone, unmodified by concomitant large vessel anastomoses, are estimated to occur in 11 to 20 percent of cases.

The study of vascular anastomoses is facilitated by stripping the amnion from the fetal surface of the placenta. Large vessel anastomoses are easily identified grossly (fig. 12-14), and can be confirmed by moving blood back and forth between the contributing vessels or highlighted by the injection of milk, colored dye (fig. 12-15), or air (fig. 12-16). The size, diameter, location (central or peripheral), and type (arteries cross over veins) of anastomoses should be recorded. Arteriovenous anastomoses are potentially more important physiologically but are more difficult to identify as they occur between capillaries deep in the villous parenchyma and therefore cannot be directly visualized. Potential sites of arteriovenous anastomoses can be suspected when an unpaired artery from one twin penetrates the chorionic plate in close proximity to an unpaired vein from the co-twin (fig. 12-17). This configuration is highly suggestive of an underlying anastomosis, as chorionic plate arteries and veins are normally paired, penetrating the chorionic plate together.

A variety of perfusion techniques to document arteriovenous anastomoses have been described. They vary in complexity, but a simple method to confirm the presence of an arteriovenous anastomosis is to inject any colored substance (milk, dye) into the arterial branch supplying a suspected anastomosis and document its return to the venous district of the co-twin (fig. 12-15). The injection of air is particularly quick and easy, and has the advantage of displacing blood from the shared placental district; the resulting pallor allows estimation of the volume of shared parenchyma (see chapter 13). Injected colored substances may be seen in vessels even after histologic processing (12,29). Injection procedures can be repeated at multiple sites in an attempt to document the

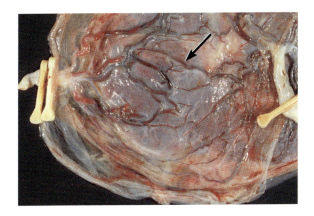

Figure 12-14

LARGE VESSEL ANASTOMOSES

Large vessel anastomoses, such as this artery-to-artery anastomosis, are common in diamnionic monochorionic (DiMo) placentas and are easily identified on gross inspection. Arteries cross over veins.

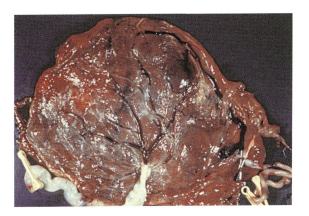

Figure 12-15

VASCULAR ANASTOMOSES

Any colored substance (here India ink) may be injected to highlight vascular anastomoses (here an artery-to-artery anastomosis).

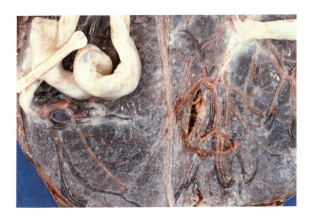

Figure 12-16

VASCULAR ANASTOMOSES

Vascular anastomoses are most easily confirmed by air injection. This DiMo placenta has a large artery-to-artery anastomosis. The vessels are pale because blood has been displaced by air. Air bubbles are seen on the left.

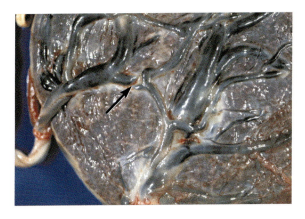

Figure 12-17

ARTERIOVENOUS ANASTOMOSES

Although arteriovenous anastomoses occur between capillaries deep in shared placental parenchyma and cannot be seen grossly, the presence of an unpaired artery penetrating the chorionic plate in the vicinity of an unpaired vein from the co-twin (arrow) is highly suggestive of underlying arteriovenous parenchymal vascular connections. Here an unpaired artery (from the umbilical cord barely visible at bottom) penetrates the chorionic plate adjacent to an unpaired, dilated vein associated with the cord at left.

number of anastomoses. It should be emphasized that all injection studies are qualitative and do not address the physiologic significance of the anastomosis: the overall balance of blood flow in vivo. Nevertheless their documentation is essential if vascular anastomosis is to be invoked as a cause of or contributor to discordant fetal growth (see below). Villous disruption results in leakage of injected material, thus compromising any injection techniques, and injection studies are generally precluded by prior fixation.

Rarely, a monochorionic placenta presents as two apparently distinct "discs," superficially resembling dichorionic separate placentas. The nature and position of the septum and the intermingling of the vascular districts with anastomosis identify these as monochorionic. The appearance of two separate discs is due to involution

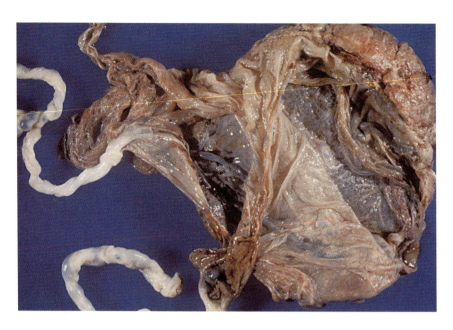

Figure 12-18

VELAMENTOUS CORD INSERTION

DiDi twin placenta with two velamentous cord insertions, one into the membranous septum.

or atrophy of the intervening villous tissue, perhaps because of factors related to the implantation site (over a uterine septum or leiomyoma) or irregular maternal blood supply (2).

Umbilical Cord, Chorionic Vascularity, and Placental Mass

Anomalies of the umbilical cord are more common in multiple than in singleton gestations (fig. 12-18). Kobac and Cohen (57) reported an incidence of velamentous cord insertion in twins that was nine times higher than in singletons. The frequency of anomalous insertion (marginal and velamentous) increases with the proximity of the twins, progressing from diamnionic separate to dichorionic fused to diamnionic monochorionic (13,34,70,99).

Anomalous cord insertion in multiples has the same significance as in singletons. Membranous vessels, especially vasa previa, are associated with compression, trauma, rupture, and fetal bleeding and thrombosis (fig. 12-19). Velamentous cords are associated with a number of additional complications including fetal malformations and low birth weight, and an increased risk of abortion, prematurity, polyhydramnios, abnormal presentation, premature rupture of membranes, and postpartum hemorrhage (48,81,103). Anomalous cord insertion may be accompanied by decreased chorionic vascularity and abnormal placental development (17,43). The placental capillary bed may be decreased in association with velamentous insertion thereby predisposing to fetal growth restriction (43). There is some evidence that velamentous cord insertion is a factor influencing twin-twin transfusion and associated early delivery (17,39,72,75).

Single artery cords are also more frequent in multiple gestations, occurring in approximately 3 percent of cases as compared to 0.53 percent of singletons (126). As in singletons, a single umbilical artery is associated with congenital malformations and impaired growth, and its frequency is greater in autopsied than in liveborn infants. The incidence of single umbilical artery is increased in velamentously inserted cords (fig. 12-19). Most twins are discordant for single umbilical artery, although concordance is greater in monozygous than dizygous twins. The length of the umbilical cord is on average 7.6 cm shorter in twins than singletons, and the incidence of hypocoiled cords is also increased (8,60,112).

The variation in the chorionic vascular pattern is the same in the placentas of multiples as in singletons. Because twins exhibit a higher frequency of anomalous cord insertion, there is a concomitant increase in variant chorionic vascular patterns. The pattern and adequacy of chorionic vascularization, the relative proportion of the chorionic surface populated by vessels from each twin, and the relative placental mass serving each twin are pertinent observations in

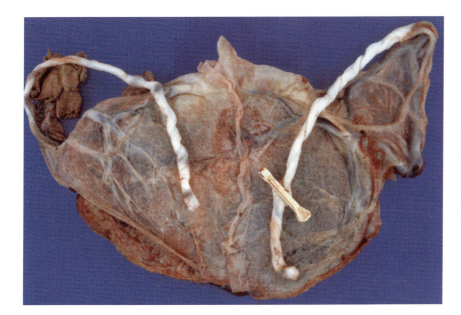

Figure 12-19

VELAMENTOUS CORD INSERTION

Velamentous cord insertion is greatly increased in multiple pregnancies. In this DiMo placenta, both cords insert velamentously. The thinner cord on the left also has a single umbilical artery, and there is an associated old clot, indicative of damage to membranous vessels.

multiple gestations. Dichorionic fused placentas may be divided and weighed. Estimates of relative placental mass in monochorionic twins should be based on the chorionic vasculature. The pattern of venous return may be a better indicator of placental supply than the arterial distribution. Not all discordantly grown twins have asymmetric placentas, and not all twins with asymmetric placentas are discordantly grown, but these associations are not uncommon. In twins with discordant placental mass, the smaller placenta is frequently associated with a lesser number of chorionic vessels. Whether the smaller placenta impairs the growth of the fetus, or both fetus and placenta are small secondary to another influence, is not always clear.

Monoamnionic Monochorionic Placentas

MoMo placentas are uncommon, accounting for less than 2 percent of twin gestations. In MoMo gestations, both twins develop within a single amnionic sac. The amnion commonly separates from the underlying chorion, and is often nearly completely detached at delivery. This finding explains why more apparently single sacs are artifactual than truly monoamnionic. Before considering a monochorionic placenta to be monoamnionic, the amnion between the cord insertions should be complete and continuous. Remnants of detached amnion and septum may be found encircling the cords or attached to the free membranes when carefully sought. Although membrane patterns are established early and persist throughout pregnancy, intragestational disruption of diamnionic septa has been reported. This suggests that at least some monoamnionic placentas may have been diamnionic originally (13,36,77).

The umbilical cords in MoMo gestations are typically very closely inserted, usually within 6 cm of each other (figs. 12-20–12-22). Rarely, there is partial cord fusion. Large vessel anastomoses are frequent but not invariable between the closely inserted cords (fig. 12-22). Arteriovenous parenchymal anastomoses also occur but are less significant clinically than in DiMo twins (see below).

Twins that share an amnionic cavity (monoamnionic) are at increased risk for cord entanglements. Entanglements around the neck or body parts of the co-twin occur in up to 22 percent of monoamnionic twins (68). Such entanglements may result not only in cord compression but in mistaken cord transection at delivery if one twin's cord is looped around its co-twin. The two cords are often entangled with each other and may be remarkably complex (fig. 12-23). Cord entanglements of all types are unquestionably a risk factor for monochorionic twins, with a reported frequency between 53 and 71 percent. Cord entanglement as a factor in fetal mortality is most common prior to 24 weeks while there is still sufficient room for fetal movement; after 30 to 32 weeks and in

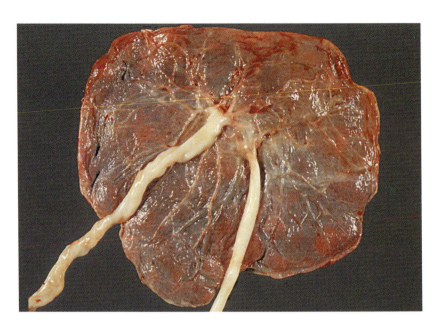

Figure 12-20

CORD INSERTION IN MONOAMNIOTIC MONOCHORIONIC PLACENTA

Close cord insertions, as seen here, are very common in monoamnionic monochorionic (MoMo) twin gestations.

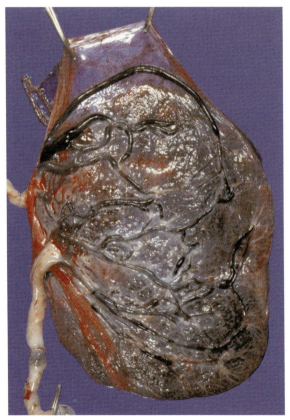

Figure 12-21

CORD INSERTION IN MONOAMNIONIC MONOCHORIONIC PLACENTA

This MoMo placenta shows marginal and velamentous cord insertions. A large membranous vessel is seen at top.

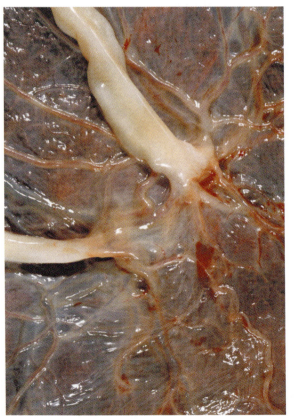

Figure 12-22

VASCULAR ANASTOMOSIS IN MONOAMNIONIC MONOCHORIONIC PLACENTA

Large vessel anastomoses are common in MoMo placentation. An artery-to-artery anastomosis is present between these closely inserted cords.

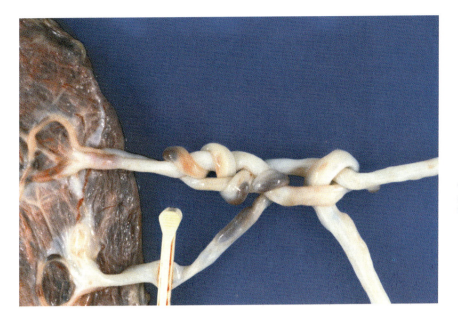

Figure 12-23

COMPLEX CORD ENTANGLEMENT IN MONOAMNIONIC MONOCHORIONIC PLACENTA

Cord entanglements are common in MoMo gestations and may be complicated, as in this case.

higher multiples, cord entanglement is less common as opportunity for movement decreases. The contribution of cord entanglement to fetal morbidity and mortality should be based on evidence of chronic vascular compromise, such as cord narrowing, grooving, edema, or thrombosis. Alternatively, entangled cords may not be a problem until the forces of labor result in acute vascular obstruction.

COMPLICATIONS OF MULTIPLE PREGNANCY

Twin-Twin Transfusion Syndrome

Vascular communications in monochorionic placentas create the potential for blood flow between the twins. When there is a net flow of blood from one twin to the other, different clinical manifestations result depending on the size, number, and type of vascular communications. Capillary-sized arteriovenous anastomoses involve the transfusion of small amounts of blood slowly over long periods of time (chronic transfusion). A large volume of blood can be transferred rapidly through large caliber chorionic plate vessels, often at the time of labor and delivery (acute transfusion). Not infrequently, both occur: an acute transfusion is superimposed on a chronic long-term process (acute on chronic transfusion). Large vessel anastomoses are likely to be bidirectional and arteriovenous connections are likely to be unidirectional.

Chronic Transfusion. *Definition and Etiology.* The chronic twin-twin transfusion syndrome is the most common form of twin-twin transfusion and is an important cause of perinatal mortality in monochorionic twins. Schatz (13, 56) proposed that the chronic twin-twin transfusion syndrome results when there is unbalanced flow of blood from one twin (the donor) to its co-twin (the recipient) through arteriovenous anastomoses deep within shared placental lobules (the "third circulation"). Chronic unidirectional diversion of blood results in anemia, relative deprivation, and growth retardation of the donor as compared to the larger, polycythemic recipient. Hypervolemia and hypertension in the recipient result in increased urine output and polyhydramnios, while hypotension and hypovolemia in the donor lead to oliguria, oligohydramnios, and decreased movement (the "stuck" twin) in the donor (18). Either twin may be hydropic. Commonly, cardiac dysfunction and congestive heart failure result in hydrops in the recipient, although the donor too, may develop hydrops on the basis of profound anemia.

Although the presence of vascular anastomoses is a necessary precondition for the development of the twin-twin transfusion syndrome, factors beyond shifts of blood may contribute. Several additional/alternative pathophysiologic mechanisms have been proposed (67). Differential serum protein concentration and colloid osmotic pressure between the twins, presumably due to chronic protein transfer from donor to recipient, may result in increased fluid absorption by the relatively hyperproteinemic recipient, with consequent edema and hydramnios. A higher concentration of atriopeptin, an atrium-derived peptide produced in response to blood volume overload, has been found in the recipient twin, presumably causing increased fetal urine production and polyhydramnios (88). Velamentous cord insertion is significantly more common in monochorionic gestations with the twin-twin transfusion syndrome (39). It has been proposed that velamentous cords are more easily compressed, resulting in decreased umbilical vein flow to the donor and enhancement of flow through arteriovenous anastomoses to the recipient. Others have speculated that polyhydramnios may contribute to umbilical and chorionic vessel compression, providing the therapeutic rationale for amniocentesis (121). The possibility that the donor twin produces growth stimuli that enhance growth of the better perfused recipient has been proposed by Vetter (119). Other factors that potentially affect flow dynamics include fetal blood pressure, heart rate, and movement.

The clinical definition of the twin-twin transfusion syndrome is imprecise. The diagnosis is complicated because twins may show asymmetric growth for reasons other than a chronic twin-twin transfusion (maternal, fetal, umbilical cord, or placental factors). A hemoglobin concentration difference of greater than 5 g/100 mL and a twin weight difference of 15 to 20 percent are considered definitive criteria by some, although similar weight and hemoglobin discrepancies are just as common in dichorionic twins without an anatomic basis for transfusion (26,71, 100). Conversely, hemoglobin concentrations in twins with the chronic twin-twin transfusion syndrome may be similar if the donor's compensatory hematopoiesis has been sufficient.

A relatively selective criterion is a recipient heart weight that is 2 to 4 times that of the donor. This feature is generally not present in any other process resulting in twin weight/growth discordance. The disparity in heart weight/size is due not only to a generalized growth differential but also to the increased cardiac work load associated with the hypervolemia, hypertension, and hyperviscosity experienced by the recipient twin. Heart size discrepancy may be the first manifestation of the chronic twin-twin transfusion syndrome, evident on ultrasound as early as 10 weeks. A difference in overall fetal size is usually apparent only later in gestation. Discrepant amnionic fluid volumes, hydrops, or congestive heart failure, and a stuck twin are other ultrasound findings very suggestive of the twin-twin transfusion syndrome.

Prevalence. The lack of uniformly applied criteria for the diagnosis of the twin-twin transfusion syndrome and the variability in its severity and clinical expression explain in part the great variation in its reported frequency, which ranges from 5 to 30 percent of monochorionic gestations. Recent studies indicate close correspondence between the number of cases of well-documented twin-twin transfusion and the number of monochorionic twin placentas with arteriovenous anastomoses without concomitant large vessel anastomoses, the specific pattern of vascular anastomoses most often associated with twin-twin transfusion (12,31,70). This occurs in 9 to 20 percent of monochorionic gestations. Superficial vascular anastomoses appear to mitigate against the effects of arteriovenous transfusion, probably by allowing transfer of blood back to the donor from the recipient. In the absence of superficial anastomoses, arteriovenous transfusions are uncompensated, resulting in marked growth discordance, hydramnios, early delivery, and high rates of perinatal mortality.

The twin-twin transfusion syndrome is not a significant cause of fetal mortality in monoamnionic twins presumably because the majority of such twins have large vessel anastomoses, which are known to modify parenchymal connections. In addition, any intra-amnionic pressure differences that potentially could affect blood flow in diamnionic twins would be equalized in monoamnionic twins. For unexplained reasons, the twin-twin transfusion syndrome is more common in females (6,8).

Gross and Microscopic Findings. After delivery, there is a marked discrepancy in the size and appearance of the infants and their corresponding placental territories (fig. 12-24). The donor twin is smaller, pale, and anemic; the recipient is heavier, edematous, plethoric, and polycythemic. Either twin may be hydropic. Classically, there is marked discordance in the size and

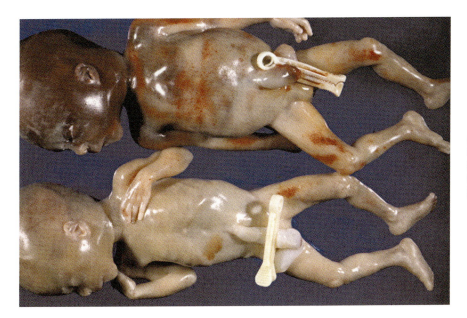

Figure 12-24

TWIN-TWIN TRANSFUSION SYNDROME

Twin-twin transfusion syndrome in which both twins died. The donor twin (bottom) is smaller and pale. The recipient twin (top) is larger and plethoric.

Figure 12-25

TWIN-TWIN TRANSFUSION SYNDROME

Marked discrepancy in size and weight of the fetal organs (especially the heart) is seen in this twin-twin transfusion syndrome, with twin death early in the second trimester. A reversal of the expected pattern, with congestion of the smaller (donor) organs and pallor of the larger (recipient) organs, suggests that the donor died first with subsequent exsanguination of the recipient into the relaxed donor circulation.

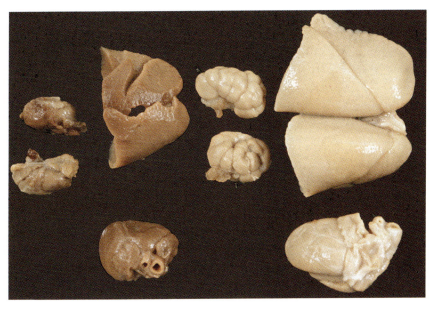

weight of the fetal organs: the organs of the recipient are larger and heavier than those of the donor (fig. 12-25). The recipient's heart, especially, is comparatively enlarged, and there is myocardial hypertrophy involving all chambers, with thickened ventricular walls. Smooth muscle mass is increased in the media of pulmonary and systemic arteries and arterioles (fig. 12-26) (37,59). Pulmonary arterial calcification, presumably related to increased cardiac output, has been described in the recipient twin (96,106). The donor heart is usually subnormal in size, and arterial muscle mass is decreased. Glomeruli are enlarged, up to twice normal size in the recipient twin, and they are either normal or reduced in size in the donor (fig. 12-27) (85,86). Discrepancies in renal tubular development and tubular dilatation have also been documented (87,92).

The placental territories of the donor and recipient twins may also be discordant (fig. 12-28). The donor's placental territory may be large, bulky, and pale, reflecting fetal anemia. The villi are large and edematous with numerous Hofbauer

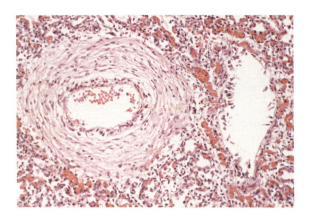 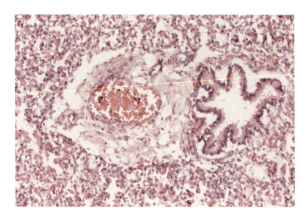

Figure 12-26

TWIN-TWIN TRANSFUSION SYNDROME

Increased smooth muscle media of recipient's pulmonary arteries (left) as compared to donor's (right).

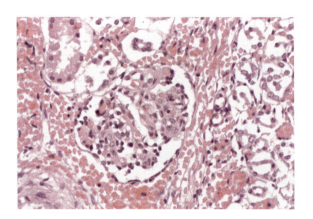 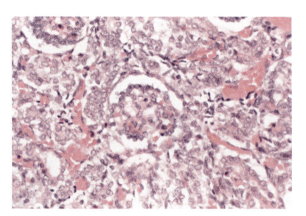

Figure 12-27

TWIN-TWIN TRANSFUSION SYNDROME

Glomeruli are much larger in the recipient twin (left) as compared to those of the donor (right).

cells and small capillaries containing nucleated red blood cells (figs. 12-29, 12-30). In other cases, the donor's placenta has been described as pale and atrophied. Amnion nodosum may be found when there is associated oligohydramnios. The recipient's placental territory is generally smaller, firm, and deep red. The villi are appropriately mature with dilated and intensely congested vessels (figs. 12-31, 12-32).

Clinical Features. Typically, the chronic twin-twin transfusion syndrome is clinically manifest in the second trimester, with acute hydramnios and growth discrepancy between the twins, but it may be suspected earlier based on the ultrasound demonstration of differential amnionic fluid volumes. Hydramnios may cause maternal discomfort or lead to respiratory compromise, and therapeutic amniocentesis may be required to relieve symptoms.

The consequences of the twin-twin transfusion syndrome are grave. Mortality rates are as high as 70 to 100 percent depending on the gestational age at diagnosis and delivery. The earlier the syndrome is manifest, the more likely the outcome will be fatal. Hydrops is also correlated with poor survival (46). When the condition develops in the second trimester, it is usually associated with preterm labor and death of one or both fetuses, or significant morbidity if the neonates survive. Both twins are at great risk.

Multiple Pregnancy

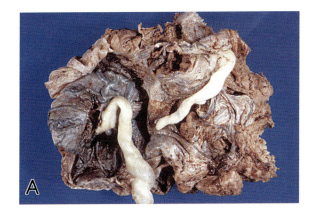

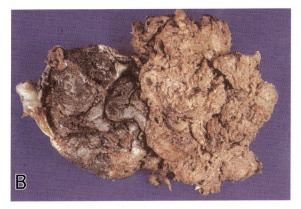

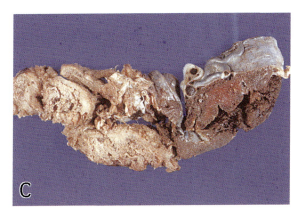

Figure 12-28

TWIN-TWIN TRANSFUSION SYNDROME

The donor's placental territory is large and pale in comparison to the recipient's territory, which is smaller and intensely congested. Fetal surface (A), maternal surface (B), and cut section (C). The twins, delivered at 32 weeks, survived but both are severely handicapped. (Figs. 12-28 through 12-32 are from the same patient.)

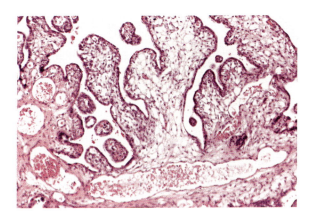

Figure 12-29

TWIN-TWIN TRANSFUSION SYNDROME

The donor villi are relatively immature, large, and edematous.

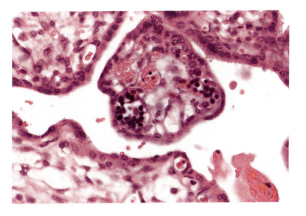

Figure 12-30

TWIN-TWIN TRANSFUSION SYNDROME

Numerous immature erythroid precursors in the donor's placental territory indicate fetal anemia.

The recipient twin is subject to cardiac failure, hemolytic jaundice, kernicterus, and thrombosis due to hemoconcentration. The donor twin may be severely anemic or hypoglycemic and is at risk for ischemic lesions. Both twins are likely to suffer from the additional complications of prematurity. Multiorgan necrotic lesions, including white matter infarcts, leukoencephalopathy, hydranencephaly, porencephaly, intestinal atresia, renal cortical necrosis, and

Placental Pathology

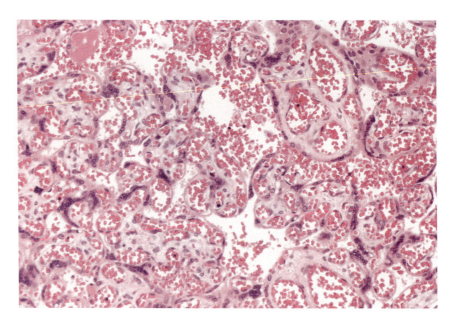

Figure 12-31

TWIN-TWIN TRANSFUSION SYNDROME

Recipient's villi are appropriately mature but intensely congested.

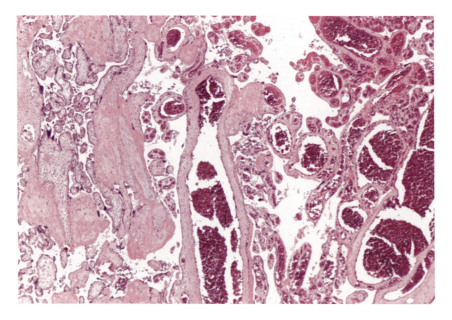

Figure 12-32

TWIN-TWIN TRANSFUSION SYNDROME

Donor (left) and recipient (right) placental territories.

aplasia cutis (fig. 12-33), may occur in either or both twins regardless of whether one, both, or neither survives (30). Initial speculation that such necrotic lesions are mediated by the transfer of thromboplastin from a dead twin to the surviving co-twin via intra-twin anastomoses has been disproved by prenatal blood sampling studies demonstrating no evidence of abnormal coagulation parameters in this setting (89,93). These lesions are now attributed to the altered hemodynamics, transitory cardiovascular compromise, and hypoperfusion associated with complex, fluctuating placental vascular connections.

Although most chronic transfusions progress, some fluctuate or even reverse. If one twin dies in utero and the transfusion ceases, the situation may resolve itself. Alternatively, the surviving twin (usually the recipient) may exsanguinate into the suddenly relaxed circulatory system of the dead co-twin (usually the donor) (see fig. 12-25). Acute hypotension, and possibly blood loss after twin death, is considered

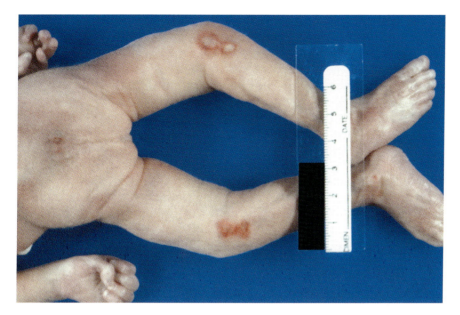

Figure 12-33

TWIN-TWIN TRANSFUSION SYNDROME

Both twins had ischemic lesions including the aplasia cutis seen here in the donor.

a likely explanation for necrotic lesions in the surviving twin, a view supported by Doppler studies showing dramatic umbilical-flow velocity changes in the surviving twin (42,53,62,66). It has been estimated that neurologic sequelae occur in as many as 27 percent of surviving twins (67). Cerebral lesions have been demonstrated sonographically in twins at birth and in utero, developing rapidly in some cases (11,49, 50,111). These observations are important in attempting to explain the high incidence of cerebral palsy in twins, reportedly five times the incidence in singletons and affecting primarily monozygous twins. Recognizing that lesions predictive of cerebral palsy are of prenatal onset is important not only in medicolegal considerations but also when contemplating the possible consequences of intentional fetal reduction for the surviving twin.

The almost uniform mortality associated with early and severe twin-twin transfusion has stimulated attempts to interrupt the process with the hope of saving at least one of the twins. Management strategies have included treatment with indomethacin to reduce fetal urine output and polyhydramnios, digoxin to treat congestive heart failure, decompressive amniocentesis to prolong pregnancy and affect fetal blood flow, division of intervening membranes, selective feticide, and laser ablation of anastomoses. The latter approach requires accurate prenatal mapping of physiologically significant arteriovenous anastomoses and their successful ablation in vivo. Although presently at the limit of technical feasibility, this procedure is reportedly successful in many cases, although most are uncontrolled, and the definition of success is a single surviving twin (27,28). Increasingly sophisticated Doppler studies are used to tailor treatment strategies to individual vascular patterns and to assess the results of intervention. Pathologic documentation of laser sites, with confirmation of anastomotic interruption and mapping of residual anastomoses, plays an important part in this emerging treatment strategy. The enthusiasm for intervention must be tempered by the knowledge that the two fetal circulations are connected and that any manipulation will potentially affect both fetuses. Given the complexity and uniqueness of the vascular anatomy, it is difficult if not impossible to predict the consequences.

Acute Transfusion. Plethora of one twin and pallor of the other do not always signify a chronic transfusion, but may instead reflect acute shifts of blood through large superficial vascular anastomoses. Significant shifts of a large blood volume may occur rapidly through these large vessel connections. Simple acute transfusions are usually diagnosed at birth. The donor is pale and the recipient plethoric, but there is no growth differential. Hemoglobin and hematocrit levels are equal in initial assessments, but eventually, fluid equilibration will unmask the anemia and the disparity between the twins. Acute transfusions may occur when one twin experiences circulatory collapse for whatever reason or when a twin exsanguinates through the unclamped cord of its delivered co-twin. Although simple clinically documented acute transfusion is rare, silent cases occurring in utero may account for the dramatic increase in cerebral palsy in like-sex twins.

Acute on Chronic Transfusion. Superimposition of acute transfusion on established chronic transfusion is more common than simple acute transfusion, and when this occurs, there is reversal of the expected pattern of pallor/plethora in the donor/recipient twins, with plethora of the smaller, original donor twin and pallor of the larger, recipient twin (fig. 12-25). Whether this pattern develops when the donor dies and the recipient's blood drains into the donor's flaccid vascular tree, or the acute transfusion occurs first, overwhelming the capacity of the donor's heart leading to death, is unknown. Both mechanisms may be operative. Acute transfusion also occurs as a complication of intervention to alleviate the affects of chronic transfusion. On occasion, an acute transfusion, fetomaternal hemorrhage, or both occur in twins with discordant growth for reasons unrelated to chronic transfusion. While this scenario may mimic an acute on chronic transfusion, lack of evidence for adaptation to chronic transfusion (no discrepancy in heart size or polyhydramnios/oligohydramnios) helps exclude chronic transfusion as a relevant contributing factor.

Asymmetric Growth

Established growth standards for twin gestations indicate that the growth curves for both dichorionic and monochorionic twins approximate those of singletons prior to 34 weeks (3,95,109). Thereafter, twins weigh progressively less than singletons as pregnancy advances. When twin growth is discordant, the larger twin approximates the growth of an age-matched singleton, and the growth rate of the smaller twin slows and may gradually decline into the range of growth restriction (small for gestational age [SGA]). In dichorionic twins, growth discordancy usually manifests around 25 weeks, but in monochorionic twins, the onset of growth discordance is more variable, commencing in some cases as early as 18 to 20 weeks.

Twin birth weight discordance is strongly associated with preterm birth, perinatal death, and postnatal morbidity (21). The majority of twins with discordant growth are dichorionic, and even among monochorionic twins, twin-twin transfusion is not the most common cause of growth discrepancy (123).

While a chronic transfusion may be a significant factor in some cases, even when it occurs, other factors may contribute as much or more to discordant growth. Cord anomalies, including velamentous insertion and single umbilical artery, are associated with decreased fetal weight, and both are much more frequent in twin gestations, increasing with the proximity of the twins (monochorionic greater than dichorionic fused greater than dichorionic separate). In one recent study, peripheral cord insertion (velamentous, marginal, and markedly eccentric) was the strongest predictor of discordant growth and SGA in dichorionic and monochorionic twins (99).

Velamentous and marginal cord insertion are thought to be the result of differential placental growth, with displacement from the site of original implantation (trophotropism), resulting from intrauterine crowding in twin gestation. Peripheral cord insertion may be accompanied by differences in placental vascularization: higher Doppler S/D ratios and lower numbers of small muscular arteries in tertiary villi have been demonstrated in the smaller of discordant twins with peripheral cord insertion.

Discordant birth weight is also associated with placental mass: smaller babies have smaller placentas (12,47). Since the fetal-placental weight ratio in smaller twins is normal to decreased, maternal vascular insufficiency is unlikely to be a major cause of impaired growth. Rather, poor placentation with asymmetric trophotropism and abnormal cord insertion, asymmetric placental volume, and decreased placental vascularization are the major causative factors in growth restriction and twin growth discordance.

These factors may explain the coexistence of oligohydramnic, growth restricted, and polyhydramnic larger twins (twin oligohydramnios-polyhydramnios sequence [TOPS]) in dichorionic gestations and in monochorionic gestations in

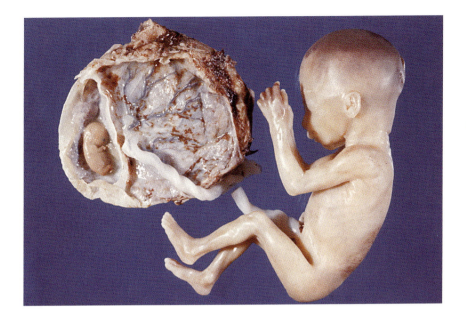

Figure 12-34

DISCORDANT DIAMNIONIC DICHORIONIC EMBRYO/ FETAL TWIN DEMISE

which twin-twin transfusion has been carefully excluded by marker erythrocyte studies (18). Theoretically, asymmetric placental development and discrepant vascular resistance may eventuate in interfetal shunts and twin-twin transfusion in some cases. Whether placental and fetal growth asymmetry reflect a generalized problem in the conceptus, or result from a primary placental problem, is unclear.

While discordant parenchymal lesions present a possible explanation for growth asymmetry, most placental disease processes involve twin placentas to a similar degree; concordance for most findings is higher than might be expected based on their prevalence in singleton placentas (100). In one recent study, the only finding significantly associated with discordant SGA twins was the presence of fibrotic avascular villi (100). This lesion, indicative of proximal fetal vascular occlusion (fetal thrombotic vasculopathy) and associated with neurologic impairment in term infants, may contribute to the increased morbidity and mortality in twins.

Intragestational Fetal Loss

Multiple fetuses have higher mortality rates at all stages of gestation and after birth. The causes of intrauterine twin death vary with gestational age but are essentially the same as in singletons (see chapter 9, Intrauterine Fetal Death), with the important addition of the specific complications of monochorionic placentation. Monochorionic twins are greatly overrepresented among twin deaths at all gestational ages, confirming the significant contribution of placentation type to twin demise (69,70).

The pathologic findings in intragestational fetal loss depend on the time of fetal death and the duration of retention in utero. One or both twins may die, concordantly or discordantly, and they may be delivered at intervals or retained and delivered together (fig. 12-34). Careful monitoring indicates that there is a high rate of loss in the earliest weeks of pregnancy. A large percentage of aborted twin embryos/early fetuses are monochorionic, and like singletons aborted at this stage, the majority are grossly abnormal, with growth disorganization and demonstrated chromosomal abnormalities. Both twins may die as embryos or one may die as an embryo and the other as a fetus.

Vanishing Twin. Twin gestations are commonly converted to singletons with the embryonic/early fetal death of one twin (vanishing twin). Levi (64) demonstrated that of twins diagnosed before 10 weeks, 71 percent were born as singletons; similar findings were reported by Robinson and Caines (102). When a twin dies early in the first trimester, it may be difficult or impossible to identify any residue. Frequently, only a flattened mass of sclerotic placenta remains as a vaguely thickened area of membranes, either adjacent to, separated from, or superimposed on the disc of the surviving co-twin (fig.

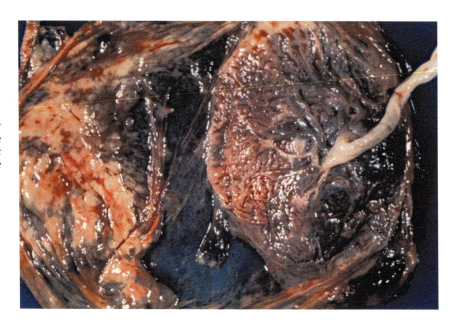

Figure 12-35

VANISHING TWIN

In this example of very early twin death (vanishing twin), the only residue is a mass of sclerotic placenta separated from the survivor's disc.

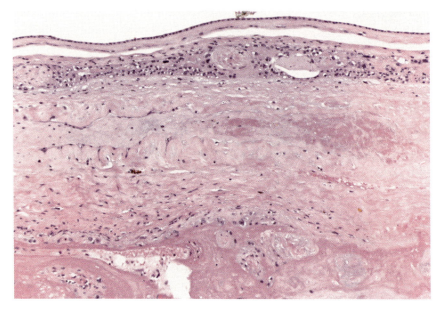

Figure 12-36

PLACENTAL REMNANT IN TWIN DEMISE

Fused DiDi septal membranes overlie the collapsed gestational sac and atrophied placenta of the dead twin. A fetal remnant was not identified.

12-35). On careful inspection, a collapsed gestational sac, sometimes containing an embryonic remnant, may be discerned (figs. 12-36, 12-37). Microscopic examination may establish the nature of the membranous septum and thus, chorionicity (fig. 12-36). When identified, the dead twin is often severely degenerated, generally providing few clues as to the cause of death (fig. 12-38). Elective reduction, usually undertaken in induced multiples early in pregnancy (10 to 12 weeks), is becoming increasingly common. While not the subject of systematic study, it is our collective impression that reduced embryonic remnants are more easily identified than those of spontaneous death (fig. 12-39).

Fetus Papyraceus. The death of a twin in the second trimester may result in delivery of both twins or delivery of the dead twin only, with the pregnancy continuing with the survivor (interval delivery). Alternatively, the dead fetus may be retained, and progressively compressed and flattened by the growth of the co-twin. Depending on the length of retention, this flattened dead twin, a fetus papyraceus, is variably altered

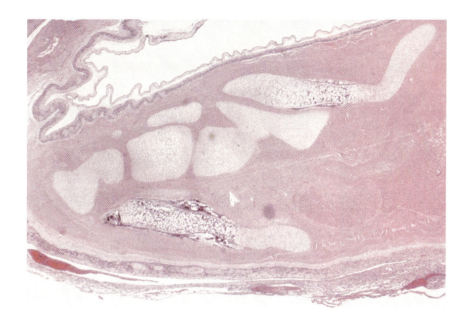

Figure 12-37

EARLY TWIN DEMISE

A necrotic fetal remnant is present beneath necrotic amnion in this case of early fetal loss.

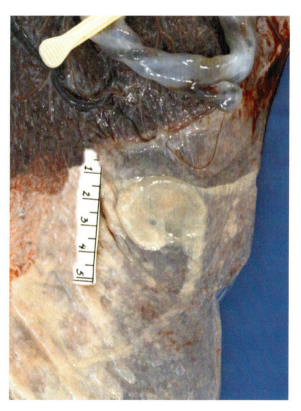

Figure 12-38

EARLY TWIN DEMISE

The fetal remnant is obvious but markedly degenerated in this case of early fetal loss.

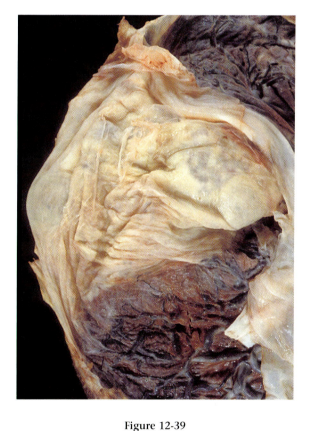

Figure 12-39

MULTIPLE PREGNANCY WITH ELECTIVE REDUCTION

After elective reduction, fetal remnants are usually relatively easily identified, as in this case in which two reduced embryos are present in the membranes. The corresponding placental territories are reduced to areas of slight thickening.

Placental Pathology

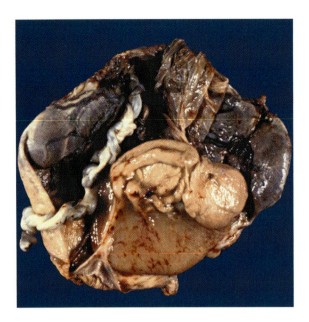

Figure 12-40

FETUS PAPYRACEUS

The fetus papyraceus is easily recognized.

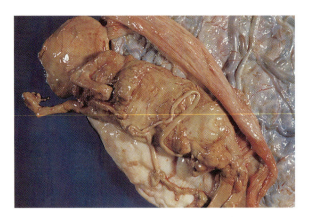

Figure 12-41

FETUS PAPYRACEUS

This fetus papyraceus exhibits more advanced degenerative changes. Its relatively firm and pale placental territory is visible beneath.

(figs. 12-40–12-43). Some are still easily recognizable and others resemble amorphous necrotic material and are easily overlooked. Specimen radiographs may reveal skeletal remnants. It has been estimated that the creation of a fetus papyraceus takes about 10 weeks, and can occur in both monochorionic and dichorionic gestations. The degree of maceration generally precludes the establishment of cause of death, although anomalous cord insertion and twin-twin transfusion syndrome have been implicated in many cases (7,55). The corresponding placenta is generally pale, thinned, and sclerotic, with avascular, fibrotic villi enmeshed in fibrin (figs. 12-43, 12-44). In some cases, it may be difficult to identify a placenta at all. In monochorionic gestations with large anastomoses, the placental territory of the dead twin may be maintained by the live one. The amnionic cavity of the fetus papyraceus is gradually compressed as the amnionic fluid is resorbed.

Survivors of Co-Twin Demise. A variety of abnormalities, including intestinal atresia, skin defects, amputations, gastroschisis, and especially brain damage, have been reported in twins surviving the in utero death of a co-twin (4,7,9,66,74,105,116,120). The risk of serious cerebral damage in surviving twins is reportedly around 20 percent and may be even higher in certain subsets (94). Monochorionic twins appear to be primarily at risk (4,11,41,51,54,63,78,94,108,116,118,122,127). At all gestational ages, the risk of cerebral palsy is higher in like-sex surviving co-twins (121). The similarity of the lesions seen in surviving co-twins to those attributed to complex vascular anastomoses in monochorionic twins suggests a similar mechanism. If so, it is unlikely that obstetric intervention, however prompt, would prevent such damage to the co-twin. Survivors of a twin death also have a higher postnatal mortality rate.

Duplication Abnormalities

Occasional monozygous twins are far from identical, and instead show marked discrepancies in size and configuration. Others show varying degrees of incomplete separation. Asymmetric and incomplete duplications include acardiac, parasitic, and conjoined fetuses. A *parasitic twin* is a variably developed fetiform mass attached to its co-twin either internally or externally (fig. 12-45). *Conjoined twins* retain their overall symmetry but are incompletely separated or possibly secondarily fused during development (114,115). Neither shows specific placental abnormalities (fig. 12-46).

Acardiac twinning is the most common asymmetric duplication anomaly, occurring in 1 percent of monochorionic twins (41). The acardius

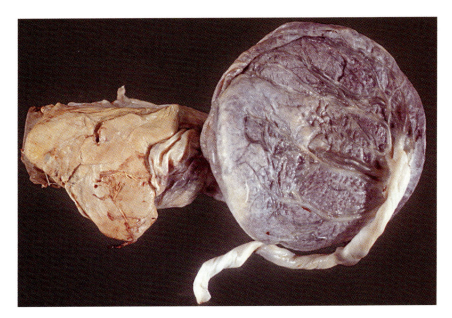

Figure 12-42
FETUS PAPYRACEUS
This fetus papyraceus is barely recognizable as such.

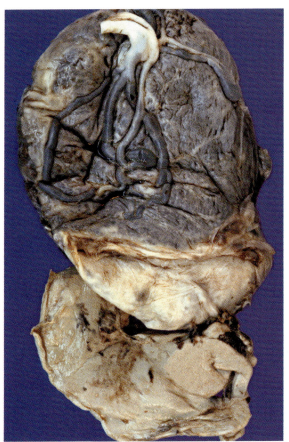

Figure 12-43
FETUS PAPYRACEUS
The placental territory of this fetus papyraceus is markedly firm and pale.

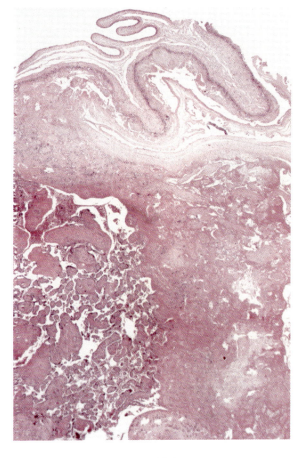

Figure 12-44
FETUS PAPYRACEUS, PLACENTA
The placental villi of the dead fetus are necrotic and enmeshed in fibrin in contrast to the viable placenta of the co-twin.

Placental Pathology

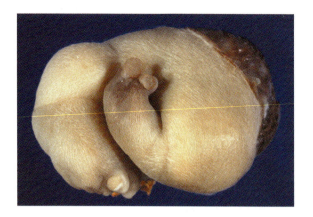 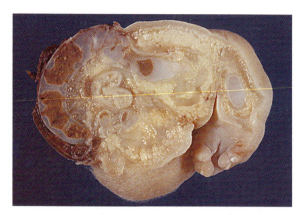

Figure 12-45

PARASITIC TWIN

Left: A parasitic twin removed from the abdominal cavity of its co-twin.
Right: Cut section.

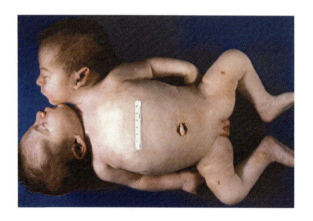 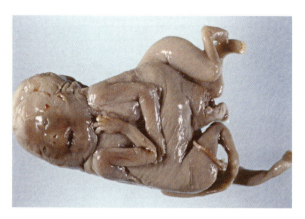

Figure 12-46

CONJOINED TWINS

Two examples of the many variants of conjoined twins.

is a grossly malformed, often bizarre fetus of variable size, appearance, and degree of organogenesis. No two are alike (44,107). Some are amorphous, shapeless masses resembling teratomas (fig. 12-47) and others are remarkably well developed (fig. 12-48). Commonly, acardiac fetuses have relatively well-developed legs and perineal structures, a trunk into which the umbilical cord inserts, and a rounded, dome-like upper body (fig. 12-49). A single body cavity may contain abdominal viscera, but thoracic structures and the heart are typically absent, although cardiac remnants or a deformed heart are identified on occasion. Organ development is highly variable: some acardiac twins demonstrate an absence of most organs, while in others, the organs are well developed. Acardiac twins may be hydropic, sometimes larger than the co-twin, with associated hydramnios (76).

Regardless of gross appearance, degree of development, or organogenesis, the essential feature common to all acardiac fetuses is their circulation, which is maintained entirely by the co-twin (the "pump" twin). Blood from the normal pump twin reaches the acardiac through an artery-to-artery anastomosis, flows through the acardiac in reverse course, then returns to the normal twin through a vein-to-vein anastomosis (fig. 12-50). The majority of acardiac twins have a single umbilical artery, although some

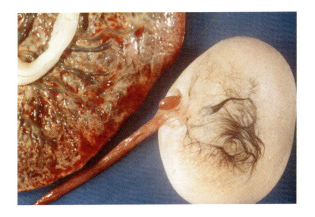

Figure 12-47

ACARDIAC FETUS

This acardiac fetus is an amorphous tissue mass with a patch of hair and an umbilical cord with a single umbilical artery.

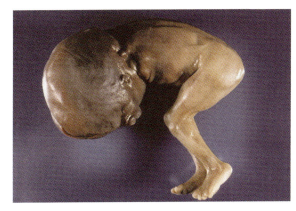

Figure 12-48

ACARDIAC FETUS

This acardiac fetus has well-developed lower extremities and head, but lacks a thoracic cavity.

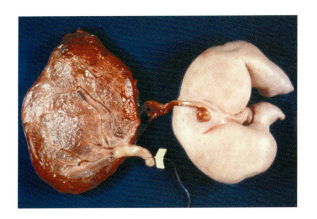
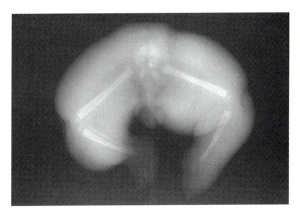

Figure 12-49

ACARDIAC FETUS

Left: This is a relatively common appearance of an acardiac fetus with a recognizable pelvis and lower extremities, and a dome-shaped upper body.
Right: A radiographic view.

have three vessel cords (82). Reverse blood flow has been documented sonographically (24,95,128). The vascular anastomoses are often quite large, occurring at the level of the umbilical cord or chorionic plate. The acardiac has no placental parenchymal vascular connections and is, therefore, analogous to a conjoined twin and not to a twin-twin transfusion. The joining of the twins at the level of the chorionic circulation is emphasized in the alternative designation, *chorangiopagus parasiticus (CAPP)*, which is preferred by some. Alternatively, the term *twin reversed arterial perfusion (TRAP)*, emphasizes the proposed vascular pathophysiology.

These specific placental vascular connections between the acardiac and normal co-twin establish the diagnosis. They occur in monochorionic placentas, either diamnionic or monoamnionic, although monoamnionic placentation is especially prevalent among acardiac twin gestations (82). Acardiac twins are greatly over-represented in triplet and higher multiple gestations (52). In diamnionic placentas, amnion nodosum may accompany the acardiac fetus.

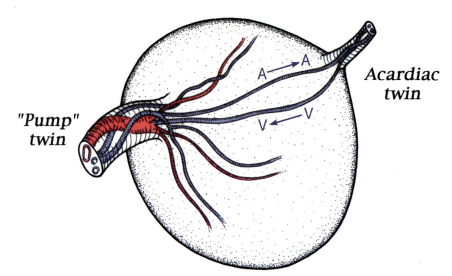

Figure 12-50

ACARDIAC FETUS

The circulation in all acardiac twins is accomplished by the co-twin ("pump" twin). Blood reaches the acardiac via a large artery-to-artery anastomosis, circulates through the acardiac in reverse direction, and returns to the pump twin via a large vein-to-vein anastomosis. Blood returning from the acardiac to the pump twin is still deoxygenated. (Modified from figure 25.89 from reference 13.)

The pump twin is at risk for cardiovascular overload. The extra work involved in circulating blood through the acardiac twin may result in cardiomegaly and high output failure, in some cases associated with hydrops and hydramnios. Pump twins also tend to be growth impaired, perhaps because blood is diverted away from the placenta toward the acardiac twin, which returns still deoxygenated. Many pump twins have congenital anomalies (108).

Strategies similar to those employed in management of the twin-twin transfusion syndrome (indomethacin, umbilical cord ligation and occlusion, selective removal, and ablation of connecting vessels) have been successful in ameliorating the effects of cardiac overload in the pump twin (5,104).

An ongoing debate is whether the acardiac fetus results from 1) primary agenesis of the heart with continued maintenance only by specific vascular connections with its co-twin; or 2) aberrant circulation as the primary event causing secondary regression of the heart. As detailed by Van Allen (117), development of an acardiac fetus requires the establishment of vascular connections in early gestation and eventual assumption of the entire circulation by the pump twin. Whether the establishment of this circulatory arrangement requires some degree of primary developmental discordance between the twins (asymmetric duplication, chromosomal abnormalities, body stalk anomalies) is unknown. Once established, the altered blood flow could result in developmental abnormalities and progressive degenerative changes in the heart and other tissues. The timing and initiation of anastomotic flow, flow volume, degree of degenerative change, and possible initial developmental discordance are all factors that could influence the ultimate form assumed by the acardiac twin.

Cytogenetic analysis of acardiac and pump twins has yielded variable results. Abnormal karyotypes have been identified in some but not all twin sets. One case of triploid acardiac/diploid twinning has been attributed to fertilization of an oocyte and its first polar body (15).

HIGHER MULTIPLE BIRTHS

Examination of placentas from higher multiple births is merely an extension of the observations applied to twins (fig. 12-51). The chorionicity, membrane relationships, cord insertion, chorionic vascularity, potential vascular anastomoses, and relative placental volumes should be assessed as in twins. Patterns of placentation vary depending on zygosity. Triplets, for example, may be monochorionic, dichorionic (fig. 12-52), or trichorionic (fig. 12-53), with all possible combinations of amnionic sacs. Multichorionic placentas are usually fused as space in the uterus is limited. Combinations of monozygous and polyzygous multiples are common.

Higher Multiple Birth Triplets

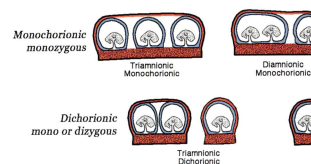

Figure 12-51
PATTERNS OF PLACENTATION IN TRIPLETS

Monozygous triplets may be monoamnionic, diamnionic, or triamnionic. Dizygous triplets may be dichorionic or trichorionic. Trizygous triplets must be trichorionic. Multichorionic placentas may be separate or fused. (Modified from fig. 4-13 from Fox H. Pathology of the placenta. Philadelphia: WB Saunders; 1997:94.)

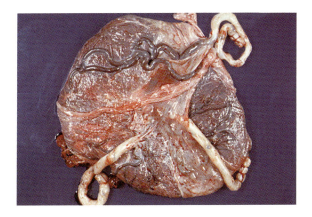

Figure 12-52
TRIAMNIONIC DICHORIONIC TRIPLET PLACENTA
Monochorionic placentas are at the bottom.

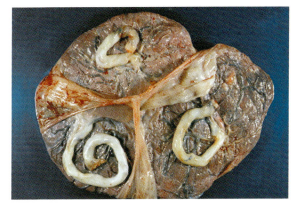

Figure 12-53
TRIAMNIONIC TRICHORIONIC TRIPLET PLACENTA

Because of the common employment of ART, the frequency of higher multiple births has increased markedly in recent years (figs. 12-54, 4-55). In many institutions, triplets and even quadruplets or quintuplets are no longer unusual. Higher multiples experience the same complications as twins—prematurity, low birth weight, congenital anomalies, increased perinatal morbidity/mortality—which are progressively problematic with increasing numbers. Acardiac fetuses are much more frequent in higher multiples than in twins. Cord entanglement is less common in monoamnionic higher order multiples, presumably due to the limited opportunity for movement in the increasingly crowded uterus.

While the outlook in higher multiple births has improved, complications are still common and the outcome is often poor. Consequently, selective fetal reduction has been advocated, and there is now a substantial body of accumulated experience. Remnants of reduced fetuses are regularly identifiable when carefully sought (1,14,65,73).

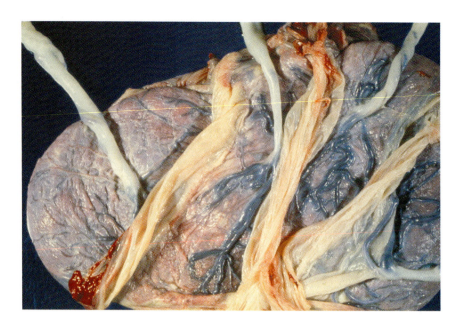

Figure 12-54

QUADRIAMNIONIC QUADRICHORIONIC QUADRUPLET PLACENTA

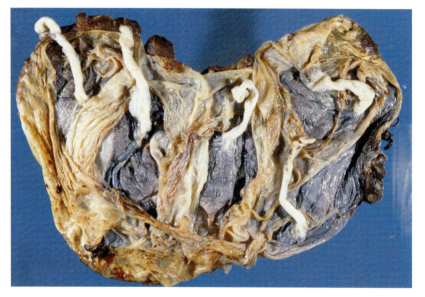

Figure 12-55

QUINTIAMNIONIC QUINTICHORIONIC QUINTUPLET PLACENTA

REFERENCES

1. Albrecht JL, Tomich PG. The maternal and neonatal outcome of triplet gestations. Am J Obstet Gynecol 1996;174:1551–6.
2. Altshuler G, Hyde S. Placental pathology case book. A bidiscoid, monochorionic placenta. J Perinatol 1993;13:492-3.
3. Ananth CV, Vintzileos AM, Shen-Schwartz S, Smulian JC, Lai YL. Standards of birth weight in twin gestations stratified by placental chorionicity. Obstet Gynecol 1998;91:917–24.
4. Anderson RL, Golbus MS, Curry CJ, Callen PW, Hastrup WH. Central nervous system damage and other anomalies in surviving fetus following second trimester antenatal death of co-twin. Report of four cases and literature review. Prenat Diagn 1990;10:513–8.
5. Arias F, Sunderji S, Gimpelson R, Colton E. Treatment of acardiac twinning. Obstet Gynecol 1998;91:818–1.

6. Bajoria R. Abundant vascular anastomoses in monoamniotic versus diamniotic monochorionic placentas. Am J Obstet Gynecol 1998;179:788–93
7. Baker VV, Doering MC. Fetus papyraceous: an unreported congenital anomaly of the surviving infant. Am J Obstet Gynecol 1982;143:234–5.
8. Baldwin VJ. Pathology of multiple pregnancy. New York: Springer-Verlag; 1993.
9. Balfour RP. Fetus papyraceous. Obstet Gynecol 1976;47:507.
10. Becker A, Busjahn A, Faulhaber HD, et al. Twin zygosity. Automated determination with microsatellites. J Prod Med 1997;42:260–6.
11. Bejar R, Vigliocco G, Gramajo H, et al. Antenatal origin of neurologic damage in newborn infants. II. Multiple gestations. Am J Obstet Gynecol 1990;162:1230–6.
12. Bendon RW. Twin transfusion syndrome: pathological studies of the monochorionic placenta in liveborn twins and of the perinatal autopsy in monochorionic twin pairs. Pediatr Pathol Lab Med 1995;15:363–76.
13. Benirschke K, Kaufmann P. Pathology of the human placenta. New York: Springer; 2000.
14. Berkowitz RL, Lynch L, Stone J, Alvarez M. The current status of multifetal pregnancy reduction. Am J Obstet Gynecol 1996;174:1265–72.
15. Bieber FR, Nance WE, Morton CC, et al. Genetic studies of an acardiac monster: evidence of polar body twinning in man. Science 1981;213:775–7.
16. Botting BJ, Davies IM, Macfarlane AJ. Recent trends in the incidence of multiple births and associated mortality. Arch Dis Child 1987;62:941–50.
17. Bruner JP, Anderson TL, Rosemond RL. Placental pathophysiology of the twin oligohydramnios-polyhydramnios sequence and the twin-twin transfusion syndrome. Placenta 1998;19:81–6.
18. Bruner JP, Rosemond RL. Twin-to-twin transfusion syndrome: a subset of the twin oligohydramnios-polyhydramnios sequence. Am J Obstet Gynecol 1993;169:925–30.
19. Bulmer MG. The biology of twinning in man. London: Oxford University Press; 1970.
20. Cameron AH. The Birmingham twin survey. Proc R Soc Med 1968;61:229–34.
21. Cooperstock MS, Tummaru R, Blakewell J, Schramm W. Twin birth weight discordance and risk of preterm birth. Am J Obstet Gynecol 2000;183:63–7.
22. Corney G, Robson EB, Strong SJ. Twin zygosity and placentation. Ann Hum Genet 1968;32:89–96.
23. Costa T, Lambert M, Teshima I, Ray PN, Richer CL, Dallaire L. Monozygotic twins with 45,X/46,XY mosaicism discordant for phenotypic sex. Am J Med Genet 1998;75:40–4.
24. Coulam CB. First trimester diagnosis of acardiac twins. Obstet Gynecol 1996;88:729.
25. Dallapiccola B, Stomeo C, Ferranti G, Di Lecce A, Purpura M. Discordant sex in one of three monozygotic triplets. J Med Genet 1985;22:6–11.
26. Danskin FH, Neilson JP. Twin-to-twin transfusion syndrome: what are appropriate diagnostic criteria? Am J Obstet Gynecol 1989;161:365–9.
27. De Lia JE, Kuhlmann RS, Cruikshank DP, O'Bee LR. Current topic: placental surgery: a new frontier. Placenta 1993;14:477–85.
28. De Lia JE, Kuhlmann RS, Harstad TW, Cruikshank DP. Fetoscopic laser ablation of placental vessels in severe previable twin-twin transfusion syndrome. Am J Obstet Gynecol 1995;172:1202–11.
29. DePaepe ME, Burke S, Luks FI, Halit P, Singer DB. Demonstration of placental vascular anatomy in monochorionic twin gestations. Pediatr Dev Pathol 2002;5:37–44.
30. Denbow ML, Battin MR, Cowan F, Azzopardi D, Edwards AD, Fisk NM. Neonatal cranial ultrasonographic findings in preterm twins complicated by severe fetofetal transfusion syndrome. Am J Obstet Gynecol 1998;178:479–83.
31. Duncan KR, Denbow ML, Fisk NM. The aetiology and management of twin-twin transfusion syndrome. Prenat Diagn 1997;17:1227–36.
32. Eberle AM, Levesque D, Vintzileos AM, Egan JF, Tsapanos V, Salafia CM. Placental pathology in discordant twins. Am J Obstet Gynecol 1993;169:931–5.
33. Ellis RF, Berger GS, Keith L, Depp R. The Northwestern University multihospital twin study II. Mortality of first versus second twin. Acta Genet Med Gemellol 1979;28:347–52.
34. Englert Y, Imbert MC, Van Rosendael E, et al. Morphological anomalies in the placentae of IVF pregnancies: preliminary report of a multicentric study. Hum Reprod 1987;2:155–7.
35. Erdmann J, Nothen MM, Stratmann M, Fimmers R, Franzek E, Propping P. The use of microsatellites in zygosity diagnosis of twins. Acta Genet Med Gemellol 1993;42:45–51.
36. Feldman DM, Odibo A, Campbell WA, Rodis JF. Iatrogenic monoamniotic twins as a complication of therapeutic amniocentesis. Obstet Gynecol 1998;91:815–6.
37. Fesslova V, Villa L, Nava S, Mosca F, Nicolini U. Fetal and neonatal echocardiographic findings in twin-twin transfusion syndrome. Am J Obstet Gynecol 1998;179:1056–62.
38. Finberg HJ. The "twin peak" sign: reliable evidence of dichorionic twinning. J Ultrasound Med 1992;11:571–7.

39. Fries MH, Goldstein RB, Kilpatrick SJ, Golbus MS, Callen PW, Filly RA. The role of velamentous cord insertion in the etiology of twin-twin transfusion syndrome. Obstet Gynecol 1993;81:569–74.
40. Fujikura T, Froehlich LA. Twin placentation and zygosity. Obstet Gynecol 1971;37:34–43.
41. Fusi L, Gordon H. Twin pregnancy complicated by single intrauterine death. Problems and outcome with conservative management. Br J Obstet Gynaecol 1990;97:511–6.
42. Gaziano E, Gaziano C, Brandt D. Doppler velocimetry determined redistribution of fetal blood flow: correlation with growth restriction in diamniotic monochorionic and dizygotic twins. Am J Obstet Gynecol 1998;178:1359–67.
43. Giles W, Trudinger B, Cook C, Connelly A. Placental microvascular changes in twin pregnancies with abnormal umbilical artery waveforms. Obstet Gynecol 1993;81:556–9.
44. Gillim DL, Hendricks CH. Holoacardius: review of the literature and case report. Obstet Gynecol 1953;2:647–53.
45. Gonsoulin W, Copeland KL, Carpenter RJ Jr, Hughes MR, Elder FF. Fetal blood sampling demonstrating chimerism in monozygotic twins discordant for sex and tissue karyotype (46,XY and 45,X). Prenatal Diagn 1990;10:25–8.
46. Gonsoulin W, Moise KJ Jr, Kirshon B, Cotton DB, Wheeler JM, Carpenter RJ Jr. Outcome of twin-twin transfusion diagnosed before 28 weeks of gestation. Obstet Gynecol 1990;75:214–6.
47. Hanley ML, Shen-Schwarz S, Ananth CV, Smulian JC, Vintzieos AM. Birthweight discordancy in twin gestations: is it related to discordancy of placental mass or histopathologic lesions? Am J Obstet Gynecol 1998;178:S83.
48. Heinonen S, Ryynanen M, Kirkinen P, Saarikoski S. Perinatal diagnostic evaluation of velamentous umbilical cord insertion: clinical, Doppler and ultrasonic findings. Obstet Gynecol 1996;87:112–7.
49. Hughes HE, Miskin M. Congenital microcephaly due to vascular disruption: in utero documentation. Pediatrics 1986;78:85–7.
50. Hurst RW, Abbitt PL. Fetal intracranial hemorrhage and periventricular leukomalacia: complications of twin-twin transfusion. AJNR Am J Neuroradiol 1989;10:S62–3.
51. Ishimatsu J, Hori D, Miyajima S, Hamada T, Yakushiji M, Nishimi T. Twin pregnancies complicated by the death of one fetus in the second or third trimester. J Matern-Fetal Invest 1994;4:141–5.
52. James WH. A note on the epidemiology of acardiac monsters. Teratology 1977;16:211–16.
53. Jou HJ, Ng KY, Teng RJ, Hsieh FJ. Doppler sonographic detection of reverse twin-twin transfusion after intrauterine death of the donor. J Ultrasound Med 1993;5:307–9.
54. Jung JH, Graham JM, Schultz N, Smith DW. Congenital hydraencephaly/porencephaly due to vascular disruption in monozygotic twins. Pediatrics 1984;73:467–9.
55. Kindred JE. Twin pregnancies with one blighted. Am J Obstet Gynecol 1944;48:642–82.
56. Kloosterman GJ. The "third circulation" in identical twins. Ned Tijdschr Verloskd Gynaecol 1963;63:395–412.
57. Kobak AJ, Cohen MR. Velamentous insertion of cord with spontaneous rupture of vasa previa in twin pregnancy. Am J Obstet Gynecol 1939;38:1063–6.
58. Kovacs BW, Kirschbaum TH, Paul RH. Twin gestations. I. Antenatal care and complications. Obstet Gynecol 1989;74:313–7.
59. Lachapelle MF, Leduc L, Cote JM, Grignon A. Fouron JC. Potential value of fetal echocardiography in the differential diagnosis of twin pregnancy with presence of polyhydramnios-oligohydramnios syndrome. Am J Obstet Gynecol 1997;177:388–94.
60. Lacro RV, Jones KL, Benirschke K. The umbilical cord twist: origin, direction and relevance. Am J Obstet Gynecol 1987;157:833–9.
61. Lambalk CB, Boomsma DI. The endocrinology of dizygotic twinning (abstract 61). Twin Res 1998;1:96.
62. Lander M, Oosterhof H, Aarnoudse JG. Death of one twin followed by extremely variable flow velocity waveforms in the surviving fetus. Gynecol Obstet Invest 1993;36:127–8.
63. Larroche JC, Droull P, Delezoide AL, Narcy F, Nessmann C. Brain damage in monozygous twins. Biol Neonate 1990;57:261–78.
64. Levi S. Ultrasonic assessment of the high rate of human multiple pregnancy in the first trimester. J Clin Ultrasound 1976;4:3–5.
65. Lipitz S, Uval J, Achiron R, Schiff E, Lusky A, Reichman B. Outcome of twin pregnancies reduced from triplets compared with nonreduced twin gestations. Obstet Gynecol 1996;87:511–4.
66. Liu S, Benirschke K, Scioscia AL, Mannino FL. Intrauterine death in multiple gestation. Acta Genet Med Gemellol 1992;41:5–26.
67. Lopriore E, Vandenbussche FP, Tiersma ES, de Beaufort AJ, de Leeuw JP. Twin-to-twin transfusion syndrome: new perspectives. J Pediatr 1995;127:675–80.
68. Lumme RH, Saarikoski SV. Monoamnionic twin pregnancy. Acta Genet Med Gemellol 1986;35:99–105.
69. Machin G, Bamforth F, Innes M, McNichol K. Some perinatal characteristics of monozygotic twins who are dichorionic. Am J Med Genet 1995;55:71–6.

70. Machin G, Still K, Lalani T. Correlations of placental vascular anatomy and clinical outcomes in 69 monochorionic twin pregnancies. Am J Med Genet 1996;61:229–36.
71. Machin GA. Some causes of genotypic and phenotypic discordance in monozygotic twin pairs. Am J Med Genet 1996;61:216–28.
72. Machin GA. Velamentous cord insertion in monochorionic twin gestation. An added risk factor. J Reprod Med 1997;42:785–9.
73. Macones GA, Schemmer G, Pritts E, Weiblatt V, Wapner RJ. Multifetal reduction of triplets to twins improves perinatal outcome. Am J Obstet Gynecol 1993;169:982–6.
74. Mannino FL, Jones KL, Benirschke K. Congenital skin defects and fetus papyraceous. J Pediatr 1977;91:559–64.
75. Mari G, Uerpairojkit B, Abuhamad A, Martinez E, Copel J. Velamentous insertion of the cord in polyhydramnios-oligohydramnios twins [abstract 102]. Am J Obstet Gynecol 1995;172:291.
76. Markavy KL, Scanlon JW, Hydrops fetalis in a parabiotic acardiac twin. Am J Dis Child 1978;132:638–9.
77. Megory E, Weiner E, Shalev E, Ohel G. Pseudo-amniotic twins with cord entanglement following genetic funipuncture. Obstet Gynecol 1991;78:915–8.
78. Melnick M. Brain damage in a survivor after in-utero death of monozygous co-twin. Lancet 1977;2:1287.
79. Menezo YJ, Sakkas D. Monozygotic twining: is it related to apoptosis in the embryo? Hum Reprod 2002;17:247–8.
80. Milham S Jr. Pituitary gonadotrophin and dizygotic twinning. Lancet 1964;14:566.
81. Monie I. Velamentous insertion of the cord in early pregnancy. Am J Obstet Gynecol 1965;93:276–81.
82. Moore TR, Gale S, Benirschke K. Perinatal outcome of forty-nine pregnancies complicated by acardiac twinning. Am J Obstet Gynecol 1990;163:907–12.
83. Myrianthopoulos NC. An epidemiological survey of twins in a large, prospectively studied population. Am J Hum Genet 1970;22:611–29.
84. Myrianthopoulos NC. A survey of twins in the population of a prospective collaborative study. Acta Genet Med Gemellol 1970;19:15–23.
85. Naeye R. Organ composition in newborn parabiotic twins with speculation regarding neonatal hypoglycemia. Pediatrics 1964;34:415–8.
86. Naeye R. Organ abnormalities in human parabiotic syndrome. Am J Pathol 1965;46:829–42.
87. Naeye RL, Blanc WA. Fetal renal structure and the genesis of amniotic fluid disorders. Am J Pathol 1972;67:95–108.
88. Nageotte MP, Hurwitz SR, Kaupke CJ, Vaziri ND, Pandian MR. Atriopeptin in the twin transfusion syndrome. Obstet Gynecol 1989;73:867–70.
89. Nicolini U, Pisoni MP, Cela E, Roberts A. Fetal blood sampling immediately before and within 24 hours of death in monochorionic twin pregnancies complicated by single intrauterine death. Am J Obstet Gynecol 1998;179:800–3.
90. Nylander PP. Perinatal mortality in twins. Acta Genet Med Gemellol 1979;28:363–8.
91. Nylander PP. Serum levels of gonadotrophins in relation to multiple pregnancy in Nigeria. J Obstet Gynaecol Br Commonw 1973;80:651–3.
92. Oberg KC, Pestaner JP, Bielamowicz L, Hawkins EP. Renal tubular dysgenesis in twin-twin transfusion syndrome. Pediatr Dev Pathol 1999;2:25–32.
93. Okamura K, Murotsuki J, Tanigawara S, Uehara S, Yajima A. Funipuncture for evaluation of hematologic and coagulation indices in the surviving twin following co-twin's death. Obstet Gynecol 1994;83:975–8.
94. Pharaoh PO, Adi Y. Consequences of in-utero death in twin pregnancy. Lancet 2000;355:1597–602.
95. Pinar H, Sung CJ, Oyer CE, Singer DB. Reference values for singleton and twin placental weights. Pediatr Pathol Lab Med 1996;16:901–7.
96. Popek EJ, Strain JD, Neumann A, Wilson H. In utero development of pulmonary artery calcification in monochorionic twins: a report of three cases and discussion of the possible etiology. Pediatr Pathol 1993;13:597–611.
97. Powers WF, Kiely JL. The risks of confronting twins: a national perspective. Am J Obstet Gynecol 1994;170:456–61.
98. Pretorius DH, Leopold G, Moore TR, Benirschke K, Sivo JJ. Acardiac twin. Report of Doppler sonography. J Ultrasound Med 1988;7:413–6.
99. Ramos-Arroyo MA, Ulbright TM, Yu PL, Christian JC. Twin study: relationship between birth weight, zygosity, placentation, and pathologic placental changes. Acta Genet Med Gemellol 1988;37:229–38.
100. Redline RW, Shah D, Sakar H, Schluchter M, Salvator A. Placental lesions associated with abnormal growth in twins. Pediatr Dev Pathol 2001;4:473–81.
101. Reynolds MA, Schieve LA, Martin JA, Macaluso M. Trends in multiple births conceived using assisted reproductive technology, United States, 1997-2000. Pediatrics 2003;111(Part 2):1159–62.
102. Robinson HP, Caines JS. Sonar evidence of early pregnancy failure in patients with twin conceptions. Br J Obstet Gynaecol 1977;84:22–5.
103. Robinson L, Jones K, Benirschke K. The nature of structural defects associated with velamentous and marginal insertion of the umbilical cord. Am J Obstet Gynecol 1983;146:191–3.

104. Rodeck C, Deans A, Jauniaux E. Thermocoagulation for the early treatment of pregnancy with an acardiac twin. N Engl J Med 1998;339:1293–5.
105. Saier F, Burden L, Cavanagh D. Fetus papyraceous: an unusual case with congenital anomaly of the surviving fetus. Obstet Gynecol 1975;45:217–20.
106. Samon LM, Ash KM, Murdison KA. Aorto-pulmonary calcification: an unusual manifestation of idiopathic calcification of infancy evident antenatally. Obstet Gynecol 1995;85:863–5.
107. Sato T. Kaneko K, Konuma S, Sato I, Tamada T. Acardiac anomalies: review of 88 cases in Japan. Asia Oceana J Obstet Gynecol 1984;10:45–52.
108. Schinzel AA, Smith DW, Miller JR. Monozygotic twinning and structural defects. J Pediatr 1979;95:921–30.
109. Senoo M, Okamura K, Murotsuki J, Yaegashi N, Uehara S, Yajima A. Growth pattern of twins of different chorionicity evaluated by sonographic biometry. Obstet Gynecol 2000;95:656–61.
110. Sepulveda W, Sebire NJ, Odibo A, Psarra A, Nicolaides KH. Prenatal determination of chorionicity in triplet pregnancy by ultrasonographic examination of the ipsilon zone. Obstet Gynecol 1996;88:855–8.
111. Sherer DM, Abramowicz JS, Jaffe, R, Smith SA, Metlay LA, Woods JR Jr. Twin-twin transfusion syndrome with abrupt onset of microcephaly in the surviving recipient following spontaneous death of the donor twin. Am J Obstet Gynecol 1993;169:85–8.
112. Soernes T, Bakke T. The length of the human umbilical cord in twin pregnancies. Am J Obstet 1987;157:1229–30.
113. Soma H, Takayama M, Kiyokawa T, Akaeda T, Tokoro K. Serum gonadotropin levels in Japanese women. Obstet Gynecol 1975;46:311–2.
114. Spencer R. Conjoined twins: theoretical embryologic basis. Teratology 1992;45:591–602.
115. Spencer R. Theoretical and analytical embryology of conjoined twins: part I: embryogenesis. Clin Anat 2000;13:36–53.
116. Szymonowicz W, Preston H, Yu VY. The surviving monozygotic twin. Arch Dis Child 1986;61:454–8.
117. Van Allen MI, Smith DW, Shepard TH. Twin reversed arterial perfusion (TRAP) sequence: a study of 14 twin pregnancies with acardius. Semin Perinatol 1983;7:285–93.
118. Van Bogaert P, Donner C, David P, Rodesch F, Avni EF, Szliwowski HB. Congenital bilateral perisylvian syndrome in a monozygotic twin with intra-uterine death of the co-twin. Dev Med Child Neurol 1996;38:166–70.
119. Vetter K. Consideration on growth discordant twins. J Perinat Med 1993;21:267–72
120. Wagner DS, Klein RL, Robinson HB, Novak RW. Placental emboli from a fetus papyraceous. J Pediatr Surg 1990;25:538–42.
121. Wax JR, Blakemore KJ, Blohm P, Callan NA. Stuck twin with cotwin nonimmune hydrops: successful treatment by amniocentesis. Fetal Diagn Ther 1991;6:126–31.
122. Weig SG, Marshall PC, Abroms IF, Gauthier NS. Patterns of cerebral injury and clinical presentation in the vascular disruptive syndrome of monozygotic twins. Pediatr Neurol 1995;13: 279–85.
123. Wenstrom KD, Tessen JA, Zlatnik FJ, Sipes SL. Frequency, distribution, and theoretical mechanisms of hematologic and weight discordance in monochorionic twins. Obstet Gynecol 1992; 80:257–61.
124. Williams K, Hennessy E, Alberman E. Cerebral palsy: effects of twinning, birthweight, and gestational age. Arch Dis Child Fetal Neonatal Ed 1996;75:F178–82.
125. Winn HN, Gabrielli S, Reece EA, Roberts JA, Salafia C, Hobbins JC. Ultrasonographic criteria for the prenatal diagnosis of placental chorionicity in twin gestations. Am J Obstet Gynecol 1989;161:1540–2.
126. Yoshida K. Absence of one umbilical artery in twins [Abstract]. Twin Res 1998;1:116.
127. Yoshida K, Soma H. Outcome of the surviving cotwin of a fetus papyraceous or of a dead fetus. Acta Genet Med Gemellol 1986;35:91–8.
128. Zucchini S, Borghesani F, Soffriti G, Chirico C, Vultaggio E, Di Donato P. Transvaginal ultrasound diagnosis of twin reversed arterial perfusion syndrome at 9 weeks gestation. Ultrasound Obstet Gynecol 1993;3:209–11.

13 EXAMINATION TECHNIQUE

PATHOLOGIST-CLINICIAN RELATIONSHIP

As with all aspects of placental pathology, a gross examination of the placenta requires interaction between the pathologist and clinician at a variety of different levels, both before and at the time of submission of a specimen for pathologic evaluation.

Logistical Considerations. Many experts believe that examination of the placenta prior to fixation is optimal. Fixation in an adequate amount (at least 2 to 3 volumes) of formalin is an acceptable alternative, especially if transportation and storage issues are problematic. If placentas are examined fresh, prompt refrigeration is essential. Prolonged refrigeration is usually not a problem and adequate histology can be obtained as long as 5 to 7 days after delivery.

Guidelines for Submission. Clinicians and pathologists should reach an understanding so that the appropriate placentas reach the pathology laboratory. Such guidelines have been published in several venues and a representative summary is shown in Table 13-1 (10,18,31). In some centers, placentas are labeled and stored in a refrigerator in the delivery room for as long as a week to ensure retrieval of placentas from those few cases that present with neonatal problems hours or days after delivery.

Clinical Scenario. Pathologists have to understand the relevant clinical issue(s) before undertaking a gross examination of the placenta. This requires a working knowledge of obstetric disease and the terminology used to describe it (including jargon and abbreviations, Table 13-2). The method of communicating this clinical information varies in different practice situations. In selected cases, direct verbal communication initiated by either the clinician or pathologist is required. For the remainder of cases, busy clinicians and pathologists need to develop a reliable format for providing the necessary information on the specimen requisition form. At University Hospitals, Cleveland, Ohio, clinicians and pathologists have designed a separate placenta record sheet, submitted along with the specimen requisition form in lieu of the clinical history, which provides the pathologist with all of the information needed (Table 13-3). We consider gestational age, maternal obstetric history (OB index [gravidity and parity]), the presence of underlying maternal disease, fetal weight, neonatal Apgar scores, and the specific questions or reasons for submission as minimum information required for a productive pathologic consultation.

APPROACH TO THE SPECIFIC CLINICAL SCENARIO

Having addressed the importance of understanding the question being asked, we now turn to an overview of the gross findings that may help provide the answer. In chapter 2, clinical outcomes were separated into three groups: preterm delivery, fetal growth restriction, and hypoxic-ischemic injury. Specific gross abnormalities seen in these, and a few other clinical scenarios, are listed below.

Table 13-1
INDICATIONS FOR PLACENTAL EXAMINATION

Neonatal	Prematurity
	Fetal growth restriction
	Unexpected adverse outcome
	Congenital anomalies
	Suspected fetal infection
	Fetal hydrops
	Fetal hematologic abnormalities
Obstetric	Intrauterine fetal death
	Maternal disease/maternal death
	Signs of maternal infection
	Gestational hypertension
	Oligohydramnios/polyhydramnios
	Antepartum hemorrhage—acute and/or chronic
	Postpartum hemorrhage
	Abnormal biophysical/ biochemical monitoring
	In utero therapy
	Abnormal placenta noted at delivery

Table 13-2
LIST OF COMMONLY USED OBSTETRICAL ABBREVIATIONS

AROM	artificial rupture of membranes
BPP	biophysical profile
BTBV	beat-to-beat variability
FGR	fetal growth restriction
GA	gestational age
GBS	group B *Streptococcus*
GDM	gestational diabetes
GDMA2	insulin-dependent gestational diabetes
IUFD	intrauterine fetal death
IUGR	intrauterine growth restriction
IVDA	intravenous drug abuse
IVF	in vitro fertilization
IVH	intraventricular hemorrhage
LAC	lupus anticoagulant
LOF	low-outlet forceps
LTCS	low transverse C-section
MSAFP	maternal serum alpha-fetoprotein
MSF	meconium-stained fluid
NIHF	nonimmune hydrops fetalis
NRNST	nonreactive nonstress test
NST	nonstress test
OA	occiput anterior
OCT	oxytocin challenge test
OP	occiput posterior
PET	preeclampsia/toxemia
PIH	pregnancy-induced hypertension
PNC	prenatal care
PPH	postpartum hemorrhage
PPHN	persistent pulmonary hypertension of the newborn
PROM	premature rupture of membranes
PPROM	prolonged premature rupture of membranes
PUBS	percutaneous umbilical blood sampling
SROM	spontaneous rupture of membranes
SVD	spontaneous vaginal delivery
Triple Check	maternal serum HCG[a], AFP, and estriol levels
TTTS	twin-twin transfusion syndrome
UC	umbilical cord
U/S	ultrasound
VAVD	vacuum-assisted vaginal delivery
VBAC	vaginal birth after C-section

[a]HCG = human chorionic gonadotropin; AFP = alpha-fetoprotein.

Preterm Delivery. 1) Findings consistent with maternal underperfusion: reduced placental weight, villous infarction, thin umbilical cord; 2) acute marginal abruption/peripheral separation: recent marginal retroplacental and/or retromembranous blood clot; 3) chronic abruption/peripheral separation: circumvallate membrane insertion, old marginal blood clot, green discoloration of the fetal surface; 4) maternal floor infarction (diffuse perivillous fibrinoid deposition): diffuse or patchy thickening of the basal plate; and 5) specific types of amnionic fluid infection: intervillous abscesses (*Listeria* infection), peripheral cord abscesses (*Candida* infection).

Fetal Growth Restriction (Intrauterine Growth Restriction). 1) Chronic abruption/peripheral separation: as above; 2) findings consistent with maternal underperfusion: as above; 3) maternal floor infarction (diffuse perivillous fibrinoid deposition): as above; 4) fetal thrombotic vasculopathy and chronic villitis: patchy areas of pale firm villous parenchyma; 5) spatial constraint: abnormal placental shape, peripheral cord insertion, marginal atrophy, giant chorangioma; and 6) maldevelopment: cystic or molar villi, single umbilical artery.

Hypoxic-Ischemic Injury. 1) Umbilical cord problems: excessive length, excessive twisting, tight knots, strictures, torn or occluded vessels at the placental insertion site; 2) fetal thrombotic vasculopathy: chorionic plate thrombi and subjacent areas of pale firm avascular villi; 3) chronic meconium exposure: green umbilical cord, deep chorionic plate staining, umbilical cord ulceration; 4) possible fetomaternal hemorrhage: multiple or large symmetric intervillous thrombi, pale villous parenchyma; and 5) abruptio placenta: central retroplacental hemorrhage with distortion of the overlying placenta, compression crater (concavity) indenting the basal plate, irregular intraplacental hemorrhages.

Other. 1) Retained placenta (placenta accreta, vaginal birth after caesarian section): incomplete or disrupted maternal surface; 2) fetal macrosomia (maternal diabetes, hydrops fetalis, metabolic storage disease, Beckwith-Wiedemann syndrome): placentomegaly (large placenta, more than 650 g; extremely large placenta, more than 1,000 g); 3) oligohydramnios sequence: amnion nodosum; 4) amnion rupture sequence: shredded

Table 13-3
CLINICAL DATA SHEET TO ACCOMPANY PLACENTA TO PATHOLOGY

Placenta Record

Sheet filled out by M.D. (Printed Name) _____

Gestational Age (Best Estimate) _____

Ob Index: G_____   Full term _____   Prem _____   Ab _____   Lvg _____

Maternal History:

Baby (weight, Apgars, malformations, other):

Any specific questions about this placenta?

---

discohesive amnion, amnionic cords encircling and constricting the umbilical cord; and 5) fetal akinesia sequence (central nervous system [CNS] disease, myopathy, or severe uterine spatial constraint): short umbilical cord.

STEPWISE HANDLING OF THE SPECIMEN

From a practical standpoint the actual physical handling of the gross specimen may vary. The procedure used by the authors is described below.

1. Employ universal precautions for preventing the transmittal of human immunodeficiency virus (HIV) and other blood-borne pathogens with every specimen. (If desired, known positive cases can be prefixed in a large volume of formalin for a period of up to 2 weeks.)

2. Work in a sufficiently large, well lit, and well-ventilated space, with a large supply of absorbent tissue pads, a nearby scale, a large centimeter ruler, scissors, smooth forceps, a large knife, scalpel or razor blades, and small containers of formalin for the fixation of untrimmed tissue blocks.

3. Remove the placenta from the container, drain, and gently remove loose blood clots over an appropriate biohazard waste receptacle.

4. Place the placental disc on the cutting surface with the membranes in anatomic position and the maternal surface down.

5. Prepare two membrane rolls approximately 3 to 4 cm in width and place in the small formalin container (fig. 13-1). Remove the remaining membranes from the placental margin.

6. Measure, remove, and section the umbilical cord. Place two sections taken from areas that are one third and two thirds of the distance from free end to insertion in the small formalin container.

7. Measure the placental disc and the shortest distance from the margin to the cord insertion site.

Placental Pathology

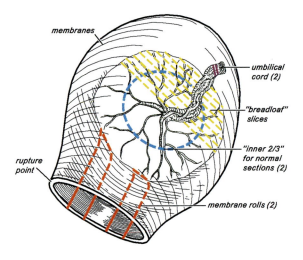

Figure 13-1

SCHEMATIC DIAGRAM OF THE PLACENTA AND MEMBRANES WITH POINT OF MEMBRANE RUPTURE INDICATED AND SECTIONING TECHNIQUE SUMMARIZED

The point of rupture refers to that point along the circular opening (which corresponds to the fully dilated cervical os in situ) that is closest to the placental disc. Normal planes of cut section are indicated by parallel yellow-green dotted lines. An inner concentric circle (blue dotted line) shows the area where full-thickness sections of normal parenchyma should be obtained. Also depicted are the marginal blocks used for preparation of membrane rolls (brown dotted lines). The minimum number of sections from each location is indicated in parentheses. These sections can be accommodated in four cassettes. Separate sections should be submitted from abnormal areas.

8. Weigh the placenta (after removal of the umbilical cord and membranes).

9. Inspect the maternal and fetal surfaces and make parallel cuts at 1- to 2-cm intervals starting at the maternal surface and extending to, but not through, the fetal surface.

10. Remove full-thickness blocks (approximately 3 to 4 cm in width) by extending the parallel cuts through the fetal surface using forceps and scissors. Place in formalin.

11. Return the sectioned placenta to its original container and fill with formalin.

12. Trim and block final tissue sections into cassettes 4 to 6 hours or more after the initial examination.

13. When new clinical data or unexpected pathologic features require further study, return to the fixed placenta after histologic examination to reexamine the gross specimen and/or submit additional tissue.

14. Discard fixed specimen after 30 days as per College of American Pathologists (CAP) guidelines.

GROSS DESCRIPTION

While varying somewhat between pathologists, the ideal gross description of the placenta should be concise, consistent from case to case, and must include certain specific synoptic elements. These key elements are as follows:

1. Presence or absence of fixative.
2. Trimmed weight of the placental disc.
3. Length and color (yellow, green, red) of the umbilical cord plus its point of insertion into the disc or membranes relative to the nearest placental margin.
4. Type of membrane insertion (marginal versus circumvallation; partial or complete).
5. Completeness of membranes.
6. Point of membrane rupture (shortest distance to the placental margin).
7. Color of the fetal surface (blue, green, brown).
8. Shape abnormalities (accessory lobes, multilobation).
9. Disruption or incompleteness of the maternal surface.
10. Specific abnormalities seen on cut section (thickening of the basal plate, mass lesions, hemorrhages).

This data provides the examining pathologist and any later reviewers with a complete image of the gross specimen to complement the findings on the microscopic slides. Other information may be needed for specific cases, but the overall goals should be brevity, completeness, and consistency of descriptive terminology. One measurement that is not currently routine, but which may assume importance in the future, is the degree of twisting of the umbilical cord. This is most conveniently measured as the number of diagonal twists in a representative 10-cm segment and expressed as "twists per centimeter" for comparisons with appropriate reference standards (6,29; see pages 195 and 321).

TECHNIQUE AND RATIONALE FOR TISSUE SAMPLING

Approaches to sampling may vary between institutions, but the same goals of consistency with respect to the number, nature, and methods of preparing and labeling blocks apply. Our approach is illustrated in figure 13-1 and described below.

Membrane Rolls (Two Rolls, One Section from Each). Membranes are sampled to assess: 1) maternal decidual arteries for vasculopathy; 2) the location and nature of inflammatory infiltrates; 3) the presence, amount, and depth of exogenous substances such as meconium, hemosiderin, or fetal squamous cells (33); and 4) diffuse pathologic changes such as amnion necrosis, fresh hemorrhage, and ischemic necrosis of the decidua.

In many cases, decidual vasculopathy is focal and most prominent near the membrane insertion. For this reason we recommend preparing two membrane rolls and including a small portion of the peripheral placenta at the center of each (fig. 13-1). An advantage of this approach is that peripheral placenta does not have to be included in the remaining sections (see below for an alternative approach).

Umbilical Cord (Two Pieces, One Section from Each). The cord is sampled to assess: 1) the number of umbilical arteries; 2) the presence or absence of inflammatory cells in vein, arteries, and/or stroma; 3) the amount of Wharton's jelly (often assessed by the cross sectional dimensions of the cord); and 4) miscellaneous findings such as spirochetes, *Toxoplasma* cysts, meconium-associated vascular necrosis, and dystrophic mineralization of the cord stroma.

Parenchyma (2 to 3 Full-Thickness Sections). The parenchyma is sampled to assess: 1) overall development of the villous trees ("accelerated" or "delayed" maturation/distal villous deficiency or immaturity [see chapter 4]); 2) features of the interhemal membrane (trophoblast and adjacent fetal capillaries): syncytial knots, deficient vasculosyncytial membranes, villous cytotrophoblast proliferation, avascular/ hypovascular villi, chorangiosis/chorangiomatosis; 3) abnormalities of the villous stroma: chronic villitis, villous edema, vascular-stromal karyorrhexis, intravillous hemorrhage, mesenchymal dysplasia; 4) circulating fetal cells: nucleated red blood cells (NRBC) with or without parvovirus inclusions, fetal leukemia; 5) intervillous space (maternal infarcts, perivillous fibrin(oid), intervillositis, primary or metastatic tumors); 6) basal plate (microscopic hemorrhage, plasma cells, superficial implantation site); and 7) chorionic plate (inflammation, thrombosis, pigment deposition, vascular necrosis).

Since gas exchange is known to be maximal in the central and basal two thirds of the placenta, random sections should be concentrated in these areas. Sections should preferably be of full thickness. If the placenta is too thick, chorionic and basal plates need to be represented on at least one slide each. Lesions, generally solid or hemorrhagic, should be sampled so as to include adjacent normal parenchyma. Only one section of each type of lesion is necessary. Two additional sections of grossly unremarkable placental parenchyma are routine; one may be sufficient if several different abnormalities need to be sampled.

According to the approach outlined above, a grossly unremarkable placenta may be sampled in as few as four cassettes: two containing a membrane roll and cord section each, and two of full-thickness parenchyma. In our lab, we submit five cassettes on virtually all singleton placentas.

MULTIPLE PREGNANCY

Placentas from twins and higher order multiple pregnancies present additional challenges for gross examination. To avoid confusion, this discussion concentrates on twin placentas. Higher order gestations (triplets, quadruplets, etc.) should be approached in the same general fashion with the following caveats.

Most higher order multiple gestations are the consequence of multiple ovulation, and hence, each placenta is likely to be diamnionic dichorionic with respect to each of the other placentas. Nevertheless, the number of membrane layers (amnions and chorion) within each dividing membrane needs to be documented, both at the time of gross examination and by subsequent histologic sections.

Additional gestational sacs ("vanishing twins," fetus papyraceus) aborted earlier in gestation remain in the uterus as missed abortions and are often identified as thickened plaques in the fetal membranes. Each should be sampled for microscopic examination.

The overall approach to twin placentas is guided by the following simple precepts which are important to consider before gross examination:

1. The primary responsibility of the pathologist is to separate monochorionic placentas

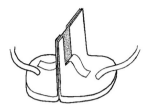
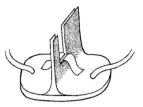
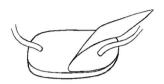

Figure 13-2

SCHEMATIC DIAGRAM OF DIFFERENT TYPES OF TWIN PLACENTAS WITH THEIR DIVIDING MEMBRANES

A: Fused diamnionic dichorionic placentas with a dividing membrane consisting of two amnions flanking two centrally fused chorions.
B: A single diamnionic monochorionic placenta with two fused amnions in the dividing membrane.
C: A single monoamnionic monochorionic placenta with artifactual peeling of the surface amnion mimicking a dividing membrane.

which are associated with a much higher rate of complications from dichorionic placentas (see chapter 12). Until recently, monochorionic twins were thought to invariably be monozygotic or identical. A recent case report has shown this not to be true, but in the overwhelming majority of cases the dictum "monochorionic placentas are monozygous" remains true (28). Chorionicity should be established before dissection by evaluation of the dividing membrane and then documentation by histologic section in the form of either a dividing membrane roll or a T section. If a dividing membrane is not identified, one needs to distinguish between a single monoamnionic monochorionic placenta and a dichorionic placenta with torn membranes (fig. 13-2). Careful inspection of the placental discs to recognize fused placentas in the latter case, understanding of the underlying anatomy, and careful reconstruction of the membrane sacs usually allow this distinction to be made.

2. Dichorionic means two placentas. Each placenta is a separate developmental, structural, and functional entity, and should be physically separated from its partner (even if intimately fused to it), individually weighed, and independently evaluated at gross examination. Dichorionic placentas virtually never have twin-twin anastomoses and an exception to this general rule should only be entertained in exceptional circumstances.

3. Monochorionic means one placenta. Monochorionic placentas are identified by evaluating the dividing membrane (or by the lack of a dividing membrane in monoamnionic gestations). The placental discs should not be separated and are weighed as one. Virtually all monozygous placentas have twin-twin anastomoses, but the number and nature of the anastomoses vary considerably and should be evaluated at the time of gross examination (see below).

4. Twin pregnancies, both monochorionic and dichorionic, are associated with higher rates of perinatal morbidity and mortality than gestational age-matched singleton pregnancies (22). This is the second major reason that all twin placentas are submitted to pathology. In some monochorionic placentas, morbidity and mortality may be due to a twin-twin vascular anastomosis (diamnionic) or cord entanglement (monoamnionic). Much more common, particularly in dichorionic twins, are abnormalities that result from competition between the fetoplacental units for maternal nutritional support in a uterus designed to carry a single gestation. This competition may be reflected in placental shape, peripheral umbilical cord insertion, and other types of suboptimal placental implantation that are detectable on gross examination and

may help to explain discordant outcomes in the delivered fetuses (23). For these reasons, it is crucial to maintain the separate identity of each placenta in the gross description and histologic sections, even if the placentas are not labeled at the time of receipt in pathology. For monochorionic twins this means taking some sections from each placenta in the area away from the region between the two umbilical cord insertions.

The authors' specific techniques for the gross examination of twin placentas are as follows:

1. Completely separated twin placentas and twin placentas connected by membranes alone are separate diamnionic dichorionic and each can be processed as a singleton. A dividing membrane role is not necessary.

2. For single or fused twin placentas, identify and pull upwards on the dividing membrane (fig. 13-2). Next, tug on the dividing membrane firmly in the direction of each umbilical cord. A true dividing membrane is anchored on both sides and will not peel off the placenta. Artifactual loosening of the surface amnion can mimic a dividing membrane, but will peel back still further with traction. Holding the membrane up, nick each side of the dividing membrane with a scalpel blade and peel the nicked edge downward with fine forceps. After peeling each side there will either be a window (two layers) or a residual opaque central layer (three layers). Also consider the following:

   a. If the membrane is initially translucent and shows only two layers after peeling, the placenta is diamnionic monochorionic. Prepare a membrane roll of the dividing membrane, remove the membranes and cords, and weigh the placenta.

   b. If no dividing membrane is present and the placental disc shows no cleavage plane extending from basal to chorionic plate, the placenta is monoamnionic monochorionic. Remove the membranes and cords and weigh the placenta.

   c. If the dividing membrane is initially opaque and shows three layers after peeling, the placentas are fused diamnionic dichorionic. Prepare a membrane roll of the dividing membranes. Remove the membranes and cords. Turn the placenta over and separate the two placentas by gentle, but firm, blunt dissection. Weigh the separated discs individually. Subsequent examination is as described above for singleton placentas.

3. Monochorionic twin placentas generally have a vascular communication. In most cases, this communication consists of surface artery-to-artery anastomoses combined with deeper parenchymal connections (artery-artery, vein-vein, artery-vein). The deep connections are generally small and not detectable by simple injection studies. It has been shown that cases with clinically significant twin-twin transfusion syndrome have much larger deep artery-to-vein anastomoses and a paucity of counterbalancing surface artery-artery anastomoses (2a).

We screen for large deep anastomoses in all monochorionic placentas. One rapid and simple way to accomplish this is as follows (fig. 13-3). Select the placenta with the thinner umbilical cord (i.e., the presumably volume-depleted donor). In sequential fashion, the 2 to 3 major arteries (arteries go over veins) are then proximally ligated and distally injected with air using a plastic syringe with a 19-gauge needle inserted at a point just after their emergence from the umbilical cord insertion site. Major anastomoses will allow air to pass freely into the opposite placenta. If the transmitted air appears in a vein having no surface continuity with the injected artery, a deep artery-vein anastomosis has been confirmed. If the first 2 to 3 injections are negative, the placenta is turned around and the major arteries of the second placenta are injected. If all injections are negative after this 5 to 10 minute exercise, clinically significant anastomoses have been virtually excluded. A more rigorous dye injection protocol has recently been described (8).

Twin placentas without gross lesions can be adequately sampled in nine cassettes: the same minimum four cassettes per placenta described above for singletons plus one dividing membrane roll.

ALTERNATIVE APPROACHES TO PLACENTAL EXAMINATION

Prefixation. By way of necessity (submission from distant sites) or preference, many pathologists examine placentas that are submitted after fixation in formalin (9). The most important consideration with this approach is the amount of formalin, which should be at least 2

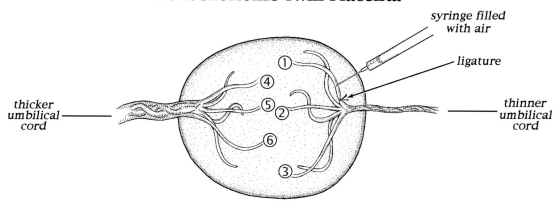

Figure 13-3

SCHEMATIC DIAGRAM DEPICTING A METHOD FOR THE RAPID EVALUATION OF TWIN ANASTOMOSES IN MONCHORIONIC TWIN PLACENTAS

Beginning with the placenta having the thinner umbilical cord, all major arteries (travelling over veins) are back ligated and injected with air. Numbers 1-6 indicate sequential injection of all major arteries in both placentas. The appearance of air in arteries or veins of the opposite placenta confirms a major unobstructed anastomosis.

to 3 volumes. Other pathologists prefer to prefix freshly received placentas in order to enhance the firmness of parenchymal lesions or decrease the risk of viral transmission to the examiner. The latter consideration, although intuitively reasonable, is not based on studies demonstrating protection.

Techniques for the examination and sampling of formalin-fixed placentas are the same as described above. Placental weight is increased by approximately 10 percent following fixation, an increase with little clinical relevance (5). In terms of ease of processing, membrane rolls are more difficult to prepare after fixation but parenchymal sections are easier. With the exception of poor fixation due to inadequate amounts of fixative, the histologic appearance is minimally altered by prefixation. A small amount of villous shrinkage with prefixation may lead to overdiagnosis of "accelerated maturation" by inexperienced observers (see chapter 6).

Orientation of the Membrane Role. Two schools of thought have emerged with respect to the preparation of membrane roles. In the one outlined above, priority is given to obtaining marginal placental tissue to assess decidual arteries, circumvallation, and marginal separation. This method incorporates a piece of marginal placenta at the center of the membrane roll. In the other school, priority is given to the site of membrane rupture to assess necrosis and degree of inflammation (4). In this method, the point of rupture forms the center of the role.

En Face Sections of the Basal Plate. Obtaining sufficient basal plate to assess abnormalities such as atherosis, persistent muscularization of basal arteries, chronic deciduitis, excessive fibrin deposition, or superficial implantation requires careful preparation of parenchymal tissue blocks. An alternative technique has been described in which en face "shave" sections are taken parallel to the basal plate (14). These sections provide an interesting perspective not usually captured in standard sections, but are not easy to cut or prepare.

SPECIAL STUDIES

Histochemical Stains. Stains for microorganisms (Gomori methenamine silver [GMS], periodic acid–Schiff [PAS], Gram, silver impregnation stains [Steiner, Warthin-Starry, Dieterle]) and hemosiderin deposition (Prussian blue, Gomori's iron stain) are useful in selected cases. Phosphotungstic acid hematoxylin (PTAH) stains may assist in identifying early fetal thrombi. Alcian blue and PAS have been used in the assessment of metabolic storage disease (25), but have little specificity in our experience. The demonstration of meconium by the Luna-Ishak stain has been advocated by at least one investigator (1).

Immunocytochemistry. Assessment of early and late antigens of cytomegalovirus is of some utility, although the ability to detect additional positive cases over and above those already identified by diagnostic inclusions is limited. CD68 staining to demonstrate the monomorphic nature of the intervillous infiltrate is useful in cases of chronic histiocytic intervillositis (7). Other lineage markers for fetal capillary endothelium (CD34), T lymphocytes (CD3), natural killer (NK) cells (CD56), plasma cells (syndecan-1), metastatic tumors (carcinoembryonic antigen [CEA], HMB45, cytokeratins), trophoblast subtypes (keratin, human chorionic gonadotropin [HCG], human placental lactogen [HPL], and placental alkaline phosphatase [PLAP]), and decidual cells (desmin) are occasionally useful.

Polymerase Chain Reaction. Placentas showing nonimmune hydrops or excessive fetal NRBCs can be evaluated for parvovirus B19 infection by polymerase chain reaction (PCR) (27). Specific fetal mutations (e.g., factor V Leiden) are identified using DNA extracted from paraffin-embedded umbilical cord tissue (30). The maternal versus paternal origin of chromosomes in cases of suspected complete or partial mole can be assessed using PCR-based microsatellite analysis of decidual and placental tissues (13,24).

Cytogenetics. The placental karyotype may be useful in cases where the fetus is either unavailable or macerated. Routine karyotyping is not generally helpful in cases of suspected confined placental mosaicism (see chapter 4) because the abnormalities are often focal and confined to cell lineages, such as trophoblast cells or amniocytes, which are not cultured by conventional techniques. Direct karyotyping of trophoblast cells and competitive genomic hybridization are more sensitive techniques for detecting confined placental mosaicism, but are unfortunately not available in most pathology laboratories (3,12). Flow cytometry or image analysis is useful for the confirmation of polyploidy in some partial (triploid or pentaploid) and complete (tetraploid) molar pregnancies (16). More specific genetic questions involving particular chromosomes (e.g., translocations) may be addressed by multicolor fluorescence in situ hybridization (FISH) (19).

Electron Microscopy. Ultrastructural examination is useful in some cases with suspected inborn errors of metabolism, particularly in the context of first trimester chorionic villous sampling (17). In rare cases, examination for viral capsids may be undertaken, but a thorough knowledge of the expected structure, size, and location of the expected structures is essential to avoid misinterpretation of artifacts (32).

Bacterial Cultures. Although many studies have demonstrated that organisms causing chorioamnionitis can be recovered from the placenta in over 95 percent of cases, this information is not generally thought to be clinically useful (11,21). The arguments against placental culture are as follows. Chorioamnionitis is a stereotyped response to any organism. Variables such as duration of infection, maternal antibody levels, and the magnitude of the fetal inflammatory response are more important than the identity of the pathogen. Most infections are caused by easily predictable, but difficult to culture, organisms such as vaginal anaerobes and mycoplasma. Identification of more virulent organisms, such as *Escherichia coli,* group B *Streptococcus,* and *Haemophilus influenzae,* from the placenta is poorly predictive of fetal infection (and hence prone to overinterpretation) and rarely alters clinical management. If placental cultures are elected, strict adherence to proper technique is essential since placentas are delivered through a nonsterile birth canal. One technique is to cauterize and incise the amnionic surface of the chorionic plate and slide the sterile culture swab between the amnionic and chorionic layers (15). An alternative is to culture the subchorionic fibrin, a technique that is likely to have decreased sensitivity, but perhaps more specificity (2). Despite these objections to routine culture, careful bacteriologic studies to delineate the pathogenic properties of specific organisms may help explain why some instances of chorioamnionitis are so injurious while others are not.

Other. In situ hybridization and various morphometric techniques to study placental architecture are beyond the scope of this publication but have been reviewed in recent publications (20,26).

REFERENCES

1. Altshuler G, Arizawa M, Molnar-Nadasdy G. Meconium-induced umbilical cord vascular necrosis and ulceration: a potential link between the placenta and poor pregnancy outcome. Obstet Gynecol 1992;79:760–6.
2. Aquino TI, Zhang J, Kraus FT, Knefel R, Taff T. Subchorionic fibrin cultures for bacteriologic study of the placenta. Am J Clin Pathol 1984;81:482–6.
2a. Bajoria R, Wigglesworth J, Fisk NM. Angio-architecture of monochorionic placentas in relation to the twin-twin transfusion syndrome. Am J Obstet Gynecol 1995;172:856–63.
3. Barrett IJ, Lomax BL, Loukianova T, Tang SS, Lestou VS, Kalousek DK. Comparative genomic hybridization: a new tool for reproductive pathology. Arch Pathol Lab Med 2001;125:81–4.
4. Bendon RW, Sander C. Examination of the placenta. In: Lewis S, Perrin E, eds. Pathology of the placenta. New York: Churchill Livingston; 1999:27–47.
5. Benirschke K, Kaufmann P. Pathology of the human placenta. New York, NY: Springer; 2000.
6. Blickstein I, Varon Y, Varon E. Implications of differences in coiling indices at different segments of the umbilical cord. Gynecol Obstet Invest 2001;52:203–6.
7. Boyd TK, Redline RW. Chronic histiocytic intervillositis: a placental lesion associated with recurrent reproductive loss. Hum Pathol 2000;31:1389–96.
8. De Paepe ME, Burke S, Luks FI, Pinar H, Singer DB. Demonstration of placental vascular anatomy in monochorionic twin gestations. Pediatr Dev Pathol 2002;5:37–44.
9. Fox H. Pathology of the placenta, 2nd ed. Philadelphia: W.B. Saunders; 1997.
10. Gersell DJ. ASCP survey on placental examination. American Society of Clinical Pathologists. Am J Clin Pathol 1998;109:127–43.
11. Hillier SL, Martius J, Krohn M, Kiviat N, Holmes KK, Eschenbach DA. A case-control study of chorioamnionic infection and histologic chorioamnionitis in prematurity. N Engl J Med 1988;319:972–80.
12. Kalousek DK, Dill FJ. Chromosomal mosaicism confined to the placenta in human conceptions. Science 1983;221:665–7.
13. Keep D, Zaragoza M, Hassold T, Redline RW. Very early complete hydatidiform mole. Hum Pathol 1996;27:708–13.
14. Khong TY, Chambers HM. Alternative method of sampling placentas for the assessment of uteroplacental vasculature. J Clin Pathol 1992;45:925–7.
15. Kundsin RB, Driscoll SG, Monson RR, Yeh C, Biano SA, Cochran WD. Association of ureaplasma urealyticum in the placenta with perinatal morbidity and mortality. N Engl J Med 1984;310:941–5.
16. Lage JM, Bagg A. Hydatidiform moles: DNA flow cytometry, image analysis and selected topics in molecular biology. Histopathology 1996;28:379–82.
17. Lake BD, Young EP, Winchester BG. Prenatal diagnosis of lysosomal storage diseases. Brain Pathol 1998;8:133–49.
18. Langston C, Kaplan C, Macpherson T, et al. Practice guideline for examination of the placenta: developed by the Placental Pathology Practice Guideline Development Task Force of the College of American Pathologists. Arch Pathol Lab Med 1997;121:449–76.
19. Lorber BJ, Grantham M, Peters J, Willard HF, Hassold TJ. Nondisjunction of chromosome-21: comparisons of cytogenetic and molecular studies of the meiotic stage and parent of origin. Am J Hum Genet 1992;51:1265–76.
20. Mayhew TM, Barker BL. Villous trophoblast: morphometric perspectives on growth, differentiation, turnover and deposition of fibrin-type fibrinoid during gestation. Placenta 2001;22:628–38.
21. Pankuch GA, Appelbaum PC, Lorenz RP, Botti JJ, Schachter I, Naeye RL. Placental microbiology and histology and the pathogenesis of chorioamnionitis. Obstet Gynecol 1984;64:802–6.
22. Powers WF, Kiely JL. The risks confronting twins: a national perspective. Am J Obstet Gynecol 1994;170:456–61.
23. Redline RW, Hassold T, Zaragoza MV. Prevalence of the partial molar phenotype in triploidy of maternal and paternal origin. Hum Pathol 1998;29:505–11.
24. Redline RW, Shah D, Sakar H, Schluchter M, Salvator A. Placental lesions associated with abnormal growth in twins. Pediatr Dev Pathol 2001;4:473–81.
25. Roberts DJ, Ampola MG, Lage JM. Diagnosis of unsuspected fetal metabolic storage disease by routine placental examination. Pediatr Pathol 1991;11:647–56.
26. Robertson EG, Neer KJ. Placental injection studies in twin gestation. Am J Obstet Gynecol 1983;147:170–4.

27. Rogers BB, Rogers ZR, Timmons CF. Polymerase chain reaction amplification of archival material for parvovirus B19 in children with transient erythroblastopenia of childhood. Pediatr Pathol Lab Med 1996;16:471–8.
28. Souter V, Kapur R, Nyhold D, et al. A report of dizygous monochorionic twins. N Engl J Med 2003;349:154–8.
29. Strong TH Jr, Jarles DL, Vega JS, Feldman DB. The umbilical coiling index. Am J Obstet Gynecol 1994;170:29–32.
30. Vern TZ, Alles AJ, Kowal-Vern A, Longtine J, Roberts DJ. Frequency of factor V (Leiden) and prothrombin G20210A in placentas and their relationship with placental lesions. Hum Pathol 2000;31:1036–43.
31. Vogler C, Petterchak J, Sotelo-Avila C, Thorpe C. Placental pathology for the surgical pathologist. Adv Anat Pathol 2000;7:214–29.
32. Wang J, Atchison RW, Walpusk J, Jaffe R. Echovirus hepatic failure in infancy: report of four cases with speculation on the pathogenesis. Perspect Pediatr Pathol 2001;4:454–60.
33. Yang SS. ADAM sequence and innocent amniotic band: manifestations of early amnion rupture. Am J Med Genet 1990;37:562–8.

14 DIAGNOSTIC ULTRASOUND IN OBSTETRICS

INTRODUCTION

Diagnostic ultrasound has had a profound influence on obstetric practice. The potential benefits of ultrasound screening of pregnant women include correct assignment of gestational age, determination of fetal number, diagnosis of uterine/adnexal pathology, detection of fetal malformations/growth disturbances, and identification of placental abnormalities. In 1984, the National Institutes of Health (NIH) published a consensus conference list of indications for sonography in pregnancy (Table 14-1) (11). At that time, the NIH also commissioned an expert panel to evaluate the efficacy of ultrasound screening of low-risk pregnancies. This ultimately resulted in the Routine Antenatal Diagnostic Imaging with Ultrasound (RADIUS) trial (15). RADIUS was a multicenter, prospective randomized controlled trial involving 15,151 pregnant women at low risk for perinatal complications. Women were randomly assigned to receive either two ultrasound examinations, one at 15 to 22 weeks and the other at 31 to 35 weeks, or ultrasound only for clinical indications. The RADIUS study revealed no significant difference in perinatal morbidity or mortality between the routinely screened pregnant women and the group scanned only for clinical indications. The trial did demonstrate that one or more clinical indications for ultrasound developed in 45 percent of low-risk women. Despite the lack of proven benefit in women with low-risk pregnancies, ultrasound imaging is now routinely employed in the management of most pregnancies, reflecting the expectations of patients, societal pressures, and the numerous clinical indications for its use.

ULTRASOUND IMAGING OF THE PLACENTA AND UMBILICAL CORD

A routine component of the ultrasound screening examination is assessment of placental location, specifically its relation to the internal cervical os. Placenta previa, a placenta that presents in front of the fetus, is not an uncommon finding in the midtrimester, occurring in as many as 1 in 20 pregnancies (fig. 14-1). The majority of these resolve spontaneously with advancing gestation so that the risk in the third trimester is approximately 1 in 200. A

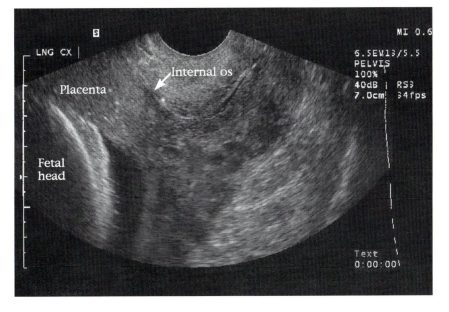

Figure 14-1

INTRAVAGINAL ULTRASOUND IMAGE OF THE MATERNAL PELVIS IN A SAGITTAL PLANE THROUGH THE CERVIX AT 33 WEEKS' GESTATION

Maternal head is at the left, her feet to right. The lower margin of the placenta extends between the fetal head and the internal os of the cervix, indicating a marginal placenta previa.

Table 14-1
INDICATIONS FOR SONOGRAPHY IN PREGNANCY[a]

Estimation of gestational age for patients with uncertain clinical dates and for confirmation of clinical dating for patients who are to undergo elective repeat cesarean delivery, induction of labor, or elective termination of pregnancy

Evaluation of fetal growth (when the patient has an identified cause for uteroplacental insufficiency, such as severe preeclampsia, chronic hypertension, chronic significant renal disease, or severe diabetes mellitus, or for other medical complications of pregnancy when fetal malnutrition is suspected [intrauterine growth restriction or macrosomia])

Vaginal bleeding of undetermined etiology during pregnancy

Determination of fetal presentation when the presenting part cannot be adequately assessed in labor

Suspected multiple gestation

Adjunct to amniocentesis (chorionic villus sampling)

Significant uterine size-clinical dates discrepancy

Pelvic mass detected clinically

Suspected hydatidiform mole

Adjunct to cervical cerclage

Suspected ectopic pregnancy or significant risk for ectopic pregnancy

Adjunct to special procedures such as chorionic villus sampling, in vitro fertilization, intrauterine transfusion

Suspected fetal death

Suspected uterine abnormality (uterine duplication malformation, significant leiomyoma)

Intrauterine contraception device localization

Ovarian follicle development surveillance

Biophysical profile for fetal well-being (after 28 weeks' gestation)

Observation of intrapartum events (e.g., version/extraction of second twin, manual removal of placenta)

Suspected polyhydramnios or oligohydramnios

Suspected abruptio placenta

Adjunct to external version from breech to vertex presentation

Estimation of fetal weight and/or presentation in premature rupture of membranes and/or premature labor

Abnormal serum alpha-fetoprotein value for clinical gestational age

Follow-up observation of identified fetal anomaly

History of previous congenital anomaly

Serial evaluation of fetal growth in multiple gestations

Estimation of gestational age in late registrants of prenatal care

[a]Modified from an NIH consensus study, reference 1.

commonly accepted definition of a low-lying placenta is one in which the placental margin is within 2 cm of the internal cervical os. Translabial and intravaginal ultrasound imaging allow definitive assessment of placental location in relation to the internal os. The risk for persistent placenta previa is increased in women who have had a previous cesarian section, which also increases the risk for abnormal placental invasion of the myometrium which can result in placenta accreta, percreta, and increta.

Clinically, placenta, accreta, percreta, and increta result in failure of the placenta to separate from the uterus following delivery of the fetus with subsequent hemorrhage that may be life-threatening. These disorders are not usually definitively diagnosed sonographically. However, certain ultrasound findings should increase

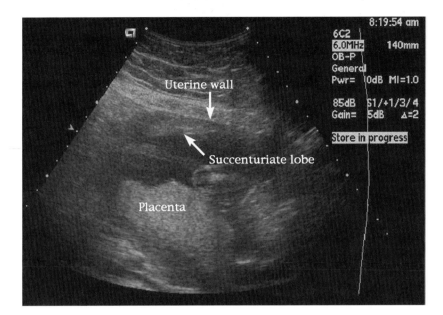

Figure 14-2

ULTRASOUND IMAGE OF A SUCCENTURIATE LOBE

The main placental mass is attached to the posterior uterine wall in the white area below (placenta), and the succenturiate lobe (arrow) is the oval pale white area above, attached to the anterior uterine wall. (See chapter 4, figs. 4-13 and 4-14, for gross pathologic correlation.)

the index of suspicion, especially in patients with clinical risk factors such as placenta previa, previous cesarian section, and advanced maternal age. These findings include absence or thinning of the normal hypoechoic (hypoechoic refers to a dark region in a sonographic image where the echoes appear less bright than the surrounding structures) zone between the placenta and myometrium of the anterior lower uterine segment, irregularity or disruption of the uterine serosa/bladder wall interface, large prominent vascular spaces in the placenta, and villous tissue extension into the bladder. While ultrasound may be useful in identifying patients at risk for abnormal implantation, the evolution of rapid magnetic resonance imaging (MRI) provides an adjunctive imaging technique capable of providing a more reliable assessment of suspected placenta accreta/increta/percreta.

Sonographic evaluation of the placenta can detect other variants of placental location and structure. A succenturiate placental lobe is identified as a portion of placenta attached to the main body of the placenta by vessels in the fetal membranes. Most succenturiate lobes are small, although they may rival the main body of the placenta in size (fig. 14-2). The umbilical cord insertion site designates the main body of the placenta. Such accessory lobes do not usually interfere with fetal growth and development. However, knowledge of their presence is important to assure all placental tissue is removed at delivery, thereby avoiding postpartum hemorrhage and infection due to retained products of conception.

Vasa previa is a rare condition (1 in 2,000 to 5,000 deliveries) that refers to the presence of umbilical cord vessels overlying the internal cervical os in front of the presenting fetal part. Rupture of these vessels may result in fetal exsanguination. Vasa previa should be considered in the setting of a velamentous cord insertion site and succenturiate lobe when the body of the placenta is located in the lower uterine segment and the lobe is on the opposite side of the internal cervical os. In patients at risk, the use of transvaginal ultrasound and color Doppler imaging are important in establishing the diagnosis. In equivocal cases, the finding of characteristic umbilical artery Doppler waveforms in vessels adjacent to the internal os is helpful in establishing the diagnosis.

Cystic areas (fluid-filled spaces which appear dark on the ultrasound image), sometimes prominent, are commonly observed when imaging the placenta (fig. 14-3). Such lesions are not always clinically significant and may correspond with such pathologic findings as perivillous fibrin deposition, subchorionic fibrin deposition, and intervillous thrombosis (18). Differentiation among these various etiologies

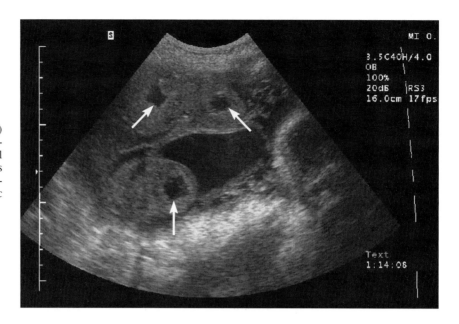

Figure 14-3

ULTRASOUND IMAGE OF INTRAPLACENTAL CYST

Three hypoechoic (dark) areas within the lighter placental mass represent intraplacental hematomas or cystic areas (arrows). (See chapter 6, figs. 6-13 and 6-16, for pathologic correlation.)

is not possible sonographically. Placental function is generally not impaired unless such lesions are large (greater than 2 to 3 cm) or numerous (more than five).

Subchorionic hemorrhage typically presents at the placental margin as a small, complex cystic area which may separate the chorion from the myometrium (fig. 14-4). This finding is common, especially in the first trimester in patients with a history of vaginal bleeding. Subchorionic hemorrhage is associated with miscarriage and preterm labor.

As the placenta matures, calcifications appear in a relatively predictable fashion. This is the basis of an attempt to "grade" placental changes and correlate the sonographic placental grade with pulmonary maturity (17). Echogenic (bright) areas in the placental substance are grade I, echogenic areas in the basal area of the placenta near the uterine wall are grade II, and indentations of the chorionic plate extending to the basal plate and larger irregular echo densities (bright areas) within the placenta constitute grade III. Due to the lack of a consistent relationship between placental grade and pulmonary maturity or fetal outcome, this scheme currently has little clinical relevance.

Placental abruption refers to premature separation of the normally implanted placenta, and is characterized by abdominal pain, vaginal bleeding, and uterine tenderness. Abruption is a clinical, not a sonographic, diagnosis. However, there are ultrasound findings that may be observed as a result of the presence of maternal blood beneath the placenta, membranes, or both. The ultrasound appearance is variable depending on the timing of the hemorrhage. Recent blood collections are relatively hyperechoic (i.e., appear brighter than surrounding structures), becoming less bright as the clot organizes. As the clot lysis, a mixed echo texture is seen. Sonographically, abruption typically extends from the margin of the placenta. As expected, the larger the size of the retroplacental hemorrhage the worse the prognosis. Detachment of more than 30 to 40 percent of the placenta from the myometrium is associated with fetal growth restriction and death.

The umbilical cord can be visualized sonographically beginning at 8 weeks' gestation, at which time the length is similar to the crown-rump length. The umbilical cord length continues to parallel fetal length throughout gestation. The normal umbilical cord contains two arteries and one vein. The umbilical vein delivers oxygenated blood from the placenta to the fetus via its connection with the left portal vein. The umbilical arteries originate from the hypogastric arteries, course immediately to the right and left of the fetal bladder, and return deoxygenated blood from the fetus to the placenta through the umbilical cord (fig. 14-5).

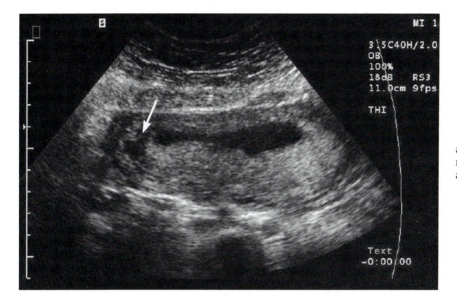

Figure 14-4

ULTRASOUND IMAGE OF SUBCHORIONIC HEMATOMA

The small, dark, hypoechoic area (arrow) toward the left margin of the placenta represents a subchorionic hematoma.

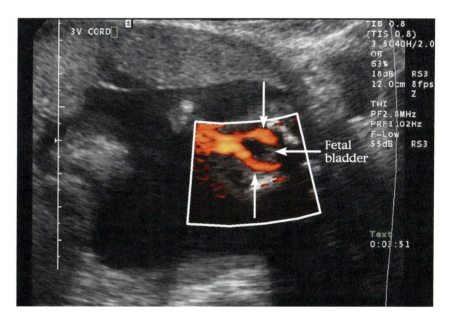

Figure 14-5

TRANSVERSE IMAGE THROUGH THE PELVIS OF AN 18-WEEK FETUS

Power Doppler image confirms the presence of two umbilical arteries (orange, marked by arrows) joining at left to enter the umbilical cord at its insertion. The fetal bladder is the dark space between the two vessels. Compare with figure 14-6.

The most common malformation of the umbilical cord is a single umbilical artery (SUA). SUA occurs in approximately 1 percent of pregnancies and is thought to result from atrophy due to thrombosis rather than primary agenesis. SUA is associated with other structural malformations and suboptimal fetal growth. Prenatal studies have reported associated structural fetal malformations in 26 to 43 percent of cases of SUA (24). SUA is detected by examining the fetal end of the cord in cross section. If there is any question regarding vessel number in the umbilical cord, color Doppler imaging may be used to document the umbilical arteries passing immediately lateral to the bladder (fig. 14-6). When observed prenatally, a SUA should prompt a search for other malformations and follow-up sonographic assessment of fetal growth.

Cysts of the umbilical cord are occasionally detected on prenatal ultrasound imaging. When located near the fetal end of the umbilical cord, such cysts often represent remnants of the omphalomesenteric duct or allantoic duct, are lined by epithelium, and may be a transient

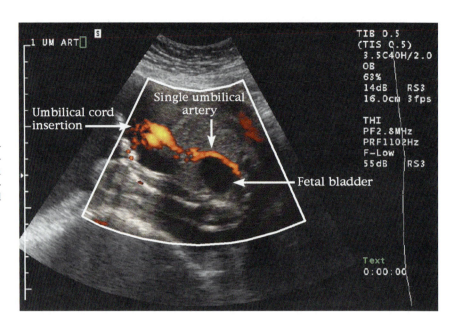

Figure 14-6

TRANSVERSE IMAGE OF THE PELVIS OF A 26-WEEK FETUS

Power Doppler image confirms that only a single umbilical artery has branched from its origin at the iliac artery, passing lateral to the bladder toward the umbilicus.

finding or persist to term. The identification of these cysts should prompt a search for malformations of the gastrointestinal and genitourinary tracts.

Umbilical cord hematomas are observed prenatally, usually following invasive diagnostic/therapeutic procedures, primarily amniocentesis and cordocentesis. Rarely, spontaneous cord hematomas occur.

Umbilical vein varices present sonographically as focal dilatations of the umbilical vein. They may occur within the fetal abdomen as well as in the cord. These varices can be large, are found in false knots of the cord, and usually have no clinical significance. Aneurysmal dilatation of surface vessels in the chorionic plate occur in mesenchymal dysplasia of the placenta, a feature of the Beckwith-Wiedemann syndrome.

ULTRASOUND IMAGING OF THE FETUS

Guidelines for the performance of the antepartum obstetrical ultrasound examination have been promulgated by the American Institute of Ultrasound and Medicine (AIUM), a multidisciplinary organization dedicated to promoting the appropriate and effective use of ultrasound imaging in clinical medicine. Standards for first and second/third trimester ultrasound examination follow.

First Trimester Ultrasound Examination

The first trimester ultrasound consists of four components.

The presence, location, and contents of a gestational sac. If a gestational sac is identified, its location (intrauterine versus extrauterine) should be documented. The definitive diagnosis of an intrauterine pregnancy requires the presence of a yolk sac or embryo in a well-defined fluid collection completely surrounded by myometrium.

The presence or absence of fetal cardiac activity. Fetal heart motion should always be observed when the crown-rump length is greater than or equal to 5 mm. An embryo heart rate less than 90 beats per minute is associated with an increased risk for fetal death.

Fetal number. This is determined by documenting the number of embryos/fetuses. This includes assessment of chorionicity in multifetal gestations.

Evaluation of the uterus, adnexa, and cul-de-sac. The presence of uterine/adnexal masses and any significant volume of free fluid in the cul-de-sac should be sought.

Second and Third Trimester Ultrasound Examination

The second and third trimester ultrasound includes seven components.

Documentation of fetal life, number, presentation, and activity. The presence or absence of fetal heart motion and activity should be reported, including a description of any abnormalities of fetal heart rate and rhythm. For multifetal gestations, chorionicity should be assessed by examining the number of placentas, thickness of the intervening membranes, and fetal genders. In monochorionic twins, there is a single placental mass, very thin dividing membrane, and like fetal genders. Monoamnionicity is suggested by failure to visualize a dividing membrane, plus intermingling of the umbilical cords. In multifetal pregnancies, fetal sizes and amnionic fluid volumes should be compared. Fetal presentation is important to note, especially in the third trimester.

Documentation of the amnionic fluid volume. This is reported as normal, increased, or decreased for gestational age. Reduced or absent amnionic fluid volume is associated with fetal growth restriction, premature rupture of the membranes, and fetal renal pathology, such as renal agenesis, multicystic dysplastic kidney, and bladder outlet obstruction. Increased amnionic fluid volume is observed with proximal gastrointestinal obstruction, fetal central nervous system malformations, and fetal macrosomia as may be observed in mothers with insulin-dependent diabetes mellitus.

Assessment of placental location. The relationship of the placenta to the internal cervical os should be documented, as should any separation of the placenta from the uterine wall, placental cysts or tumors, and the number of vessels in the umbilical cord.

Assignment of gestational age. This is designated at the initial ultrasound examination and should not normally be readjusted on the basis of subsequent examinations. If a prior ultrasound has been performed, the appropriateness of the interval fetal growth should be noted. In the second and third trimesters, gestational age is usually assigned using a combination of cranial and limb measurements. These typically include the biparietal diameter (BPD), head circumference (HC; derived from a combination of the BPD and occipitofrontal diameter), and femur length (FL). Gestational age is unable to be accurately assigned sonographically in the third trimester due to biologic variation among the biometric parameters.

Estimated fetal weight (EFW). The EFW is calculated using the abdominal circumference plus one or more of the other biometric parameters (BPD, HC, FL), using one of a number of published formulas for prediction of fetal size. The range of error for most formulas is approximately 10 percent. Fetal weight estimation is less reliable in gestations which are large or small for gestational age. The abdominal circumference is the best predictor of fetal size but the least reliable predictor of gestational age.

Evaluation of the uterus and adnexa. The presence, location, and size of uterine/adnexal masses should be documented. Uterine assessment should include evaluation of the cervix for shortening or dilation, which can be associated with an increased risk of preterm delivery.

Survey of fetal anatomy. This should include, but not necessarily be limited to the following.

Intracranial anatomy, including cerebral ventricles and posterior fossa (cerebellum and cisterna magna). This is to detect malformations such as hydrocephaly/ventriculomegaly, anencephaly, encephalocele, and holoprosencephaly. Posterior fossa abnormalities include Dandy-Walker malformation and obliteration of the cisterna magna with displacement of the cerebellar hemispheres, as is usually observed in cases of open neural tube defects (figs. 14-7, 14-8).

Spine. Rule out open defects of the spine and abnormal position of the spine as may be seen with scoliosis and kyphosis.

Four-chamber view of the heart. Note specifically the position of the heart in the thorax, overall cardiac size, the size of the ventricles and the atria, and the integrity of the septum and cardiac valves. This view is designed to rule out major structural cardiac malformations, such as hypoplastic ventricles, large septal defects, and atrioventricular canal defects. The four-chamber view of the heart does not allow exclusion of other major cardiac anomalies including conotruncal abnormalities (tetralogy of fallot and truncus arteriosus) and transposition of the great vessels. This view is also designed to detect major space-occupying lesions of the thorax, such as cystic adenomatoid malformations, pulmonary sequestrations, and congenital diaphragmatic hernia (figs. 14-9–14-11).

Stomach. Failure to visualize the stomach may be associated with proximal gastrointestinal

Placental Pathology

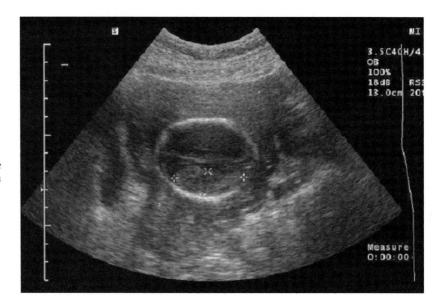

Figure 14-7

TRANSVERSE IMAGE THROUGH THE HEAD OF A 19-WEEK FETUS WHOSE MOTHER WAS BEING TREATED FOR ACUTE LEUKEMIA

The area delineated by the crosses is consistent with an intracranial hemorrhage.

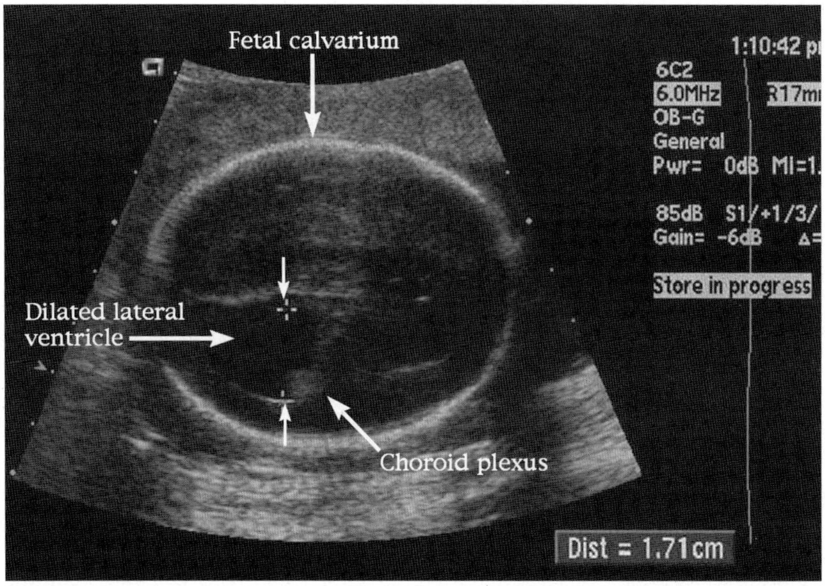

Figure 14-8

PRIMARY HYDROCEPHALUS IN A 21-WEEK FETUS

The lateral cerebral ventricular margins marked by the arrows measure 17 mm apart (normal is less than 10 mm). The pale white area (arrow) is the choroid plexus, dangling from the medial margin of the ventricle.

lesions, such as esophageal atresia. A smaller than expected stomach may be due to tracheoesophageal fistula.

Kidneys and urinary bladder. This allows detection of renal agenesis and genitourinary malformations and obstructions, including hydronephrosis, multicystic dysplastic kidney, duplex collecting system, ureterovesical junction obstruction, and distal bladder outlet obstruction as may occur with posterior urethral valves (fig. 14-12).

Cord insertion site/anterior abdominal wall. Ventral wall defects, including gastroschisis and omphalocele, are detected and distinguished from one another by examining the site of the umbilical cord insertion into the fetal abdominal wall (figs. 14-13, 14-14).

The above recommendations are considered to be minimum guidelines for a basic or screening obstetric ultrasound examination conducted for any of the common indications specified in Table 14-1. A comprehensive or targeted ultrasound examination is warranted when an increased risk for fetal pathology is identified. Indications for a targeted ultrasound

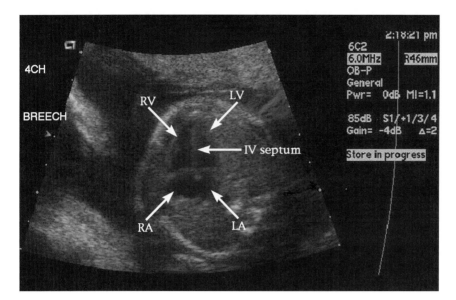

Figure 14-9

FOUR-CHAMBER VIEW THROUGH THE NORMAL FETAL HEART AT 22 WEEKS

There is concordance in the size of the hypoechoic (dark) ventricles (RV, LV) and atria (RA, LA), absence of septal defects, and separation of the two atrioventricular valves. The normal septa and valves form an echogenic (pale white) cross in the center of the heart. Compare with the atrioventricular canal defect in figure 14-10.

Figure 14-10

ATRIOVENTRICULAR CANAL DEFECT IN A 26-WEEK FETUS WITH TRISOMY 21

In this four-chamber view of the heart, the dark space in the center results from the defects in the upper portion of the ventricular septum, the lower portion of the atrial septum, and the single atrioventricular valve orifice. Compare with figure 14-9.

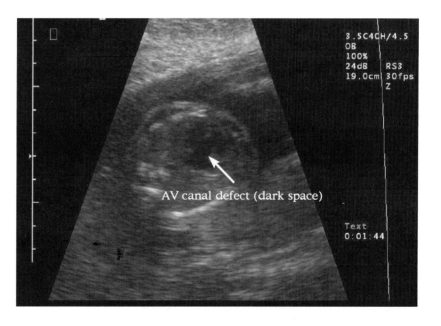

examination include abnormal findings on a screening ultrasound, an abnormal maternal serum screen for fetal neural tube defects and/or chromosome disorders, previous child with or significant family history of congenital malformations, and advanced maternal age. A targeted examination connotes interpretation by a physician with special expertise in the diagnosis and management of fetal malformations. The components of this more extensive evaluation include examination of the limbs, digits, face, cardiac outflow tracks and, when appropriate, cardiac color Doppler and flow velocity studies.

Ultrasound is increasingly utilized as a screening tool for fetal aneuploidy, in which case a host of ultrasound markers are sought in addition to the examination of the major organs. Ultrasound findings associated with an increased risk of Down's syndrome include a thickened nuchal skin fold, echogenic intracardiac focus, hyperechoic bowel, pyelectasis, relatively shortened femur and humerus, and an elevated BPD/FL ratio (7).

Placental Pathology

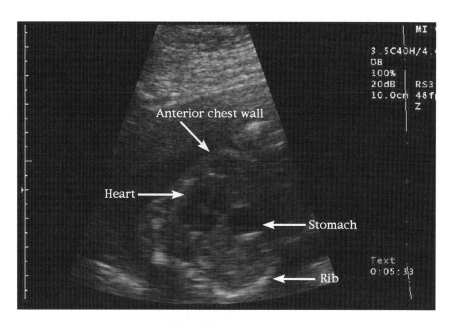

Figure 14-11

TRANSVERSE IMAGE THROUGH THE CHEST OF A 21-WEEK FETUS

The heart (at left) is displaced into the right hemithorax by the stomach (lower right), indicating a left-sided diaphragmatic hernia.

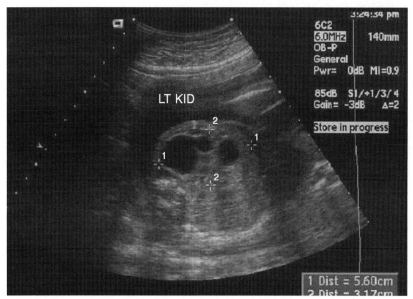

Figure 14-12

TRANSVERSE IMAGE THROUGH THE ABDOMEN OF A 26-WEEK FETUS

An enlarged left kidney contains multiple noncommunicating cysts of various sizes, consistent with a multicystic dysplastic kidney. The renal outline is marked by the four crosses and the cysts are represented by the rounded dark spaces within the kidney.

DOPPLER ULTRASOUND IN ASSESSMENT OF THE GROWTH-RESTRICTED FETUS

Fetal growth restriction is a condition of considerable clinical significance. Fetuses so affected are at increased risk for hypoxemia, acidemia, preterm delivery, and death (9). Neonatal sequelae include metabolic abnormalities, polycythemia, intraventricular hemorrhage, and neurologic damage. Recent evidence also suggests that changes in lipid metabolism in the growth-restricted fetus increase the risk for hypertension, stroke, and diabetes in these individuals as adults (3).

A variety of maneuvers are used in the assessment and management of the growth-restricted fetus. Chief among these is Doppler velocimetry, which provides a qualitative assessment of blood flow velocity.

Doppler interrogation of the umbilical artery was first reported in 1977 and since then has been one of the most vigorously evaluated of all tests of fetal well being (13). An ultrasound

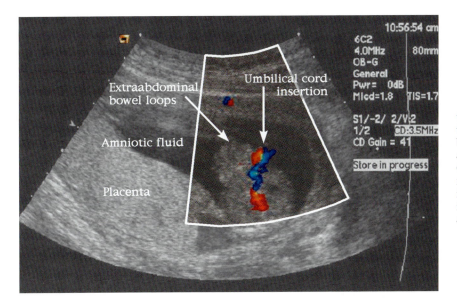

Figure 14-13

GASTROSCHISIS DEFECT IN A 15-WEEK FETUS

This transverse image through the abdomen demonstrates multiple loops of extra-abdominal bowel (arrow) herniated through a right paraumbilical defect. Color Doppler image shows the normal insertion of the umbilical cord into the abdominal wall immediately adjacent to the abdominal wall defect.

Figure 14-14

LARGE OMPHALOCELE IN A 34-WEEK FETUS

This transverse image through the fetal abdomen illustrates extrusion of most of the liver through a large ventral wall defect (margins of defect marked by arrows). The cord inserts into the dome of the omphalocele, not into the body wall, as it does in gastroschisis (see fig. 14-13).

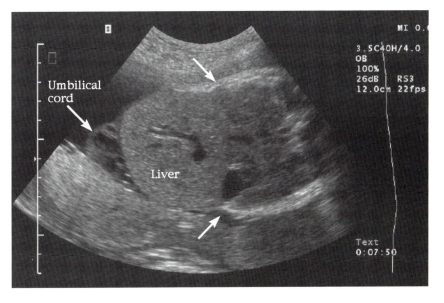

beam traversing a blood vessel is scattered by the movement of numerous cells moving at different rates. The subsequent Doppler signal is a combination of many frequencies and is proportional to the speed of the scatterer. This combination of frequencies is analyzed by computer and converted into a flow velocity waveform which represents the flow profile within a vessel. Due to a variety of technical limitations, the absolute velocity of blood flow cannot be reliably measured. In its stead, analysis of the flow waveform shape, which demonstrates the relationship between the systolic and diastolic components of blood flow in a vessel, is the preferred technique for evaluation of many vascular beds. A typical Doppler waveform illustrates the peak systolic velocity, the end-diastolic velocity, and the mean Doppler shift frequency.

A variety of indices have been employed to describe the profile of flow waveforms. All are designed to provide a quantitative description of the waveform to allow classification. The indices available on most commercial ultrasound equipment include: 1) systolic/diastolic (S/D) ratio, sometimes referred to as the A/B ratio; 2)

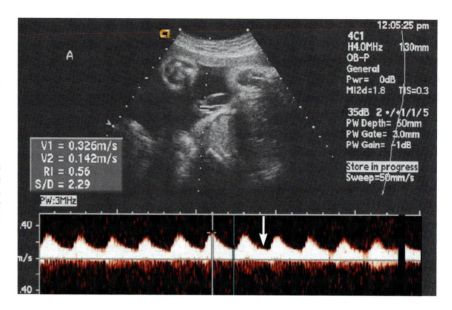

Figure 14-15

UMBILICAL ARTERY DOPPLER SYSTOLIC/DIASTOLIC (S/D) RATIO IN A NORMALLY GROWN TWIN OF A DICHORIONIC TWIN GESTATION

The height of the wave peaks indicates systolic flow and the height of the troughs indicates continuing diastolic flow (arrow). The S/D ratio of 2.29 in this twin is normal.

pulsatility index (PI) = S – D/A; and 3) resistance index (RI), also known as the Pourcelot's index = S – D/S. In these calculations, S is the peak systolic frequency, D is the end-diastolic velocity, and A is the mean value of the waveform over the cardiac cycle. These indices are derived from the maximum Doppler shift waveform and are highly correlated. The S/D ratio is the simplest to calculate and the most commonly used. The PI requires determination of the mean waveform height but is useful in describing a range of flow waveform shapes in cases where there is absent or reversed end-diastolic flow. As a rule, a low pulsatility waveform suggests low distal resistance and a high pulsatility waveform is observed in association with high vascular resistance (12,20,27).

Given that the arterial Doppler waveform reflects arterial flow velocity, it can be appreciated that downstream impedance has a major influence on waveform configuration and the aforementioned indices of measurement. Vasodilation reduces impedance and wave reflection while vasoconstriction has the opposite effect.

In normal pregnancies, the placenta is a low-resistance circuit with continuous forward flow throughout the cardiac cycle. As gestation advances, there is continuing angiogenesis, reduced vascular impedance, and a progressive increase in the end-diastolic velocity. This manifests as a decrease in the S/D ratio, PI, and RI (16).

Fetal growth restriction is often associated with uteroplacental vascular abnormalities that result in increased vascular impedance and abnormal umbilical artery flow velocity waveforms. While there is no absolute threshold for what is considered an abnormal Doppler index, an umbilical artery Doppler S/D ratio greater than 3.0 beyond 30 weeks' gestation is generally considered pathologic (figs. 14-15, 14-16) (13). As the umbilical artery S/D ratio increases, the birth weight percentile decreases (8,14). Absent end-diastolic flow is associated with obliteration of fetal stem vessels, while reversed end-diastolic flow is a manifestation of more extreme vascular pathology, including villous stromal hemorrhage and abnormal terminal villi (21,26). Evaluation of pregnancies with fetal growth restriction has demonstrated that increased impedance to flow in the uterine and umbilical arteries is associated with fetal hypoxemia and acidemia (23).

Multiple randomized controlled trials have demonstrated that Doppler ultrasound evaluation of the umbilical artery in high-risk pregnancies (primarily those with hypertension or suspected fetal growth restriction) is associated with a significant reduction in antenatal hospital admissions, inductions of labor, and perinatal mortality (1,22). An American College of Obstetricians and Gynecologists Clinical Management Guideline and subsequent expert opinion on in-

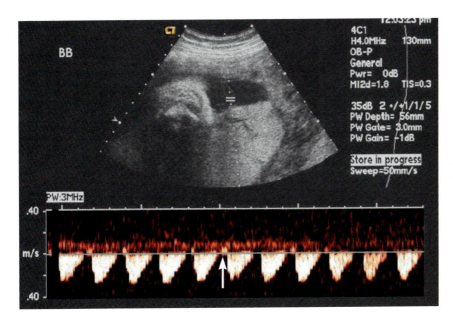

Figure 14-16

UMBILICAL ARTERY DOPPLER WAVEFORM IN A GROWTH-RESTRICTED TWIN

Other twin from the same pregnancy as in figure 14-15. Note the absence of any continuing flow between the systolic peaks (arrow). This indicates cessation of blood flow through the cord during diastole (absent end-diastolic flow). Placental lesions associated with growth restriction include especially decidual vasculopathy (chapter 6) and fetal thrombotic vasculopathy (chapter 6). (See also the discussion of growth restriction in chapter 3.)

trauterine growth restriction acknowledge the utility of umbilical artery velocimetry in the evaluation and management of fetal growth restriction (2,25). Doppler ultrasound imaging of the umbilical artery is useful in distinguishing between the normal, or constitutionally, small fetus and the pathologically small or growth-restricted fetus. Absent or reversed end-diastolic flow is predictive of fetal hypoxemia and possible acidemia while normal umbilical flow velocity waveforms likely reflect a small normal fetus. However, the precise role of Doppler ultrasound in optimizing the timing of delivery is not well defined and is currently the subject of a multicenter clinical trial (the Growth-Restriction Intervention Trial [GRIT], coordinated through the University of Leeds, UK).

While the relationship between abnormal umbilical artery Doppler flow velocity waveforms, preeclampsia and intrauterine growth restriction, and poor obstetric outcome is well established, the use of routine Doppler sonography in unselected or low-risk pregnancies has been more recently addressed. In theory, the application of Doppler velocimetry to low-risk pregnancies would allow identification of pregnancies in which there has been failure to maintain the normal low-impedance uterine and umbilical circulations prior to a clinical diagnosis of fetal compromise or uteroplacental insufficiency. A recent analysis of five trials including 14,338 women concluded that routine Doppler ultrasound in low-risk pregnancies conferred no benefits on mother or baby (10).

The uterine and umbilical arteries were the original targets of Doppler ultrasound. Its subsequent application to interrogation of fetal arterial and venous circulations has provided an additional tool for monitoring alterations in the regional blood flow which characterize fetal adaptation to placental dysfunction. In hypoxic fetuses, there is an initial redistribution of blood flow to the brain and heart. Decreased resistance to blood flow to the brain (brain sparing) manifests as a decrease in the PI of the middle cerebral artery. Fetal maladaptation to hypoxia may be associated with cardiac dysfunction, resulting in venous circulatory changes. Such changes are presumed to be secondary to reduced cardiac output due to myocardial hypoxia/ischemia. Impaired cardiac function is associated with increased venous velocities in the inferior vena cava and ductus venosus. Umbilical venous pulsations are a manifestation of significantly increased central venous pressure resulting from cardiac dysfunction and increased circulatory afterload. The above changes are associated with fetal acidemia (5,6,19).

Fetal growth restriction presenting in the third trimester is more likely to be associated with mild placental dysfunction and normal or minimally abnormal umbilical arterial Doppler studies. Absent or reduced end-diastolic flow is unlikely at greater than 32 to 34 weeks' gestation since this Doppler finding is associated with more severe placental vascular abnormalities resulting in earlier onset growth disturbance and decompensation. Arterial Doppler alterations occur weeks prior to fetal compromise while venous Doppler changes occur more proximate to fetal deterioration (4).

In summary, Doppler evaluation of the umbilical artery is a useful technique for the identification of the small fetus whose growth restriction is a result of placental vascular abnormalities that impede the delivery of oxygen and nutrients to the fetus. In such cases, the diastolic component of the Doppler flow waveform is reduced, resulting in an increased S/D ratio and PI. The absence or reversal of end-diastolic flow connotes progressive placental dysfunction and increased risk of fetal hypoxia. Abnormal studies of the umbilical artery are now often followed by Doppler interrogation of the fetal arterial and venous circulations. Specifically, a decrease in the PI of the middle cerebral artery is presumed to represent centralization, or brain sparing. Changes in the venous system are more ominous. An increase in venous velocities and umbilical venous pulsations are thought to reflect evolving cardiac dysfunction and impending fetal deterioration and possible death. While the utility of Doppler ultrasound in the identification of the fetus that merits more rigorous surveillance is not in dispute, its application to the ongoing evaluation of these at-risk pregnancies is the subject of clinical trials. Ideally, the information gained from these investigations will further define the timing and sequence of Doppler flow changes in fetal vessels and guide the clinician in striking the optimum balance between maximizing time in utero and proceeding with delivery prior to onset of fetal acidemia and death.

REFERENCES

1. Alfirevic Z, Neilson JP. Doppler ultrasonography in high-risk pregnancies: systematic review with meta-analysis. Am J Obstet Gynecol 1995;172:1379–87.
2. American College of Obstetrics and Gynecologists. Intrauterine growth restriction. ACOG Practice Bulletin 12. Washington, D.C.: ACOG; 2000.
3. Barker DJ, Gluckman PD, Godfrey KM, Harding JE, Owens JA, Robinson JS. Fetal nutrition and cardiovascular disease in adult life. Lancet 1993;341:938–41.
4. Baschat AA. Integrated fetal testing in growth restriction: combining multivessel Doppler and biophysical parameters. Ultrasound Obstet Gynecol 2003;21:1–8.
5. Baschat AA, Gembruch U, Harman CR. The sequence of changes in Doppler and biophysical parameters as severe fetal growth restriction worsens. Ultrasound Obstet Gynecol 2001;18:571–7.
6. Baschat AA, Harman CR. Antenatal assessment of the growth restricted fetus. Curr Opin Obstet Gynecol 2001;13:161–8.
7. Benacerraf B. Ultrasound evaluation of chromosomal abnormalities. In: Callen PW, ed. Ultrasonography in obstetrics and gynecology. Philadelphia: W.B. Saunders; 2000:38–67.
8. Berkowitz GS, Chitkara U, Rosenberg J, et al. Sonographic estimation of fetal weight and Doppler analysis of umbilical artery velocimetry in the prediction of intrauterine growth retardation: a prospective study. Am J Obstet Gynecol 1988;158:1149–53.
9. Bernstein IM, Horbar JD, Badger GJ, Ohlsson A, Golan A. Morbidity and mortality among very-low-birth-weight neonates with intrauterine growth restriction. The Vermont Oxford Network. Am J Obstet Gynecol 2000;182(Pt 1):198–206.
10. Bricker L, Neilson JP. Routine Doppler ultrasound in pregnancy. Cochrane Database Syst Rev 2000;2:CD001450.
11. Consensus Conference. The use of diagnostic ultrasound imaging during pregnancy. JAMA 1984;252:669–72.
12. Deane C. Doppler ultrasound: principles and practice. In Nicolaides KH, ed. Placental and fetal Doppler. New York: Parthenon Pub. Group; 2000:3–23.
13. Divon MY, Ferber A. Doppler evaluation of the fetus. Clin Obstet Gynecol 2002;45:1015–25.
14. Divon MY, Guidetti DA, Braverman JJ, Oberlander E, Langer O, Merkatz IR. Intrauterine growth retardation—a prospective study of the diagnostic value of real-time sonography combined with umbilical artery flow velocimetry. Obstet Gynecol 1988;72:611–4

15. Ewigman BG, Crane JP, Frigoletto FD, LeFevre ML, Bain RP, McNellis D. Effect of prenatal ultrasound screening on perinatal outcome. N Engl J Med 1993;329:821–7.
16. Goldkrand JW, Moore DH, Lentz SU, Clements SP, Turner AD, Bryant JL. Volumetric flow in the umbilical artery: normative data. J Matern Fetal Med 2000;9:224–8.
17. Grannum PA, Berkowitz RL, Hobbins JC. The ultrasonic changes in the maturing placenta and their relation to fetal pulmonic maturity. Am J Obstet Gynecol 1979;133:915–22.
18. Harris RD, Alexander RD. Ultrasound of the placenta and umbilical cord. In: Callen PW, ed. Ultrasonography in obstetrics and gynecology. Philadelphia: Saunders; 2000:597–625.
19. Marsal K. Intrauterine growth restriction. Curr Opin Obstet Gynecol 2002;14:127–35.
20. Maulik D. Hemodynamic interpretation of the arterial Doppler waveform. Ultrasound Obstet Gynecol 1993;3:219–27.
21. Mitra SC, Seshan SV, Riachi LE. Placental vessel morphometry in growth retardation and increased resistance of the umbilical artery Doppler flow. J Matern Fetal Med 2000;9:282–6.
22. Neilson JP, Alfirevic Z. Doppler ultrasound for fetal assessment in high-risk pregnancies. Cochrane Database Syst Rev 2000;2:CD000073.
23. Nicolaides KH, Bilardo CM, Soothill PW, Campbell S. Absence of end diastolic frequencies in the umbilical artery: a sign of fetal hypoxia and acidosis. BMJ 1988;297:1026–7.
24. Persutte WH, Hobbin J. Single umbilical artery: a clinical enigma in modern prenatal diagnosis. Ultrasound Obstet Gynecol 1995;6:216–29.
25. Resnik R. Intrauterine growth restriction. Obstet Gynecol 2002;99:490–6.
26. Salafia CM, Pezzullo JC, Minior VK, Divon MY. Placental pathology of absent and reversed end-diagnostic flow in growth-restricted fetuses. Obstet Gynecol 1997;90:830–6.
27. Thompson RS. Blood flow velocity waveforms. Semin Perinatol 1987;11:300–10.

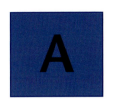

APPENDIX: PLACENTAL WEIGHTS AND MEASURES

THE VALUE OF PLACENTAL MEASUREMENTS

The recorded weight of any placenta is necessarily imprecise. The amounts of fetal and maternal blood remaining at the time it is weighed cannot be evaluated. Storage in a refrigerator is accompanied by a progressive, but variable, loss of weight, depending upon the amount of blood that drains from it. Published tables of placental weights vary considerably (compare Appendices 2, 3, 6, and 7, below). There appears to be a trend toward heavier placentas in more recent data. Placental weights increase after formalin fixation.

Based upon these variable data, Fox (3) concluded that placental weights have no value. Considered out of the context of the clinical and pathologic data, this is certainly correct. Pathologists habitually weigh every organ they get, placentas included. The value of any organ weight is crude at best, and out of context it has no independent meaning. Consider the information that a heart weighs 200 g. In isolation, the fact is useless. If we are provided some additional knowledge, such as, the patient is a 1-year-old child—or alternatively, is a 20-year-old athlete, very different prospects come to

Appendix 1A
UMBILICAL CORD LENGTHS FOR NORMAL FETUSES AT DEVELOPMENTAL AGES 8 TO 18 WEEKS[a]

Fetal Age (weeks)	Number[b]	Cord Length (cm)	95% Confidence Interval (cm)
8	3	6.4	5.2 – 7.7
9	6	8.0	7.0 – 9.1
10	7	9.7	8.7 – 10.6
11	8	11.3	10.5 – 12.1
12	15	12.9	12.2 – 13.6
13	12	14.5	13.9 – 15.1
14	12	16.1	15.5 – 16.7
15	8	17.7	17.1 – 18.4
16	9	19.4	18.6 – 20.1
17	9	21.0	20.5 – 21.4
18	3	22.6	21.5 – 23.7

[a]Table II.5 from Kalousek DK, Fitch N, Paradice BA. Pathology of the human embryo and previable fetus: an atlas. New York: Springer; 1990:228.
[b]Number of cases.

Appendix 1B
PLACENTAL WEIGHTS FOR NORMAL FETUSES AT DEVELOPMENTAL AGES 8 TO 18 WEEKS[a]

Fetal Age (weeks)	Number[b]	Placental Weight (g)	95% Confidence Interval (g)
8	2	1.6	0.0 – 3.7
9	7	15.2	13.3 – 17.0
10	10	28.8	27.2 – 30.4
11	9	42.4	41.1 – 43.8
12	14	56.1	54.8 – 57.3
13	17	69.7	68.4 – 71.0
14	15	83.3	81.8 – 84.8
15	12	96.9	95.2 – 98.6
16	11	110.5	108.5 – 112.5
17	14	124.2	121.8 – 126.5
18	4	137.8	135.0 – 140.5

[a]Table II.6 from Kalousek DK, Fitch N, Paradice BA. Pathology of the human embryo and previable fetus: an atlas. New York: Springer; 1990:228.
[b]Number of cases.

APPENDIX 1
A: Umbilical cord lengths for normal fetuses at developmental ages 8 to 18 weeks.
B: Placental weights for normal fetuses at developmental ages 8 to 18 weeks. These tables are especially helpful for evaluating placentas at earlier gestational ages, which are not covered in most other series (6).

Appendix 2A

PERCENTILES, MEANS, AND STANDARD DEVIATIONS FOR PLACENTAL WEIGHTS BY GESTATIONAL AGE[a]

Gestational Age (weeks)	N[b]	Mean	SD	\multicolumn{9}{c}{Percentile}
				3	5	10	25	50	75	90	95	97
22	19	189	89		99	107	130	166	206	285	499	
23	16	190	41			127	168	188	208	262		
24	16	190	42			128	157	192	222	252		
25	26	197	70		105	128	153	184	216	299	400	
26	22	226	100		107	138	179	200	259	281	570	
27	22	240	77		119	130	166	242	310	332	381	
28	41	223	66	103	128	140	173	214	261	321	361	371
29	37	269	96	124	135	161	214	252	309	352	496	629
30	42	324	88	185	190	208	269	316	374	433	502	570
31	57	314	105	142	152	175	246	313	360	417	479	579
32	69	325	77	161	214	241	275	318	377	436	461	465
33	117	351	83	190	224	252	286	352	413	446	475	504
34	160	381	84	221	260	283	322	382	430	479	527	558
35	260	411	99	232	250	291	344	401	471	544	600	626
36	538	447	110	270	291	320	369	440	508	580	628	679
37	1103	467	107	303	324	349	390	452	531	607	660	692
38	2469	493	103	320	335	365	420	484	560	629	675	706
39	3932	500	103	330	350	379	426	490	564	635	683	713
40	4114	510	100	340	360	390	440	501	572	643	685	715
41	1982	524	100	358	379	403	452	515	583	655	705	738
42	321	532	99	370	388	412	460	525	592	658	700	771

[a]Data derived from reference 2 with assistance from biostatistician Jane McCall.
[b]Number of placentas at each placental age; SD = standard deviation.

APPENDIX 2

A–C: Placental mean trimmed weights and percentiles by gestational age and fetal-placental weight ratios by gestational age. Data is compiled from 15,463 deliveries. The patient mix included a diversity of ethnic, racial, and demographic groups at the Baystate Medical Center, Springfield, Massachusetts. Placentas were weighed fresh, after removal of cords and membranes. Placentas from intrauterine death or obvious growth dysregulation (such as triploidy) and incomplete placentas were excluded (2).

A: Mean placental weights, standard deviations, and percentiles by gestational age. Small placentas in the 3rd to 5th percentile ranges are especially likely to be pathologic. Those at the 95th to 97th percentiles deserve attention, but neonatal morbidity is less common.

mind and the pathologist's attention level would undergo a quantum leap.

In our experience, the placental weight may be useful when considered in the context of gestational age and other clinical data. For instance, no matter which table or graph provided below is utilized, a placenta with no identifiable lesions at 36 weeks' gestation that weighs 400 g probably functioned normally, and requires no extra concern on the basis of weight alone. Another placenta at 36 weeks' gestation that weighs only 200 g—not a rare experience—requires some explanation. If no obvious reason is apparent, a closer look is

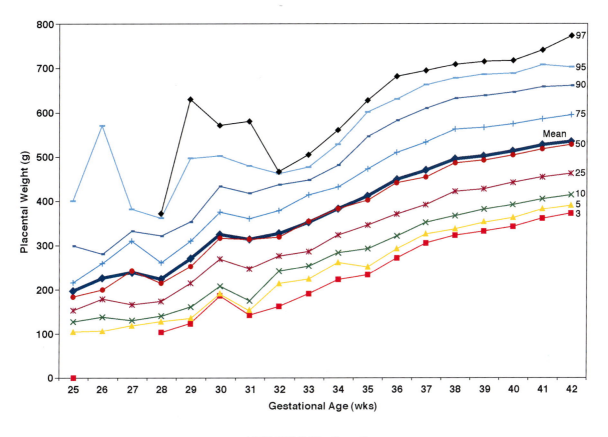

APPENDIX 2 (Continued)

B: Graphic representation of the percentile data in Appendix 2A. Data derived from reference 2 with assistance from biostatistician Jane McCall. Percentiles are listed at the right margin.

worthwhile. Some missing but significant historical data or a subtle pathologic process may need attention. Preeclampsia? Anticardiolipin antibodies? Fetal growth restriction? Confined placental mosaicism? Likewise, a 650-g placenta at 40 weeks may exceed the 90th percentile, but the only reliable correlate is a fetal weight over 4 kg. On the other hand, placentas that weigh more than 800 g, and especially those greater than 1,000 g, are almost certainly pathologic. The diagnostic possibilities of excessive weight include hydrops, uncontrolled gestational diabetes mellitus, Beckwith-Wiedemann syndrome, metabolic storage diseases, and massive perivillous fibrin deposition. A marked abnormality of placental weight should serve as a reminder to look again and think, and most successful pathologists are grateful for reminders.

Because of the discrepancies in recorded weights, we have commented with each set of tables upon the methods employed by each group of investigators and included our opinions about how to use the tables.

Distribution of cord coil index in 120 consecutive unselected pregnancies from the Permanente Medical Group. There is normally about one complete twist (coil)/5 cm of cord. The normal coil index is 0.2 coils/cm. The variations in coil index in an unselected group of patients are tabulated above. An overcoiled cord (OCC) has an index equal to 0.3 coils or more/cm, and an undercoiled cord (UCC) has an index of 0.1 or less. Principal clinical correlations with both OCC and UCC in this series were fetal death, intolerance to labor, intrauterine growth restriction, chorioamnionitis, thrombosis of chorionic plate vessels or cord, and cord stenosis.

Appendix 2C
FETAL-PLACENTA WEIGHT RATIO PERCENTILES BY GESTATIONAL AGE[a]

Gestational Age (weeks)	N[b]	Mean	SD	Percentile 3	5	10	25	50	75	90	95	97
22	19	2.9	0.8		1.0	1.0	2.0	2.4	3.6	3.9	4.3	
23	16	3.3	0.7				2.4	2.9	3.6	4.5		
24	16	3.4	1.0				2.0	2.6	4.0	4.6		
25	26	4.0	1.4		1.7	2.3	3.2	3.8	4.6	6.0	7.4	
26	22	4.1	1.2			2.1	2.8	3.4	3.7	4.8	5.2	7.7
27	22	4.5	1.1			2.6	3.0	3.3	3.6	4.5	6.0	7.1
28	41	4.8	1.0	2.3	2.5	3.6	3.9	4.2	4.7	6.5	6.6	6.9
29	37	5.2	1.4	1.9	2.5	3.7	4.4	5.0	5.7	7.5	8.0	9.2
30	42	5.2	1.1	2.7	3.1	3.6	4.5	5.1	5.8	6.8	6.9	7.6
31	57	5.5	1.1	3.3	4.1	4.4	4.7	5.4	6.2	6.9	7.3	8.2
32	69	5.9	1.2	3.2	4.1	4.4	5.0	5.8	6.8	7.7	7.9	8.4
33	117	6.0	1.1	4.3	4.5	4.7	5.2	6.0	6.6	7.7	8.2	8.7
34	160	6.2	1.0	4.4	4.7	5.0	5.5	6.1	6.7	7.5	7.9	8.2
35	260	6.4	1.2	4.5	4.7	5.0	5.6	6.3	7.2	8.0	8.6	9.1
36	538	6.6	1.1	4.8	4.9	5.3	5.8	6.4	7.3	8.1	8.4	8.8
37	1103	6.8	1.1	4.9	5.1	5.4	6.0	6.7	7.4	8.2	8.8	9.1
38	2469	6.9	1.1	5.1	5.2	5.6	6.1	6.8	7.5	8.3	8.9	9.2
39	3932	7.1	1.1	5.2	5.4	5.7	6.3	7.0	7.7	8.5	9.1	9.4
40	4114	7.2	1.1	5.3	5.5	5.8	6.4	7.1	7.9	8.6	9.1	9.5
41	1982	7.2	1.1	5.4	5.6	5.9	6.5	7.1	7.8	8.6	9.1	9.4
42	321	7.1	1.1	5.3	5.5	5.9	6.4	7.1	7.8	8.5	8.9	9.1

[a]Data derived from reference 2 with assistance from biostatistician Jane McCall.
[b]Number of placentas at each placental age; SD = standard deviation.

APPENDIX 2 (Continued)
C: Fetal-placental weight ratios, mean, standard deviations, and percentiles by gestational age.

Appendix 3A
MEAN WEIGHTS AND PERCENTILES FOR SINGLETON PLACENTAS[a]

Gestational Age (weeks)	90th Percentile	75th Percentile	Mean Singleton Placental Weight (g)	25th Percentile	10th Percentile	Number of Cases
21	172	158	143	128	114	3
22	191	175	157	138	122	6
23	211	193	172	151	133	7
24	233	212	189	166	145	9
25	256	233	208	182	159	19
26	280	255	227	200	175	14
27	305	278	248	219	192	9
28	331	302	270	238	210	16
29	357	327	293	259	229	11
30	384	352	316	281	249	12
31	411	377	340	303	269	14
32	438	403	364	325	290	24
33	464	428	387	347	311	30
34	491	453	411	369	331	32
35	516	477	434	391	352	44
36	542	501	457	412	372	36
37	566	524	478	432	391	32
38	589	547	499	452	409	62
39	611	567	519	470	426	103
40	632	587	537	487	442	193
41	651	605	553	502	456	87

[a]Table 1 from Pinar H, Sung CJ, Oyer CE, Singer DB. Reference values for singleton and twin placental weights. Pediatr Pathol Lab Med 1996;16:903.

APPENDIX 3

A: Table of mean trimmed weights and percentiles for singleton placentas with increasing placental ages (11). The data were collected at a large urban hospital at sea level. Term placentas were from normal deliveries and preterm placentas included only those from uncomplicated deliveries. Placentas associated with intrauterine fetal death, growth restriction, preeclampsia, chronic hypertension, antiphospholipid antibody syndrome, prolonged membrane rupture, congenital anomalies, amnionic fluid infection syndrome, maternal tobacco or drug use, gestational or preexisting diabetes mellitus, asphyxia, oligohydramnios, polyhydramnios, hydrops, and marked meconium staining were specifically excluded. Placentas with pathologic lesions such as infarcts, perivillous fibrin deposits, thrombi, and chorioangiomas greater than 1 percent of placental volume were also excluded. Gestational ages were calculated as the number of completed weeks between the first day of the last menstrual period and the day of delivery. In our experience, the greater weights listed below the 10th percentile in this table are less likely to identify significant pathology than the ranges provided in the weight curves published by Boyd et al. (Appendix 2) and by Naeye (Appendix 7).

Placental Pathology

APPENDIX 3
(Continued)

B: Graphic representation of data in Appendix A. (Fig. 1 from Pinar H, Sung CJ, Oyer CE, Singer DB. Reference values for singleton and twin placental weights. Pediatr Pathol Lab Med 1996;16:903.)

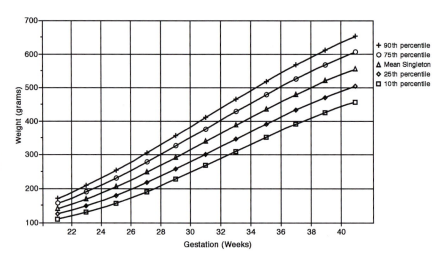

Appendix 4
MEAN WEIGHTS AND PERCENTILES FOR TWIN PLACENTAS[a]

Gestational Age (weeks)	90th Percentile	75th Percentile	Mean Twin Placental Weight (g)	25th Percentile	10th Percentile	Number of Cases
19	263	239	212	185	161	2
20	270	245	218	190	166	3
21	286	260	231	202	176	2
22	310	282	251	219	191	5
23	343	311	276	241	210	2
24	382	346	307	267	232	3
25	426	386	341	297	257	5
26	475	430	380	330	284	4
27	528	478	421	365	314	8
28	584	527	464	401	345	7
29	641	579	509	439	377	12
30	700	631	554	478	409	17
31	758	683	600	516	441	13
32	815	734	644	554	472	29
33	870	783	687	590	503	27
34	923	830	727	624	531	53
35	971	873	764	656	558	52
36	1014	912	798	684	582	66
37	1051	945	827	708	602	58
38	1082	972	850	728	619	54
39	1105	993	868	743	631	38
40	1118	1005	879	753	639	47
41	1123	1009	882	756	642	12

[a]Table 2 from Pinar H, Sung CJ, Oyer CE, Singer DB. Reference values for singleton and twin placental weights. Pediatr Pathol Lab Med 1996;16:904.

APPENDIX 4

Table of mean trimmed weights and percentiles for twin placentas with increasing placental ages (11). Both dichorionic and monochorionic placentas were included, with no distinction between the two. The same pathologic and clinical exclusions as in Appendix 3 apply to this group as well. Also excluded were triplets and higher orders of multiple gestation, and twins discordant for weight.

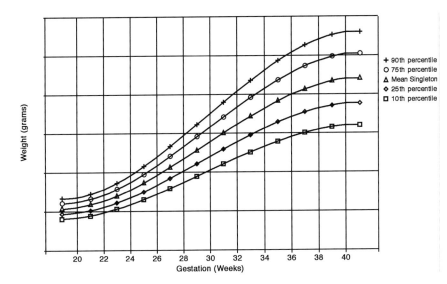

APPENDIX 5

Graphic representation of data in Appendix 4. (Fig. 2 from Pinar H, Sung CJ, Oyer CE, Singer DB. Reference values for singleton and twin placental weights. Pediatr Pathol Lab Med 1996;16:903.)

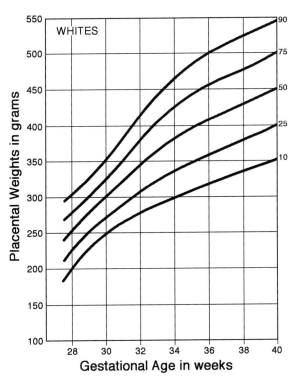
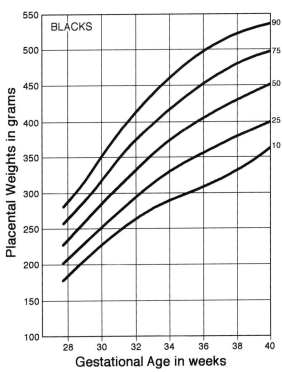

APPENDIX 6

Left and Right: Placental weight percentile curves at increasing gestational ages, compiled from the Collaborative Perinatal Study of the National Institute of Neurological and Communicative Disorders and Stroke. The data were collected from 12 medical school–affiliated hospitals in different regions of the United States between 1959 and 1966 (9).

The trimmed weights have been recorded by many different observers. They are lower than those tabulated in Appendices 2 and 3, and could represent differences in case selection and technique, and generational changes. The 90th percentile curve is lower than our current experience suggests; the 90th percentile weights in Appendices 2 and 3 are probably more relevant today. Weights below the 10th percentile curve represent a more reliable indicator of placental pathology, in our experience. Posting this curve at the signout bench is useful. It is easy to consult, serves as a reminder that one should know the computed gestational age of any placenta being studied, and that placental weights below this 10th percentile curve, especially, need some explanation. (Figs. 1 and 2 from Naeye RL. Do placental weights have clinical significance? Hum Pathol 1987;18:389.)

Appendix 7
MEAN DIFFERENCES (IN GRAMS AND PERCENT) BETWEEN FRESH AND FIXED WEIGHTS BY DAYS IN FORMALIN[a]

Days	Number[b]	Mean (g)	Min (g)	Max (g)	S.E.[c] (g)	Mean (%)	Min (%)	Max (%)
all days	106	28.3	0	80	2.0	5.8	0.0	17.0
1	23	26.8	0	70	4.8	5.3	0.0	13.5
2	6	30.3	15	50	5.7	5.6	2.9	8.9
3	25	36.1	4	80	4.4	7.3	0.6	17.0
4	15	28.5	7	58	4.2	6.0	1.1	12.6
5	13	23.5	0	75	5.5	4.8	0.0	13.6
6	24	23.8	2	70	3.8	5.1	0.4	14.4

[a]Data derived from reference 2 with assistance from biostatistician Jane McCall.
[b]Number of cases.
[c]S.E. = Standard error.

APPENDIX 7

Placental weight changes, measured daily after formalin fixation. The table lists mean differences in daily weight measurements of the same placentas, weighed fresh and after fixation in formalin of up to 1 week. Weights are expressed in grams, with minimum and maximum variance in grams and as percentage change.

Placentas were first drained of excess blood, trimmed of cord and membranes, weighed immediately, and then daily after fixation. The fixed placentas were removed from the containers, drained by gravity over a sink, blotted on an absorbent pad, and then weighed.

Appendix 8A
LEARNING CASES: HISTOLOGIC FEATURES WITH TIME-RELATED ONSET[a]

Histologic Feature	Time of Fetal Death Before Delivery (Cases with Histologic Feature)						
	<6 h (N=15)	6-24 h (N=13)	24-48 h (N=5)	2-7 d (N=5)	7-14 d (N=4)	14-28 d (N=4)	>28 d (N=5)
Intravascular karyorrhexis	0%	85%	100%	100%	100%	100%	100%
Extensive villous fibrosis	0%	0%	0%	20%	50%	100%	100%
Stem vessel luminal abnormalities							
Multifocal (10-25% of stem villi)	0%	0%	0%	60%	100%	50%	0%
Extensive (>25% of stem villi)	0%	0%	0%	20%	0%	50%	100%
Cord stromal necrosis	7%	31%	0%	60%	75%	67%	100%
Cord vascular necrosis	0%	0%	0%	0%	50%	33%	100%
Stromal "dusty" calcification	7%	0%	20%	40%	75%	75%	40%
Trophoblast basement membrane calcification/thickening	13%	0%	0%	40%	100%	50%	40%

[a]Table 2 from Genest DR. Estimating the time of death in stillborn fetuses: II. Histologic evaluation of the placenta: a study of 71 stillborns. Obstet Gynecol 1992;80:587.

APPENDIX 8

A: Evolution of placental histologic features after intrauterine fetal death. The progression of the vascular karyorrhexis, luminal fibrosis, and extensive villous fibrosis had the most significant predictive values (4). This sequence of changes may also be useful for dating the time of segmental vascular occlusion in cases of fetal thrombotic vasculopathy.

Appendix 8B

HISTOLOGIC FEATURES IN THE TEST SET:
ANALYSIS AS DIAGNOSTIC TESTS FOR SPECIFIC DEATH-TO-DELIVERY INTERVAL[a]

Tissue Feature	N[b]	Death-to-Delivery Time	Sensitivity	Specificity	Positive Predictive Value
Good Predictors					
Kidney: loss of tubular nuclear basophilia	44	4 h	0.971	0.889	0.971
Liver: loss of hepatocyte nuclear basophilia	41	≥24 h	1.000	0.920	0.889
Myocardium: inner half loss of nuclear basophilia	39	≥24 h	0.938	1.000	1.000
Myocardium: outer half loss of nuclear basophilia	38	≥48 h	1.000	0.964	0.909
Bronchus: loss of epithelial nuclear basophilia	47	≥96 h	1.000	0.973	0.909
Liver: maximal loss of nuclear basophilia	46	≥96 h	0.909	1.000	1.000
GI[c] tract: maximal loss of nuclear basophilia	47	≥1 wk	0.900	1.000	1.000
Adrenal: maximal loss of nuclear basophilia	40	≥1 wk	1.000	1.000	1.000
Trachea: chondrocyte loss of nuclear basophilia	37	≥1 wk	0.889	1.000	1.000
Kidney: maximal loss of nuclear basophilia	49	>4 wk	1.000	0.976	0.875
Intermediate Predictors					
GI epithelium: loss of nuclear basophilia	44	>8 h	0.930	0.800	0.900
Adrenal: fetal cortical loss of nuclear basophilia	39	≥24 h	0.813	0.957	0.929
Pancreas: maximal loss of nuclear basophilia	32	≥36 h	0.714	1.000	1.000
GI tract: transmural [4+] nuclear loss of basophilia	43	≥72 h	1.000	0.909	0.769
Lung: alveolar wall loss of nuclear basophilia	48	≥2 wk	1.000	0.949	0.800
Poor Predictors					
Bronchus: mucosal epithelial detachment	35	≥18 h	1.000	0.588	0.720
Bronchus: cartilage matrix loss of basophilia	40	≥24 h	0.941	0.625	0.640
Thymus: cortical lymphocyte karyorrhexis	30	≥24 h	1.000	0.429	0.429
Thymus: lymphocyte nuclear loss of basophilia	29	≥48 h	1.000	0.880	0.571
Kidney: glomerular nuclear loss of basophilia	39	≥48 h	1.000	0.821	0.688
Adrenal: adult cortical nuclear loss of basophilia	42	≥72 h	1.000	0.875	0.714
Lung: maximal nuclear loss of basophilia	49	>8 wk	1.000	0.976	0.875
Cerebral cortex: neuronal nuclear loss of basophilia	37	>8 wk	0.750	0.970	0.750

[a]Table 5 from Genest DR, Williams MA, Greene MF. Estimating the time of death in stillborn fetuses: I. Histologic evaluation of fetal organs: an autopsy study of 150 stillborns. Obstet Gynecol 1992;80:581.
[b]N = number of cases.
[c]GI = gastrointestinal.

APPENDIX 8 (Continued)

B: Evolution of histologic changes in fetal organs after intrauterine fetal death (5). Correlation of the placental pathology of a stillborn with postmortem organ changes may be valuable in some cases in order to make a distinction between pathologic vascular lesions in the placenta and the regressive changes related only to intrauterine fetal death (see 8A).

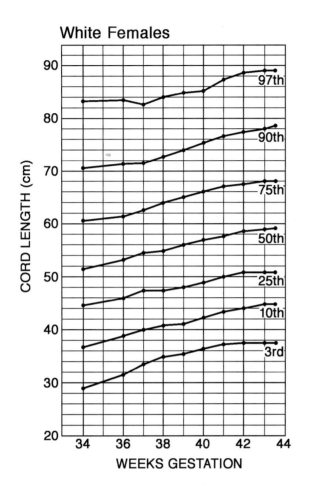
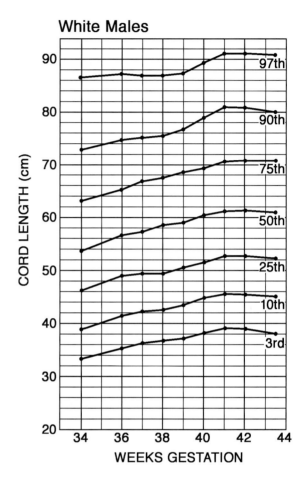

APPENDIX 9

A: Umbilical cord length by gestational age in white males from 34 to 43 weeks in the United States (8). (Fig. 1 from Mills JL, Harley EE, Moessinger AC. Standards for measuring umbilical cord length. Placenta 1983;4:423–6.)

B: Umbilical cord length by gestational age in white females in the United States. Male cords are significantly longer (p <0.0001). Cord lengths vary widely from shortest to longest in the same age groups. These data, like those in Appendix 6, were compiled from the Collaborative Perinatal Project.

Measurement of a short umbilical cord is only valuable when the entire cord can be accounted for. Portions of a cord sent for blood gas analysis often result in a false impression of a short cord based on measurement in the pathology laboratory. Umbilical cord length greater than 70 cm is considered excessively long and is associated with increased morbidity and mortality (1). Cords greater than 90 cm are associated with adverse outcome more often than not. (Fig. 2 from Mills JL, Harley EE, Moessinger AC. Standards for measuring umbilical cord length. Placenta 1983;4:423–6.)

Appendix 10
UMBILICAL CORD DIAMETER AND AREA ACCORDING TO GESTATIONAL AGE[a]

Week of Gestation (Weeks + Days)	Cases (n)	Umbilical Cord Diameter Mean (mm)	SD[b] (mm)	Umbilical Cord Area Mean (mm^2)	SD (mm^2)
10+0-10+6	6	3.19	0.40	8.11	2.06
11+0-11+6	8	3.65	0.41	11.40	4.87
12+0-12+6	8	3.68	0.53	11.70	3.16
13+0-13+6	12	4.37	0.43	15.10	2.77
14+0-14+6	13	5.10	0.39	20.50	3.00
15+0-15+6	15	5.95	0.73	26.62	7.35
16+0-16+6	24	6.47	0.81	33.04	10.58
17+0-17+6	21	7.23	0.79	38.96	9.81
18+0-18+6	18	7.87	0.74	49.12	12.90
19+0-19+6	25	8.68	1.07	55.39	15.07
20+0-20+6	20	9.47	1.48	65.01	18.13
21+0-21+6	18	10.73	1.55	80.54	21.04
22+0-22+6	23	10.93	1.58	87.45	22.96
23+0-23+6	12	12.23	1.62	104.54	22.23
24+0-24+6	20	13.14	1.72	127.88	24.33
25+0-25+6	20	13.44	1.74	128.00	27.32
26+0-26+6	18	14.34	1.80	139.03	38.44
27+0-27+6	15	14.06	1.99	143.02	44.99
28+0-28+6	13	14.34	2.07	143.40	40.95
29+0-29+6	22	16.25	2.01	186.36	49.26
20+0-30+6	23	16.24	2.12	186.65	44.56
31+0-31+6	21	16.45	2.21	187.50	43.17
32+0-32+6	21	16.59	2.42	187.95	51.66
33+0-33+6	22	16.72	2.49	189.98	48.20
34+0-34+6	24	16.72	2.57	192.53	49.15
35+0-35+6	21	16.27	2.67	182.65	47.04
36+0-36+6	20	16.53	2.30	181.70	42.02
37+0-37+6	22	16.01	1.99	181.56	42.48
38+0-38+6	18	15.85	1.82	163.07	39.30
39+0-39+6	17	14.48	1.60	149.44	37.11
40+0-40+6	9	15.59	1.41	146.77	35.66
41+0-42+0	8	14.42	1.50	139.07	24.64

[a]Table 2 from Raio L, Ghezzi F, Di Naro E, Gomez R, Franchi M, Mazor M, Bruhwiler H. Sonographic measurement of the umbilical cord and fetal anthropometric parameters. Eur J Obstet Gynecol Reprod Biol 1999;83:133.
[b]SD = Standard deviation of the mean.

APPENDIX 10

Umbilical cord diameter and cross-sectional area by gestational age (12). Determinations were based upon in vivo ultrasound measurements of normal fetuses in normal gestations.

Appendix 11
DISTRIBUTION OF CORD COIL INDEX IN 120 CONSECUTIVE UNSELECTED TPMG[a] PREGNANCIES[b]

Cord Coil Index	N[c]	(%)
0.0 - 0.049	2	(1.7)
0.05 - 0.099	7	(5.8)
0.1 - 0.149	15	(12.5)
0.15 - 0.199	20	(16.7)
0.2 - 0.249	36	(30.0)
0.25 - 0.299	16	(13.3)
0.3 - 0.349	14	(11.7)
0.35 - 0.399	5	(4.2)
0.4 - 0.449	3	(2.5)
0.45 - 0.499	2	(1.7)
Total	120	(100)

[a]TPMG = The Permanente Medical Group.
[b]Table 2 from Machin GA, Ackerman J, Gilbert-Barness E. Abnormal umbilical cord coiling is associated with adverse perinatal outcomes. Pediatr Dev Pathol 2000;3:464.
[c]N = number of cases.

APPENDIX 11

Distribution of cord coil index in 120 consecutive unselected pregnancies from the Permanente Medical Group. There is normally about one complete twist (coil)/5 cm of cord. The normal coil index is 0.2 coils/cm. The variations in coil index in an unselected group of patients are tabulated above. An overcoiled cord (OCC) has an index equal to 0.3 coils or more/cm, and an undercoiled cord (UCC) has an index of 0.1 or less. Principal clinical correlations with both OCC and UCC in this series were fetal death, intolerance to labor, intrauterine growth restriction, chorioamnionitis, thrombosis of chorionic plate vessels or cord, and cord stenosis.

REFRENCES

1. Baergen RN, Malicki D, Behling C, Benirschke K. Morbidity, mortality, and placental pathology in excessively long umbilical cords: retrospective study. Pediatr Dev Pathol 2001;4:144–53.
2. Boyd T, Gang D, Lis G, Juozokas A, Pflueger S. Normative values for placental weights (N=15463) [Abstract]. Mod Pathol 1999;12:1P.
3. Fox H. Pathology of the placenta, 2nd ed. London: W.B. Saunders; 1997:473.
4. Genest DR. Estimating the time of death in stillborn fetuses: II. Histologic evaluation of the placenta; a study of 71 stillborns. Obstet Gynecol 1992;80:585–92.
5. Genest DR, Williams MA, Greene MF. Estimating the time of death in stillborn fetuses: I. Histologic evaluation of fetal organs; an autopsy study of 150 stillborns. Obstet Gynecol 1992;80:575–84.
6. Kalousek DK, Fitch N, Paradice BA. Pathology of the human embryo and previable fetus: an atlas. New York: Springer-Verlag; 1990.
7. Machin GA, Ackerman J, Gilbert-Barness E. Abnormal umbilical cord coiling is associated with adverse perinatal outcomes. Pediatr Dev Pathol 2000;3:462–71.
8. Mills JL, Harley EE, Moessinger AC. Standards for measuring umbilical cord length. Placenta 1983;4:424–6
9. Naeye RL. Do placental weights have clinical significance? Hum Pathol 1987;18:387–91.
10. Perrin EV, Sander CH. Introduction: how to examine the placenta and why. New York: Churchill Livingston; 1984.
11. Pinar H, Sung CJ, Oyer CE, Singer DB. Reference values for singleton and twin placental weights. Pediatr Pathol Lab Med 1996;16:901–7.
12. Raio L, Ghezzi F, Di Naro E, et al. Sonographic measurement of the umbilical cord and fetal anthropometric parameters. Eur J Obstet Gynecol Reprod Biol 1999;83:131–5.

Index*

A

Abortion, 207
    Early spontaneous, 207
        Chromosomal abnormalities, 208, **208**, **209**, 213, **216**, **217**
        Chronic intervillositis, 212, **214**, **215**
        Hydatidiform mole, 210, **211**, **219-221**
        Hydropic abortion, 210, **218**, **219**
        Immune rejection, 209
        Maternal coagulopathies, 209
        Special techniques for diagnosis, 221
        Tissue examination and pathology, 209, **210-222**
    Elective, 207, **271**
    Late spontaneous abortion, 222
        Etiology, 223
        General features, 223
        Pathology, 223, **223-225**
    Recurrent spontaneous, 36
    Therapeutic, 207
Abruption, 35, 38, 128
    Chronic, 129
    Chronic abruption-oligohydramnios sequence, 130
    Marginal, 130, **134**
    Ultrasound examination, 298
Acardiac twins, 240, 272, **275**, **276**
Accelerated maturation, 33, 121, **123**
Accessory lobe, 54, **55**
Acute atherosis, 118, **122**
Acute fatty liver of pregnancy, 34
ADAM complex, 171
Adenoma, 241
    Hepatocellular, 241, **241**
Allantoic duct remnants, 180, **181**
Amnion, normal, 1
Amnion nodosum, 169, **170**, **171**
Amnion rupture sequence, 171
Amnionic adhesion malformation syndrome, 171
Amnionic band disruption complex, 171
Amnionic bands, 171, **172-175**
Amnionic fluid, 42
    Meconium-stained, 42
    Hydramnos/polyhydramnios, 42, 169
    Oligohydramnios, 42, 169
    Ultrasound examination, 301
Amnionic webs, 187
Anatomy, placental, normal, 1
    Amnion, 1
    Anchoring villi, 6, **7**
    Basal plate, 6, **7**
    Chorionic plate, 4, **4**, **5**
    Developmental anatomy, *see* Developmental anatomy
    Functional, *see* Functional anatomy
    Interhemal membrane, 5
    Margin, 8, **9**
    Membranes, 8, 163
    Membranous chorion, 1
    Stem villi, 4, **5**, **6**
        Terminal villous unit, 5, **6**
        Trophoblast, 2, **8**
        Umbilical cord, 3, **3**, 179
    Yolk sac, 2, **2**
Anemias, fetal, 232
    And fetal hydrops, 232
    Fetomaternal hemorrhage, 235
    Hemoglobinopathies, 232, **233**
    Parvovirus anemia, 232, **234**, **235**
    Twin-twin transfusion, 235
Anemias, maternal, 35
    Sickle cell anemia, 35
    Thalassemias, 35
Aneurysms, umbilical cord, 197
Anti-D gammaglobulin (Rhogam), 229
Arterial perfusion
    Fetoplacental, 17
    Maternal, 17
Asphyxia, perinatal/intrapartum, 40
Assisted reproductive techniques (ART), 249
Atherosis, decidual, 118, **122**
Avascular terminal villi, 141

B

Basal plate, normal, 6, **7**
Battledore cord insertion, *see* Marginal cord insertion
Beckwith-Wiedemann syndrome, 60, 62, 66

---

*Numbers in boldface indicate table and figure pages.

Birth asphyxia, *see* Hypoxic-ischemic injury
Blastocyst trophectoderm, 10
Bradycardia, 37
Breus mole, 127

C

Candida sp, 86, **88**
Cardiac anomalies, congenital, and fetal hydrops, 232
Cardiotocogram, 37
Cerebral palsy, 38
    Coxsackie virus infection, 39
    Cytomegalovirus infection, 39
    Intrauterine bacterial infection, 39
    Leukomalacia, 39
    Prematurity, 39
    Thrombotic events, 39
    Toxoplasmosis, 39
Cerebral vascular accident, maternal, 34
Chagas' disease, 92, **93**
Cholesterol ester storage disease, 66
Chorangiocarcinoma, 61
Chorangioma, 26, 38, 61, 239
    Angiomatous type, 61, **63**
    Cellular type, 61, **63**
    Etiology, 61
    General features, 61
    Nonspecific trophoblast hyperplasia, 61, **64**
    Pathology, 61, **63, 64**
Chorangiomatosis
    Localized, 61, **62**, *see also* Chorangioma
    Multifocal, 64
Chorangiopagus parasiticus, 275
Chorangiosis, villous, 62, *see also* Villous chorangiosis
Chorioamnionitis
    Acute, 25, 75
        Causative organisms, 85
        Clinical chorioamnionitis, 76, **77**
        Etiology, 77
        Fetal inflammatory response, 76
        General features, 75
        Histologic, 36, 75
        Maternal inflammatory response, 75
        Pathology, 78, **79-84**
        Stages of fetal response, 82, **83-86**
        Stages of maternal response, 79, **80-82**
        With peripheral funisitis, 86, **88**
    Chronic, 107, **109**
    Clinical, 36
    Necrotizing, 79, **81**
    Subacute, 84, **87**
Chorionic intervillositis, 212, **214, 215**
Chorionic plate, normal, 4, **4, 5,** 10
Chorionic-type intermediate trophoblast, 164
Chorionic vasculitis, 82
Chorionitis, acute, 79, **81**
Choristoma, 241
Chromosomal abnormalities, 68
    Etiology, 69
    Fetal hydrops, 236
    General features, 68
    Pathology, 69, **70**
Circulation
    Disorders of, 118, *see individual disorders and*
        Vasculopathy
        Fetal, 141
        Maternal, 135
    Fetal and maternal, normal, **118, 119**
Circummargination, 48
Circumvallation, 47, **48-50**
Coagulopathy, 34
Clotting disorders, placental, 117, *see also*
    Intraplacental clotting
Confined placental mosaicism, 25, 69, 225
Conjoined twins, 272, **274**
Cord, *see* Umbilical cord
Coxsackie virus infection, 39
Cystic adenomatoid malformation, congenital, 236
Cysts, placental, 175
    Subamnionic fibrin cysts, 175, **176**
    Ultrasound examination, 297, **298**
Cysts, umbilical cord
    Ultrasound examination, 299
Cytogenetics, 291
    and fetal death, 208, **208–211, 213, 216, 217**
Cytomegalovirus
    Fetal hydrops, 235
    Cerebral palsy, 39
    Placentitis, 92, 95, **96**

D

Decidual perivasculitis, chronic, 36
Decidual vasculopathy, 118
    Acute atherosis, 118, **122**
    Distal villous hypoplasia, 121, **123**
    General features, 118
    Hypertrophic, 121, **122**

Pathology, 120, **122**, **123**
Preeclampsia, 120, **123**
Spiral artery thrombi, 118
Trophoblastic knots, 121, **123**
Deciduitis, chronic, 108, **110**
Delayed villous maturation, 60
Delivery, preterm, 24
Dermatopathic melanosis of the placenta, 243
Developmental anatomy, 9
Arterial plugs, 12
Blastocyst trophectoderm, 10
Chorionic plate and body stalk, 10
Implantation, 12, **13**
Late implantation, 14, **14**, **15**
Membrane formation, 15, **16**
Mesenchymal villi, 11, **12**
Nidation and maternal capillary circulation, 10, **10**
Placental growth, 16
Placental weights, 311, **311-318**
Stem villi, 12, **13**
Syncytiotrophoblast, 10
Terminal villogenesis, 16
Trophoblast proliferative units, 16
Umbilical cord, 179, **179**
Villous stromal vasculogenesis, 10, **11**, **12**
Develpmental disorders, placenta, 47
Fetal vascular disorders, 61
Genetic disorders, 65
Membrane disorders, 47
Placental migration disorders, 54
Uterine implantation disorders, 49
Villous development disorders, 59
Diabetes mellitus, 35
Dichorionic placenta, 250, **251-255**
Disruption, 47
Distal villous hyperplasia, 59
Etiology, 59
General features, 59, **59**
Pathology, 59, **60**
Distal villous hypoplasia, 33, 59, 121, **123**, see also
Peripheral villous hypoplasia
Distal villous immaturity, 60
Etiology, 60
General features, 60
Pathology, 60
Dizygous twins, 249
Doppler ultrasound, 304, **305-307**
Down's syndrome

Fetal hydrops, 236
Ultrasound examination, 303

E

Eclampsia, 33
Electron microscopy, 291
Electronic fetal monitoring, 37
Fetal heart rate monitor (cardiotocogram), 37
Embryonic death, see Abortion, early spontaneous
Encephalopathy, hypoxic-ischemic, 40
Endocrinopathy, maternal, 36
Endothelial cushions, 141, 156
Eosinophilic vasculitis, 109, **110**
Erythroblastosis, 41, 229
Eschericha coli, 90, 291
Essential hypertension, 34
Examination techniques, 283
Clinical findings, 282
Indications for, **283**
Multiple pregnancy, 287, **288**
Special studies, 290
Specimen handling, 285, **286**
Tissue sampling, 286
Extramembranous pregnancy, 172

F

Factor V Leiden mutation, 34
Fetal death, histologic changes
In fetal organs, 319
In placenta, 318
Fetal growth restriction, 25, 38, 59
Ultrasound examination, 304
Fetal heart rate monitor, 37
Fetal hydrops, see Hydrops
Fetal-maternal hemorrhage, 127, 128
Fetal-placental weight ratios, 314
Fetal stem artery thombosis, 141
Fetal stem vessel thrombi, see Fetal thrombotic vasculopathy
Fetal thrombotic vasculopathy, 26, 35, 38, 141
General features, 141
Pathology, 142, **143-152**
Fetal vascular narrowing, 151
And intrauterine growth restriction, **152**, **153**
Fetus papyraceus, 270, **272**, **273**
Fibrinous vasculosis, 141, 156
Fluorescence in situ hybridization (FISH), 209, 221, 226, 291

Functional anatomy, 17
    Fetoplacental arterial perfusion, 17
    Fetoplacental venous return, 17
    Maternal arterial perfusion, 17
    Maternal physiology, 19
    Maternal venous drainage, 18
    Membranes and labor, 18
    Syncytiotrophoblast, 19
    Umbilical cord dynamics, 18
Funisitis
    Necrotizing, 82, **84**
    Peripheral, 86, **88**
Fusobacterium sp, 84, **87**
Furcate cord insertion, 186

G

Galactosialidosis, 66, **67**
Gangliosidoses, 66
Gastroschisis, 175, **176**
Gaucher's disease and fetal hydrops, 236
Genetic disorders, 65
    Chromosomal abnormalities, 68, *see also*
        Chromosomal abnormalities
    Mesenchymal dysplasia, 66, **68**
    Metabolic storage diseases, 65, *see also* Metabolic
        storage diseases, placenta
Germinal matrix hemorrhage, 39
Glitterinfarcts, 135
Growth hormone (GH), 19

H

Habitual abortion, 36
HELLP syndrome, 33, 34
Hemangioma
    Placental, 239
    Umbilical, 197, **198**
Hematoma, maternal, 127
Hematoma, placental, 35
    Intraplacental, 117, **120**, 127, **127**, 129
    Marginal, 128, **130**, 134
    Massive subchorial, 127, **127**, 128
    Placental abruption, 128
    Retroplacental, 128, **130-133**
    Subchorial, 127
    Umbilical, 196, **197**
Hematoma, umbilical, 196, **197**, **198**
Hemolytic disease of the newborn, 229
Hemorrhagic endovasculitis, 141, 151
    General features, 151
    Pathology, 153, **154**, **155**
Hemosiderin deposition, 49, 50, 132, **132**, **133**
Hepatoblastoma, congenital, 242, **243**
Hepatocellular adenoma, 241, **241**
Herpes simplex virus
    Fetal hydrops, 235
    Placentitis, 96, **99**
Heterotopic adrenal cortex, 241, **242**
Heterotopic liver, 241, **242**
Histiocytic intervillositis, chronic, 26, 36
Histochemical stains, 290
Human chorionic gonadotropin (HCG), 19, 208
Human placental lactogen (HPL), 19
Hydatidiform moles, 33
    And abortion, 210, **211**, **219-221**
Hydramnios, 42, 264
Hydropic abortion, 210, **218**, **219**
Hydrops, 33, 229
    Fetal hydrops, 229
    Immune hydrops, 229, 242
    Nonimmune hydrops, 229, 232, **232**
        Cardiovascular etiology, 232, **233**
        Chromosomal disorders, 236
        Fetal anemias, 232, **233**
        Fetal infections, **234**, 235, **235**
        Fetal tumors, 236
        Pulmonary lesions, 236
    Placental hydrops, 229, **230**, **231**
Hydrops fetalis, 229
Hypertension and pregnancy, 34
    Essential hypertension, maternal, 34
Hypertrophic decidual vasculopathy, 121
Hypoxic-ischemic injury, 26, 40, **40**
    Causing circulatory disruption, 27
    Causing neurologic impairment, 27

I

I-cell disease, 66, **66**
Immunocytochemistry, 291
Implantation, 12, **13**, 14, **14**, **15**
    Disorders of, 49
        Placenta accreta, increta, percreta, 51, **51**, **52**
        Placenta previa, 49
    Superficial, 53, *see also* Superficial implantation
In situ hybridization, 291
Incompetent cervix, 36
Increased umbilical vascular resistance, 151

Infantile sialic acid storage disease, 66
Infarct, placental, 35, **121**, 123, **124**, **125**
Infection, placenta, 75, *see individual disorders*
    Acquired at delivery, 100
    With no inflammation, 99
Inflammation, placenta, 75, **76**
    Anatomic location, **76**
    Etiology, **76**
    Gestational age, **77**
    Idiopathic lesions, 101
Insertion disorders, umbilical cord, 57
    Aberrant membrane vessel, 57, **58**
    Furcate insertion, 186, **186**
    Interposition, 183, **184**
    Marginal insertion, 57, **58**, 185, **185**, **186**
    Membranous insertion, 57, **57**
    Tethered insertion, 187, **187**
    Peripheral insertion, 57, **58**
    Velamentous insertion, 182, **183**, **184**
Insulin-like growth factor, 17, 60
Interhemal membrane, 5
Intervillositis
    Acute, with intervillous abscesses, 87
        Etiology, 89
        General features, 88
        Pathology, 89, **89**, **90**
    Chronic, with malarial pigment, 96, **100**
    Massive chronic, 107, **107**, **108**
Intervillous abscesses, 87, **89**, **90**
Intraplacental clotting, 117, **119**
    Hematoma, 117, **120**
    Infarct, 117, **121**
    Perivillous fibrin deposition, 117
    Placental separation, **120**
Intrauterine fetal death, 207, *see also* Abortion, late spontaneous
Intrauterine growth restriction, 38, 49, 151, **152**, **153**
Intrauterine infection, 39
Intraventricular hemorrhage, 39

K

Kleihauer-Betke test, 128, 129
Kline's hemorrhages, 127
Knots
    Trophoblastic, 121, **123**
    Umbilical, 192, **193**, **194**

L

Labor, normal, 18
Leiomyoma, 36, 52, **52**
    Intraplacental, 239, **239**, **240**
Leukemia
    Congenital, 242
    Maternal, 244
Leukomalacia, 39
    Periventricular, 40
Limb-body wall complex, 171
Listeria, *monocytogenes*, **76**, 86, 89, **89**, 284
Liver, heterotopic, 241, **242**
Long chain 3-hydroxyacyl-CoA dehydrogenase (LCHAD) deficiency, 34, 136
Luteinizing hormone, 19
Lymphoma, 244
Lymphoplasmacytic deciduitis, 36

M

Malaria, placenta, 97, **100**
Malignant melanoma, 244, **245**
Marginal cord insertion, 57, **58**, 185, **185**, **186**
Marginal separation, 25
Massive chronic intervillositis, 107, **107**, **108**
Massive chronic villitis, 224, **225**
Massive perivillous fibrinoid deposition (maternal floor infarct), 26, 38, 135
    General features, 135
    Pathology, 136, **136-141**
Maternal floor infarct, *see* Massive perivillous fibrinoid deposition
Maternal underperfusion, 25
Meconium, 42
    Induced necrosis, 198
    Staining, 164, **165-167**
Meconium aspiration syndrome, 42, 164
Melanosis, dermatopathic, 243
Membranes, placental
    Anatomy, 8, 163, **163**
    Amnion nodosum, 169, **170**, **171**
    Amnionic bands, 171, **172-175**
    Cysts, 175
        Subamnionic fibrin cysts, 175, **176**
    Developmental abnormalities, 47
        Circumvallation/cirummargination, 47, **48-50**
        Placenta membranacea, 47, **48**
    Extramembranous pregnancy, 172

Formation, 15, **16**
Gastroschisis, 175, **176**
Inflammation, 168
Interhemal membrane, 5
Labor, 18
Meconium staining, 164, **165-167**
Physiology, 163, **163**
Squamous metaplasia, 168, **168**, 170
Mesenchymal dysplasia, 66
    Beckwith-Wiedemann syndrome, 66
    Etiology, 66
    General features, 66
    Pathology, 67, **68**
Metabolic storage diseases, 65
    Cholesterol ester storage disease, 66
    Galactosialidosis, 66, **67**
    Gangliosidoses, 66
    I-cell disease, 66, **66**
    Infantile sialic acid storage disease, 66
    Sialidosis, 66
    Type IV mucopolysaccharidosis, 66
Metastases, 244, **245**, **246**
Migration disorders, placenta
    Peripheral cord insertion, 57, **57**, *see also*
        Insertion disorders, umbilical cord
    Shape abnormalities, 54, **56**, *see also*
        Multilobation, placenta
Miscarriage, 207, *see also* Abortion, late spontaneous
Monochorionic placenta, 250, **252-256**
Monozygous twins, 249, **250**
MTHFR gene mutation, 34, **136**, **139**, **140**, 142, 209
Mucopolysaccharidosis, type IV, 66
Multilobation, placenta, 54, **55**
    Accessory lobe, 54, **55**
Multiple pregnancy, 249, *see also* Twin gestation
    Complications, 261, **263-267**, **269-276**
    Higher multiple births, 276, **277**, **278**
    Twin gestation, 249, **250-256**
    Ultrasound examination, 287, **288**, **290**

N

Neonatal encephalopathy, 26, 40
Neoplasms, placental, 239
    Congenital, 242
    Maternal, 243
Neuroblastoma, congenital, 242
Nevi, congenital, 243, 244
Nucleated red blood cells (NRBC), 28, 41, 60

O

Oligohydramnios, 42, 169
Omphalomesenteric remnants, 180, **181**
Oncofetal fibronectin, 8

P

Parasitic twin, 272, **274**
Peripheral villous hypoplasia, 59, **123**
Periventricular leukomalacia, 40
Perivillitis, acute, 90, **90**
Perivillous fibrin deposition, 117
Placenta accreta, increta, percreta, 51, **52**
    Etiology, 51
    General features, 51
    Pathology, 52
    Ultrasound examination, 296
Placenta membranacea, 47, **48**
Placenta monochorionic/dichorionic, 250, **251-256**
Placenta previa, 49
    Etiology, 49
    General features, 51
    Pathology, 51
    Ultrasound examination, 295, **295**
Placental lesions, **24**, 27, **27**
    Pathway of injury, 29, **30**
    Physiologic consequences, 29
    Subcategorization, 28
Placental weights
    8-18 weeks, **311**
    22-42 weeks, **312**, **315**
    formalin fixation effect, **318**
    percentiles, **313**, **315**, **317**
    twins, **316**, **317**
Placentitis, chronic, TORCH, 92
    Etiology, 92, **93**
    General features, 92
    Pathology, 94
Plasmodium falciparum, 97
Polyhydramnios, 42
Polymerase chain reaction, 291
Post-term pregnancy, 37
Preeclampsia, 33
    And acute atherosis, 118, **123**, **124**
    Etiology, 34, 53, 54, 119
Pregnancy-induced hypertension, 33
Premature delivery, 207
Premature rupture of membranes, 37
Prenatal/perinatal injury, 23, 23

Outcomes, 23
    Fetal growth restriction, 25
    Hypoxic-ischemic injury, 26
    Preterm delivery, 24
  Placental lesions, **23**
  Risk factors, **23**, 24
Preterm birth, 37
Preterm labor, 37
Products of conception, 207
Pulmonary infarcts, maternal, 34
Pulmonary sequestration, 236

R

Recurrent pregnancy loss, 36
Rett's syndrome, 39
Retroplacental hemorrhage, 25
Rubellavirus, 92, 235

S

Sacrococcygeal teratoma, 242
Septal cyst, 7, **7**
Sialidosis, 66
Single umbilical artery, 26, 189, **191**, **192**
  Congenital malformations, 190
  Low birth weight, 192
  Perinatal mortality, 192
  Ultrasound examination, 299, **300**
Small for gestational age, 38
Specimen handling, 285
Spiral artery thrombi, 118
Spontaneous abortion, recurrent, 36
Squamous metaplasia, 168, **169**, 170
Stains, histochemical, 290
Stem villi, *see* Villi
Stillbirth, 222, *see also* Abortion, late spontaneous
Storage disorders, metabolic, *see* Metabolic storage diseases
Streptococcus, group B, 77, **86**, 90, 100, 291
Subamnionic fibrin cysts, 175, **176**
Subamnionic hematoma, 157, **157**
  Ultrasound examination, 298, **299**
Subchorionitis, 79, **80**
Succenturiate lobe, 55
  Ultrasound examination, 297, **297**
Superficial implantation, 53
  Etiology, 53
  General features, 54
  Pathology, 54, **54**, **55**

Syncytiotrophoblast, 10, 19
Syphilis
  Fetal hydrops, 235
  Placentitis, 92, **94**, **95**

T

T-cell vasculitis, 109, **110**
Tenney-Parker change, 121
Teratomas, 240
  Sacrococcygeal, 242
Terminal villous deficiency, 59
Thrombocytopenia, fetal/neonatal, 41
Thrombophilia, maternal, 34, 36
Thromboses, deep vein, maternal, 34
Thyrotoxicosis and fetal hydrops, 236
Tissue sampling techniques, 286
TORCH infections, 92, 225
Toxoplasma gondii, 92
Toxoplasmosis
  Fetal hydrops, 235
  Cerebral palsy, 39
  Placentitis, 95, **95**, 98
Treponema pallidum, 92, 235
Triplets, 276, **277**
Trisomy 13, 210, **213**
Trophoblast, 2, **8**, 16
  Chorionic-type intermediate, 164
Trophoblastic knots, 121, **123**
Trypanosoma cruzi, 92, **93**
Turner's syndrome
  Fetal hydrops, 236
Twin gestation, 249
  Chorionic vascularity, 258
  Chorionicity, 250, **251-255**
    Monoamnionic monochorionic, 259
  Complications, 261
    Asymmetric growth, 268
    Co-twin demise, 269, **269-271**
    Duplication abnormalities, 272, **274-276**
    Fetus papyraceus, 270, **272**, **273**
    Twin-twin transfusion syndrome, 261, **263-267**
    Vanishing twin, 269, **270**
  Etiology, 249
  Examination techniques, 287, **288**, 290
  Placentation, 249, **250**
  Umilical cord, 258, **258-261**
  Vascular anastomoses, 254, **256**, **257**
  Zygosity, 249

Twin reversed arterial perfusion, 275
Twin-twin transfusion syndrome, 261, **263-267**
    Acute transfusion, 267
    Acute on chronic transfusion, 268
    Chronic transfusion, 261

U

Ultrasound, diagnostic, 295
    Doppler assessment, 304, **305-307**
    Fetus, 300
    Indications, 296, **296**
    Placenta, 295, **297-300**
    Umbilical cord, 295, **297-300**
Umbilical arteritis, 82, **83**
Umbilical cord
    Abnormal torsion, 193, **195**
    Anatomy, normal, 3, **3**, 179
    Aneurysms, 197
    Cord coil index, **321**
    Cord diameter, 189
    Cord length, 187
        Long cord, 188, **189**
        Normal length, **311**
        Short cord, 187, **188**
    Development, normal, 179, **179**
    Diameter, cross section area
        10-42 weeks, **321**
    Hemangioma, 197, **198**
    Hematoma, 196, **197**
    Insertion disorders, 57, 182, *see also* Insertion disorders
    Knots, 192, **193**, **194**
    Length
        8-18 weeks, **311**
        34-44 weeks, **320**
    Meconium-induced necrosis, 198
    Numerical variation, 181
        Single umbilical artery, 26, 189, *see also* Single umbilical artery
        Supernumerary vessels, 192
    Rupture, 199
    Segmental thinning, 197, **199**
    Stricture, 196, **196**
    Thrombosis, 198, **200**
    Ulceration, 198, **199**
    Ultrasound examination, 298, **299**
    Vestigial remnants, 180
Umbilical perivasculitis, 82, **83**
Umbilical phlebitis, 82, **83**

V

Vanishing twin, 269, **270**
Varicella-zoster placentitis, 96, **99**
Vasa previa, 182
    Ultrasound examination, 297
Vascular disorders, fetal, *see* Vasculopathy
Vasculogenesis, 10, **11**
Vasculopathy
    Fetal, 61
        Chorangioma/chorangiomatosis, 61, *see also* Chorangioma
        Multifocal chorangiomatosis, 64
        Villous chorangiosis, 62, **65**
    Maternal, 38, 118
        Decidual vasculopathy, 118, *see also* Decidual vasculopathy
        Hematomas, 127, *see also* Hematomas
        Infarcts, **121**, 123, **125**, **126**
        Spiral artery thrombi, 118
Vasculosyncytial membrane, 5
Velamentous cord insertion
    Etiology, 57, 184
    General features, 182
    Multiple gestation, 258, **258**, **259**, 268
    Pathology, 183, **183**, **184**
Venous vascular return
    Fetoplacental, 17
    Maternal, 17
Vernix granulomas, 172, **174**, **175**
Vestigial remnants, 180
    Allantoic remnants, 180, **181**
    Omphalomesenteric remnants, 180, **182**
    Yolk sac remnants, 3, 182, **182**
Villi
    Anchoring, 6, **8**
    Development, 11, **12**, **13**
    Mesenchymal, 11, **12**
    Stem, 4, **5**, **6**, 12, **13**
Villitis
    Acute, 90, **91**
    Chronic, 26, 38
    Chronic histiocytic, 107, **107**
    Chronic with villous necrosis, 90
        Etiology, 91

General features, 90
Pathology, 91, **92**, **93**
Fibrosclerosing, 94
Histiocyte-predominant, 94
Of unknown etiology, 101
Etiology, 101
General features, 101
Pathology, 101, **102-106**
Villogenesis, 16
Villous chorangiosis, 62
Etiology, 62
General features, 62
Pathology, 64, **65**
Villous disorders, 59
Hypoplasia, 59, **59**
Immaturity, 60, **60**

Villous hydrops, 35, 94
Villous infarct, 123
Villous stromal vasculogenesis, 10, **11**, **12**
Vitelline vessel remnant, 4, 182

W

Weight tables, **311-322**
Weights and measures of placenta, 311
Weights, effects of formalin fixation, **318**
Wharton's jelly, deficient, 189, **189**

Y

Yolk sac remnant, 3, 182, **182**

Z

Zygosity, 249